CONTRIBUTORS

KEITH W. DEANS, R.Ph., B.S., Pharm.D.
Associate Professor of Clinical Pharmacy, Ferris State College, Big Rapids, Michigan, and Clinical Pharmacist, Butterworth Hospital, Grand Rapids, Michigan

MELISSA BIANCO TOBIN, M.S.N., R.N.
Head Nurse, ICU, Mary Hitchcock Memorial Hospital, Hanover, New Hampshire; formerly Clinical Coordinator, MICU, Graduate Hospital, Philadelphia, Pennsylvania

JOHN VANRIPER, B.S.N., R.N.
Staff Nurse, Cardiac Catheterization Laboratory, University of Michigan Hospitals, Ann Arbor, Michigan

SHARON VANRIPER, M.S., R.N., C.C.R.N.
Assistant Head Nurse, Cardiology Unit, University of Michigan Hospitals, Ann Arbor, Michigan

BONNIE WESORICK, R.N., M.S.N.
Clinical Nurse Specialist, Butterworth Hospital, Grand Rapids, Michigan, and Research Associate Professor, Grand Valley State College, Allendale, Michigan

KATHLEEN M. WHITE, R.N., M.S., C.C.R.N.
Clinical Nurse Specialist, Critical Care and Trauma, Methodist Medical Center, Dallas, Texas

LINDA ANN YACONE, R.N., B.S., C.C.R.N.
Critical Care Educational Coordinator, Halifax Medical Center, Daytona Beach, Florida

Gloria Oblouk Darovic, R.N., C.C.R.N., C.E.N.
Nurse Clinician and Instructor in Clinical Care
Chicago, Illinois

Foreword by
Robert J. Henning, M.D., F.A.C.P., F.A.C.C., F.C.C.P.

Hemodynamic Monitoring

Invasive and Noninvasive Clinical Applications

W.B. Saunders Company
Philadelphia London Toronto
Sydney Tokyo Hong Kong

W. B. Saunders Company: West Washington Square
Philadelphia, PA 19105

Library of Congress Cataloging-in-Publication Data

Darovic, Gloria O.

Hemodynamic monitoring.

1. Cardiovascular system—Diseases—Diagnosis.
2. Hemodynamics. 3. Patient monitoring.
I. Title. [DNLM: 1. Hemodynamics. 2. Monitoring, Physiologic—methods. WG 106 D224h]

RC683.D27 1987 616.1′0754 87–4799

ISBN 0–7216–1064–1

Editor: Dudley Kay
Designer: Terri Siegel
Production Manager: William Preston
Manuscript Editor: Esther Weiss
Illustrator: Sharon Iwanczuk
Illustration Coordinator: Peg Shaw
Cover Designer: Sharon Iwanczuk
Indexer: Alexandra Weir

Hemodynamic Monitoring:
Invasive and Noninvasive Clinical Applications ISBN 0–7216–1064–1

Last digit is the print number: 9 8 7 6 5 4 3 2

To my family and especially my daughter, Elizabeth Marie

FOREWORD

Proper cardiovascular catheterization and hemodynamic monitoring involve several discrete and equally important steps. These steps include the correct techniques for the insertion and manipulation of catheters and related instruments within the circulation, the collection through such instruments of samples and signals carrying hemodynamically relevant information, the extraction of information through the processing of raw data, and the interpretation and application of the hemodynamic information in the care of critically ill patients. When properly performed and interpreted by critical care practitioners, cardiovascular catheterization and hemodynamic monitoring provide invaluable information regarding cardiopulmonary function and enable the early detection of disease states. However, considerable error may occur with each step in the catheterization and monitoring process, thereby exposing the patient to significant risks from therapeutic misadventures.

This textbook on bedside hemodynamic monitoring provides basic, practical information on the technical aspects of cardiovascular catheterization, the proper techniques for the calibration of equipment and collection of raw data, and the correct interpretation of the processed information. In addition, considerable attention is given by the authors to the presentation of fundamental physiological concepts, thereby providing a solid foundation for discussion of cardiopulmonary pathophysiology and the hemodynamic profiles of the common cardiopulmonary abnormalities that occur in critically ill patients. This approach facilitates, for the critical care practitioner, the understanding of logical therapeutic interventions based on the correct interpretation of abnormal hemodynamic measurements.

The authors are to be commended for providing us with a remarkably clear, concise, and authoritative text that covers the wide scope of the clinical application of hemodynamic monitoring in critical care.

ROBERT J. HENNING, M.D., FACP, FACC, FCCP
Case Western Reserve School of Medicine

PREFACE

The introduction of bedside hemodynamic monitoring has had a revolutionary impact on evaluation and management of the critically ill. Incorrect insertion and management of these devices, however, are associated with high risk to the patient. Additionally, the clinician's inability to interpret the information, relate it to the specific clinical situation, and act appropriately renders these invasive devices a useless liability.

The purpose of this text is to provide a concise, comprehensive, and clinically applicable reference for physicians, nurses, respiratory therapists, and paramedical personnel whose patients require invasive and/or noninvasive hemodynamic monitoring.

This text also stresses the importance of integrating hemodynamic parameters with physical assessment and laboratory findings. Diagnosis, intervention and therapy of shock states, and commonly encountered cardiopulmonary disorders are discussed with emphasis on the individuality of patient response and the need to avoid a "recipe book" approach to patient care.

GLORIA OBLOUK DAROVIC

ACKNOWLEDGEMENTS

- It is with pleasure that I express gratitude to the numerous people who directly or indirectly helped in the production of this text:
- To the contributors for the effort and cooperation given under considerable time constraint,
- To the artists, production people, and editors (especially Dudley Kay) at W. B. Saunders,
- To Mary Katheryn Lauer and Dr. Henry J. L. Marriott for their friendship and support throughout the laborious writing of this book,
- To the Cardiac Catheterization Laboratory staff of Foster G. McGaw Hospital of Loyola University in Chicago and Cheryl Finkl and Roberta Bischoff of Medical Center Hospital in Largo, Florida, for their cooperation in obtaining good pressure tracings,
- To Dr. David J. Hale, Dr. Robert Henning, and Dr. Stephen Ayres for their kindness in reviewing many of the chapters,
- To Barbara J. Agnew, Nurse Consultant in Hemodynamic Monitoring, and Lucianne Robinson, Department of Hemodynamics, Cedars-Sinai Medical Center, Los Angeles, respected counselors, mentors, and generous contributors of pressure tracings,
- To the following reviewers:

Edwina McConnell, RN, PhD
Nursing Consultant
Madison, Wisconsin

Paula M. Midyette, RN, MSN
Baptist Medical Center—Montclair
Birmingham, Alabama

Wendy S. Mitchell, RN, BSN
University of Washington Hospital
Seattle, Washington

Colleen Pfeiffer, RN, MSN
William S. Middleton Veterans Memorial Hospital
Madison, Wisconsin

Anna Louise Scandiffio, RN, BSN
The Good Samaritan Hospital
Baltimore, Maryland

CONTENTS

Introduction

1

Those who have been involved in critical care over the past 20 years have witnessed tremendous advances in monitoring physiologic and hemodynamic parameters. Devices now commonly used provide immediately available pressure measurements in systemic and pulmonary circulations, central veins, pulmonary capillary bed, and right and/or left atrium (which normally reflects the filling pressure of the respective ventricles). With the information gleaned from these devices, one can also calculate cardiac index, oxygen transport, and tissue oxygen consumption. Nevertheless, these numerical values have several limitations. This chapter focuses on the limitations of these values as well as other important factors that contribute to "total patient care."

THE NUMERICAL VALUES (LIMITATIONS)

A state of health is maintained by a very complex, synchronous and intricate balance of multiple systems function. An altered physiologic state, such as disease or injury, complicates physiology as the organism attempts to maintain homeostasis through the utilization of multiple alternate physiologic pathways. Because the very complex and marvelous machinery of the human body cannot be counted on to behave uniformly in all situations in all people, isolated monitoring or laboratory values ("numbers") are useless unless they are evaluated in context with the total patient picture.

No computer or monitoring device can tell how the cardiac output, whether high or low, is distributed or if specific organ system needs are being met. For example, septicemia is an all too commonly encountered disease which, in its early stage, is characterized by a *maldistribution* of a normal or increased cardiac output. Calculation of the arteriovenous oxygen content difference reveals that oxygen is not being metabolized normally by the body tissue but does not indicate which of the tissue beds is most or least deprived. In any clinical circumstance, the maintenance of organ function depends on adequate regional blood flow and oxidative metabolism, which can only be evaluated by bedside clinical observation of skin color and temperature, capillary refill, quality of pulses, level of mentation, and urine output.

Another important consideration is the appropriateness of the "numbers" and their effect on the patient. For example, in health a heart rate of 70 beats per minute is typically considered normal and desirable. In the presence of hypovolemic shock, however, it reflects a maladaptive response to intravascular volume loss and may herald impending hemodynamic disaster. Unfortunately, hemodynamic or metabolic stability is not guaranteed because the patient's "numbers" are "good" regardless of how good is defined. If the patient looks clinically "bad" despite "good" numbers, the patient's condition is bad.

Should a crisis situation develop, time and personnel are commonly devoted to attempts to obtain "numbers" to aid in assessment and documentation of the severity of the patient's condition. For example, if a patient suddenly becomes hypotensive and an arterial line is not available, frequent attempts are made to obtain cuff blood pressure measurements. Given the best of circumstances, such as a quiet, unhurried environment, muffled Korotkoff sounds that wax and wane in intensity are difficult to auscultate. In a noisy, crowded crisis situation, accurate auscultation of arterial pressure may be impossible. Compounding this difficulty, when stroke volume is low or peripheral vascular resistance is increased, the auscultated blood pressure is known to substantially underestimate the true intra-arterial pressure. Therefore, rather than wasting time and manpower attempting to hear that which is poorly audible and, if heard, is of uncertain accuracy anyway, it is far more productive to give remedial therapy and note the patient's clinical response to therapy. A statement on the chart such as "blood pressure difficult to obtain by auscultation, radial pulses imperceptible, femoral pulses weak bilaterally, skin and mucous membranes pale, extremities cool to touch, patient obtunded and restless" clearly documents the severity of the perfusion crisis. With indications of patient improvement, such as a return of color, normalization of the sensorium, and presence of peripheral pulses, a normalizing arterial pressure may again be audible, reasonably accurate, and worth documenting.

THE PATIENT

Most patients who are candidates for invasive hemodynamic monitoring have known, suspected, or coexisting cardiovascular disease. It is reasonable, therefore, to focus attention on the performance of the anatomically or physiologically troubled heart. The patient facing acute life-threatening illness, major surgery, or trauma, however, is also typically overwhelmed with feelings of fear, insecurity, and entrapment as well as a loss of personal control. The very nature of the critical care environment with its peculiar-looking equipment, animated oscilloscope lights, hissing ventilators, gurgling chest tube drainage systems, and many alarms that join in a discordant symphony of frightening sounds seems to reflect the personal fear of the patient: "I really must be sick. Otherwise, I wouldn't be in a place like this." The accompanying feelings of helplessness, hopelessness, anxiety, and depersonalization all have the potential to produce or exacerbate physiologic aberrations. To enhance recovery, it is imperative, therefore, to care for the emotional and spiritual heart as well as the physical heart. No formula is available to accomplish this. Rather, the care giver must provide deliberate attention and possess sensitivity and intuition.

Patient situations and responses are not alike. Nevertheless, holding the patient's hand during insertion of intravascular catheters or chest tubes and including the patient in bedside dialogue during procedures when possible may be significant contributions to the patient's sense of well-being in the critical care environment. In addition, attentively listening to what the patient says and/or helping with the expression of fears, hopes, anxieties, or frustrations with statements like "You seem weary," or "I get the feeling that you're feeling frustrated, angry, frightened," etc., may open the door to an outpouring of pent-up emotions.

Sometimes the critically ill patient is rendered speechless by the nature of the disease or, more commonly, by insertion of an artificial airway. This imposes another stress as the patient is unable to give voice to feelings and basic requests. What might be interpreted by hospital personnel as restlessness or random, purposeless, or confused behavior may be an attempt to communicate a basic need. The following excerpt from a letter written by the sister of a young, very ill septicemic patient who was the recipient of many critical care support/monitoring devices exemplifies this problem.[1]

> I wish he could tell me how he feels. The other day, he was trying very hard to get his hand free to do something. Everyone thought he was trying to pull something out. A nurse got brave and freed the restraint and all he'd wanted was to get his hair, now far too long, out of his eye.

THE CARE GIVER

At the information-sending end of the monitoring equipment is a physiologically unstable and often frightened, lonely human being. It remains the responsibility of the care giver at the information-receiving end of the monitoring equipment to look after both the compelling physiological and psychological needs of the patient—an awesome responsibility.

Preparation for that responsibility mandates that the care giver receive specialized training in the art and science of critical care—a specialty whose basic requirements are as unique and complex as the physical equipment required for patient care. A care giver who does not possess adequate technical skills and levels of understanding of physiology, pathophysiology, and therapeutics negates the purpose of critical care—to obtain the best possible outcome for the acutely ill or injured patient.

Preparation for patient care does not stop with the completion of a critical care course. The established body of knowledge relating to critical care is immense; there always remains a great deal of information to learn to strengthen one's skills or provide a new insight into currently understood principles. It is the continuing responsibility of the professional critical care practitioner to keep current as new concepts in disease prevention, pathogenesis, and management continually unfold.

As practitioners of the art and science of healing, we frequently witness the entrance and exit of life as well as some of its most poignant, intimate, and critical moments. It is befitting that we do so with sensitivity and with great skill.

REFERENCE

1. Richardson M: To Paul, Wherever You May Be, unpublished.

Pulmonary Anatomy and Physiology

2

The function of the pulmonary system is the exchange of oxygen from atmosphere to blood to cells and carbon dioxide from cells to blood to atmosphere. Four processes related to lung function and gas exchange include: ventilation: bulk movement of gas in and out of the lungs; distribution of those gases throughout the upper airways and tracheobronchial tree; diffusion: passive two-way transfer of respiratory gases from the alveoli, plasma, and red blood cells; and perfusion/transport: movement of blood through the pulmonary capillaries and ultimate delivery to body tissue.

VENTILATION

Ventilation is the cyclic, rhythmic movement of the diaphragm and structures of the chest wall, which results in the bulk movement of gases in and out of the lungs.

The structures involved in ventilation include twelve ribs, the sternum, and the thoracic vertebrae that form the body cage of the thorax; and the ventilatory muscles which act to expand or contract the volume of the thoracic cavity. These muscles include the diaphragm, the primary muscle of ventilation; the external and internal intercostal muscles; and the muscles of the abdomen. The major accessory muscles of ventilation include the scalene, sternocleidomastoid, trapezius, and pectoralis muscles. Patients recruit the accessory muscles when adequate ventilation cannot be achieved by normal breathing, such as occurs with upper or lower airway obstruction. Overall, the structures of the rib cage have a tendency toward outward expansion.

The two lungs fill a large part of the thoracic cavity. The right lung has three lobes: upper, middle, and lower. The left lung has two: upper and lower. The primary bronchi and pulmonary vessels enter each lung at its mediastinal surface, known as the hilum. Otherwise, the lungs lie free in their pleural cavities.

The pleural space is a potential space created by a visceral pleura attached to the lung and a parietal pleura attached to the chest wall. A film of fluid in the pleural space facilitates friction-free movement of the lungs during ventilation. The pressure within the intrapleural space remains subatmospheric and averages minus 4 to minus 8 mm Hg. This negative pressure acts as a suction holding the elastic lungs, which have a tendency toward inward recoil, adherent to the chest wall.

Mechanics of Ventilation

At rest, the recoil properties of the lung and chest wall are equal but oppositely directed. Pressures at the nares and mouth, tracheobronchial tree, and alveoli are atmospheric, 760 mm Hg. Lung volume is static and there is no air flow. *During inspiration*, the external intercostal muscles contract, the ribs are moved outward and upward, and the dome-shaped diaphragm contracts to descend and flatten. These actions increase the dimensions and volume of the thoracic cavity. Adherent to the inside of the chest wall, the lungs follow the outward excursion of the chest and expand. Pressures within the tracheobronchial tree and alveoli become subatmospheric, 755 to 757 mm Hg, and air is sucked into the lungs. This negative intrathoracic pressure also creates a vacuum for venous blood, thus increasing venous return to the heart and cardiac output by the Starling effect (the greater the ventricular filling volume at end-diastole, the greater the subsequent force of contraction and stroke volume). *During expiration*, the external intercostal muscles relax, the elastic recoil properties of the lungs pull the chest wall to a contracted position, and the diaphragm relaxes and ascends to its resting domed shape. The volume of the thoracic cavity is thus reduced, and pressures within the tracheobronchial tree and alveoli exceed atmospheric pressure, 763 to 765 mm Hg. Air then flows out of the lungs owing to the pressure gradient. The ventilatory apparatus, the thorax, acts as a simple bellows pump. Expanding the size and volume of the thorax pulls air in, while contracting it forces air out.

Control of Ventilation

Total body oxygen consumption and carbon dioxide production are matched by adjustments in ventilation that are entirely dependent on nervous system function. In the brain, the upper pons (pneumotaxic center), lower pons (apneustic center), and medulla alternately discharge inspiratory and expiratory signals to the muscles of ventilation. Chemoreceptors in these central respiratory structures are influenced by the effect of the arterial carbon dioxide level on the pH of the cerebral spinal fluid. The normal arterial CO_2 concentration is in the range of 35 to 45 mm Hg; normal arterial pH is 7.35 to 7.45. Increasing levels of carbon dioxide, which result in systemic and cerebral spinal fluid acidosis, increase the rate and depth of breathing.

Conversely, a lowered carbon dioxide concentration and increased pH blunt the ventilatory drive.

The peripheral chemoreceptors located at the bifurcation of the carotid artery (carotid bodies) and aortic arch (aortic bodies) indirectly stimulate the central ventilatory centers in the presence of increased arterial carbon dioxide, acidemia, low perfusion states, anemia, and hypoxemia. In addition, local acidemic stimulation of the carotid chemoreceptors increases pulmonary vascular resistance and bronchiolar tone.

A chronically elevated carbon dioxide level in the range of 65 to 75 mm Hg, seen, for example, in chronic obstructive pulmonary disease (COPD), desensitizes the central ventilatory center to hypercarbia (elevated $PaCO_2$). Persons with chronic severe hypercarbia rely on the peripheral hypoxic drive to maintain ventilation. Administration of oxygen in an amount to eliminate the hypoxic drive (a PaO_2 greater than 55 to 60 mm Hg) may result in an apneic patient.

The lung contains receptors that are sensitive to stretch. Stimulation of the bronchial receptors of the Hering-Breuer reflex results in inhibition of inspiration with lung expansion beyond 1.5 liters. This protects the lung from excessive inflation.

Sensory nerves called "J" receptors, located in alveolar walls adjacent to capillaries, become stimulated when pulmonary capillaries become congested with blood or when lung tissue becomes edematous. Excitation of J receptors increases the rate of breathing and is thought to contribute to the sensation of dyspnea and to be the cause of the tachypnea that occurs before any other clinical signs of pulmonary edema become apparent.

Distribution

Distribution is the delivery of fresh air to the gas exchanging units (alveoli) via the upper airways and tracheobronchial tree. This is facilitated by ventilation and insures maximum gas partial pressure levels at the alveolus for efficient diffusion across the alveolar-capillary membrane.

Structures of the upper airway include the nose, pharynx, and larynx. The lower airway consists of the trachea; bronchi; and the basic pulmonary unit, the acinus (Fig. 2–1). This structure contains the terminal bronchioles, respiratory bronchioles, alveolar ducts, atria, alveolar sacs, and alveoli.

The portion of inhaled gases that fills the spaces of the upper airway and tracheobronchial tree is not exposed to blood and does not participate in gas exchange. This volume of gas is regarded as *anatomic dead space* ventilation and is approximately equal to 1 ml per 450 grams (1 pound) of ideal body weight. For example, the tidal volume of a normal adult at rest is approximately 500 ml. Of this inhaled air, approximately 150 ml does not reach the alveoli. In health, the ratio of dead space to tidal volume is approximately 0.3. That is, one third of the inhaled air normally does not participate in gas exchange. Dead space volume may increase if there is ventilation but no perfusion to alveoli, such as occurs with pulmonary embolism. This wasted

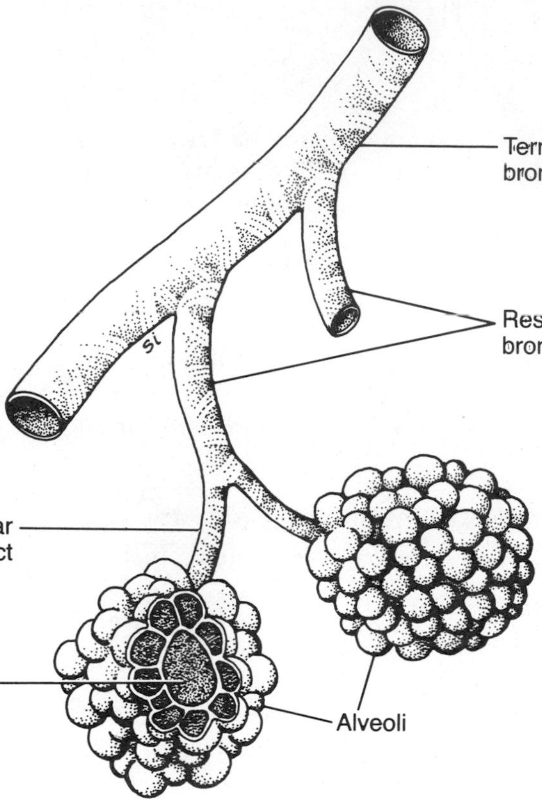

FIGURE 2–1. The acinus, the basic pulmonary unit, begins just distal to the terminal bronchiole.

ventilation is termed *alveolar dead space* and, if significant, may result in hypoxemia. Together, anatomic and alveolar dead space are referred to as *physiologic dead space*. Because alveolar dead space volume (the poorly perfused alveoli in the apices of both lungs) is insignificant in health, physiologic dead space volume is normally equal to anatomic dead space volume.

A moist mucous blanket lines the passages of the upper airways and tracheobronchial tree, providing an important cleansing and defense mechanism for the lungs. In the upper airways, mucus moves downward from the nose and sinuses to the pharynx where it is swallowed. Through upward movement of the mucous blanket toward the pharynx, captured debris and particulate matter are cleared from the lungs. Factors such as dehydration, smoking, alcohol ingestion, or a high inspired oxygen fraction may impair clearance, rendering the lungs more susceptible to infection.

Factors That Affect the Efficiency of Ventilation, Distribution of Gases, and Work of Breathing. *Resistance* (elastance) refers to the tendency of the structures of the lungs and thorax to resist distending forces. This is expressed in terms of cm H_2O pressure per liter of gas flow on lung inflation and can be related to airway, lung, and chest wall resistance to ventilation. For example, if it takes 20 cm H_2O pressure to deliver a 600 ml tidal volume to a normal adult, approximately 8 cm H_2O pressure is required to overcome airway resistance. If, however, the overall radius of the airways is reduced by one half due to bronchial swelling, bronchospasm, or mucous plugging, airflow resistance will be increased 16 times. In the spontaneously breathing person, this will produce a marked increase in the work of breathing and interfere with the adequate distribution of fresh air to alveoli and exit of exhaled gases. If the patient is being mechanically ventilated, higher peak inspiratory pressures will be required to deliver the prescribed tidal volume, and the possibility of alveolar hyperinflation and air trapping increases.

In the same person, about 5 cm H_2O pressure is required to overcome the resistance of the lung, which exerts a force in an expiratory direction, to expansion. If the patient develops pulmonary edema, atelectasis or pulmonary fibrosis, lung resistance to expansion increases.

Finally, about 7 cm H_2O pressure is required to overcome the resistance of the chest wall. Spasm or swelling of the muscles of the thorax due to trauma (especially in muscular persons), circumferential deep partial or full-thickness thoracic burns, extreme obesity, or external binders may significantly increase chest wall resistance to expansion.

Compliance refers to the distensibility or expansibility of the lungs and thorax and is measured in terms of the volume of gas, from end-expiration to end-inspiration, that can move into the lung for each unit of pressure change. This is measured in ml of lung expansion per cm H_2O pressure. In the normal person, the lungs expand approximately 130 ml for each 1 cm H_2O increase in alveolar pressure. However, just as a balloon tends to resist expansion at the onset of inflation when it is small and then becomes progressively more distensible (more volume moves in per unit of pressure) as it expands, so do the lungs resist expansion at the onset of inspiration and then become progressively more distensible as alveoli enlarge and expand. Because of the enlargement of the air spaces distal to the terminal bronchioles characteristic of pulmonary emphysema, the lungs of the emphysematous patient are highly compliant. Conversely, the lungs of the patient with massive, diffuse atelectasis are noncompliant.

In essence, compliance is the opposite of resistance. The very stiff lungs of the patient with adult respiratory distress syndrome (ARDS) are said to be highly resistant or noncompliant. On the other hand, the very nonelastic, distensible lungs of the emphysematous patient are highly compliant or nonresistant.

DIFFUSION

Diffusion is the passive two-way transfer of respiratory gases from the alveoli, plasma, and hemoglobin molecule mediated by gas pressure gradients.

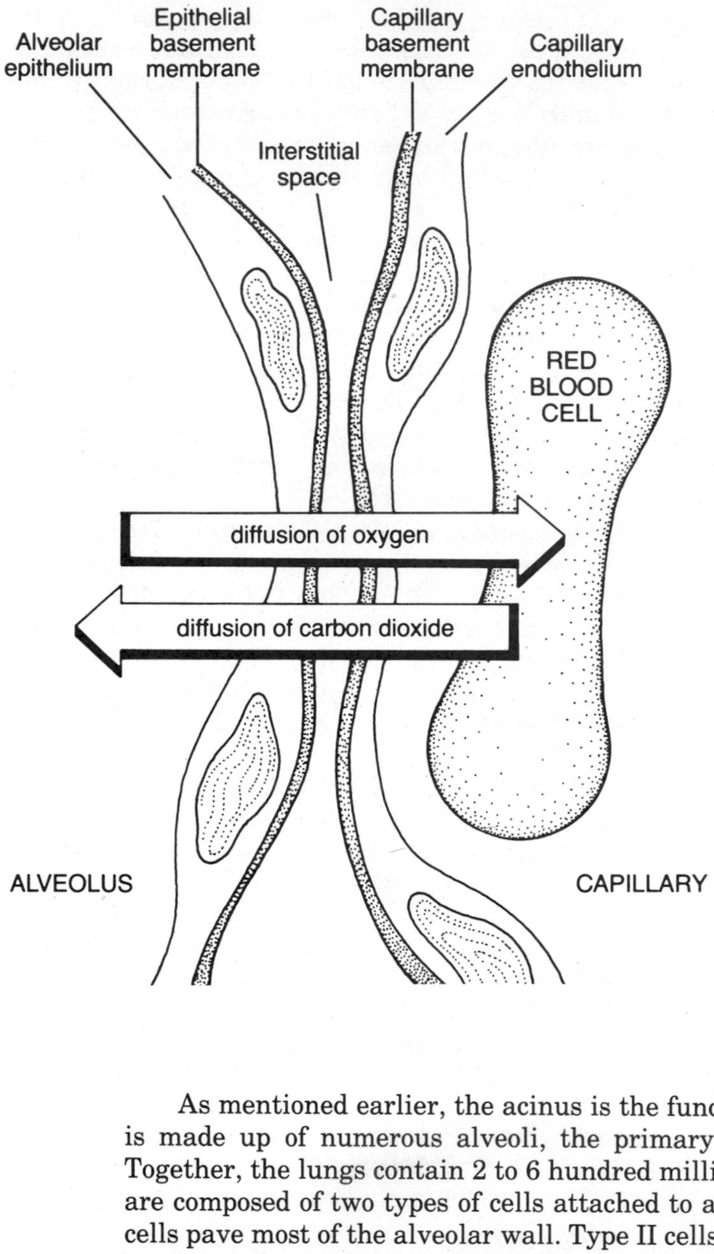

FIGURE 2–2. The alveolar-capillary membrane over which reciprocal diffusion of oxygen and carbon dioxide occurs.

As mentioned earlier, the acinus is the fundamental pulmonary unit and is made up of numerous alveoli, the primary structures of gas exchange. Together, the lungs contain 2 to 6 hundred million alveoli. The alveolar walls are composed of two types of cells attached to a basement membrane. Type I cells pave most of the alveolar wall. Type II cells produce surfactant, a surface tension-reducing agent that plays a major role in preventing alveolar collapse. Each alveolus is embraced by and wedded to an almost solid network of pulmonary capillaries. The alveolar-capillary interface (membrane) consists of the alveolar cell wall, a basement membrane, the interstitial connective tissue, a capillary basement membrane, and a capillary endothelial cell wall (Fig. 2–2).

The following factors affect gaseous diffusion across the alveolar-capillary membrane:

The thickness of the alveolar-capillary membrane—The rate of diffusion through the membrane is inversely proportional to the thickness of the membrane. Increased thickness (as in pulmonary edema or fibrosis) has the potential to interfere with the diffusion of gases. True diffusion blocks are rarely seen clinically, as it is unusual for the membrane to be thick enough to prevent equilibration of gases.

The surface area of the alveolar-capillary membrane—Normally this approximates 70 square meters (the size of a tennis court) in the average adult. Any condition that decreases the surface area (pneumothorax, COPD, pneumonectomy) produces a deficit in the exchange of gases.

The diffuse coefficient for the movement of each gas across the alveolar-capillary membrane—This relates to the individual gas's solubility in the membrane and inversely to the square root of its molecular weight. Carbon dioxide diffuses through the membrane about 20 times more rapidly than oxygen. For this reason, hypercarbia due to impaired diffusion is rare; however, impaired diffusion may produce significant hypoxemia.

The pressure gradient between the partial pressure of gases in the alveoli and the partial pressure of gases in plasma—The weight of the ocean of gases that surrounds our planet exerts a force equal to 760 mm Hg at sea level. This is termed atmospheric pressure and is the sum of all the various pressures of gases that make up the atmosphere. The pressure exerted by one gas alone is termed the partial pressure as it accounts for only part of the total atmospheric pressure. Since the atmosphere contains 21 percent oxygen, the partial pressure of oxygen in the atmosphere is 159 mm Hg (21 percent of 760 mm Hg equals 159 mm Hg). As air enters the respiratory tract, it becomes fully saturated with water and mixes with the carbon dioxide that is exiting the alveoli. This reduces the partial pressure of oxygen in the alveolus to 100 mm Hg. Table 2–1 is a comparison of alveolar and ambient gas partial pressures.

A large gas pressure gradient exists across the alveolar-capillary membrane. The partial pressure of oxygen in venous blood is 40 mm Hg while alveolar oxygen partial pressure is 100 mm Hg. The large pressure gradient (60 mm Hg) almost fully saturates the red blood cell with oxygen when it is one third past the alveolar-capillary membrane. Mixed venous blood has a $PvCO_2$ (partial pressure of carbon dioxide in venous blood) of about 47 mm Hg while alveolar CO_2 is 40 mm Hg. Driven by the pressure gradient, some of the carbon dioxide is yielded up to the alveolus, where it will ultimately be exhaled into the air.

TABLE 2–1. Comparison of Alveolar and Ambient Gas Partial Pressures

	Ambient Partial Pressure (mm Hg)	*Alveolar Partial Pressure (mm Hg)*
Nitrogen	592	573
Oxygen	159	100
Carbon dioxide	3	40
H_2O (as vapor)	3	47
Trace	3	

When oxygenated blood reaches the capillary bed, its PO_2 is about 90 to 100 mm Hg whereas the PO_2 in the interstitial space is about 40 mm Hg. This large pressure gradient causes oxygen to diffuse from the blood into the interstitial space. Because the cells are constantly metabolizing oxygen, the intracellular PO_2 is less than that of the surrounding interstitial space and averages about 23 mm Hg, but may be as low as 4 mm Hg. The pressure gradient of approximately 17 mm Hg (40 mm Hg interstitial PO_2 minus 23 mm Hg intracellular PO_2 = 17 mm Hg) causes oxygen to diffuse into the cells.

PERFUSION/TRANSPORT

PERFUSION

Perfusion is the means by which blood is brought to the alveolar-capillary membrane for removal of carbon dioxide, oxygenation, sustenance of lung tissue, and delivery to the left heart for transport to the body cells.

The lungs receive a dual blood supply. Coming directly from the aorta, the bronchial arteries provide an arterial blood supply to the supporting tissues of the lungs. The major portion of blood flow through the lungs is delivered by the right ventricle through the pulmonary arteries. This is approximately 5 liters per minute while the person is at rest.

Pulmonary Blood Flow and Perfusion Pressures. From the right ventricle, blood flows into the pulmonary trunk, which then divides into the right and left main arterial branches. These branches continue to divide into two subdivisions for approximately 24 successive generations, ultimately forming the pulmonary capillary network. At rest, blood transit time across the pulmonary capillary bed is approximately 1 second and decreases as cardiac output increases. The pulmonary arteries are very thin and distensible and have larger diameters than do the systemic arteries. These characteristics increase vascular compliance and allow the pulmonary circulation to accommodate the output of the right ventricle, which is equal to the output of the left ventricle, the chamber that serves the large systemic circulation. Further, owing to pulmonary arterial compliance, blood flow in the lungs can increase four to six times normal before pulmonary arterial pressures rise significantly. Under normal conditions, both lungs contain approximately 450 ml of blood, 70 ml of which is in the pulmonary capillaries.

Pressures in the pulmonary circulation are as follows:

Right ventricular (RV)	systolic pressure:	15–25 mm Hg
	diastolic pressure:	0–8 mm Hg
Pulmonary artery (PA)	systolic pressure:	15–25 mm Hg
	diastolic pressure:	8–15 mm Hg
Pulmonary capillary pressure:		6–12 mm Hg
Pulmonary venous pressure:		4–12 mm Hg

Pulmonary Vascular Resistance. Pulmonary vascular resistance (the opposition to blood flow through the pulmonary vasculature) is normally low due to the highly distensible, elastic character of the pulmonary vessels. Pulmonary vascular resistance (PVR) can be calculated clinically using the pulmonary artery catheter. PVR is calculated from the average (mean) pressure gradient across and blood flow through the pulmonary vascular channel. Resistance is expressed as units of force or dynes sec per cm^{-5}. (See Chapter 9, "Pulmonary Vascular Resistance.") An increase in PVR elevates the pulmonary artery systolic and diastolic pressures; conversely, decreased PVR is associated with decreased pulmonary artery systolic and diastolic pressures. Factors that influence PVR include:

1. The autonomic nervous system—This has minimal effect on the pulmonary vasculature. Parasympathetic dominance causes only a slight decrease in pulmonary vascular resistance; sympathetic dominance results in only a slight increase in pulmonary vascular tone.

2. Pulmonary arterial hypoxemia—This has a potent constrictor effect on the pulmonary vasculature. This is in direct contrast to the hypoxemia-induced vasodilation seen in systemic vascular beds. Hypoxemia-induced pulmonary vasoconstriction is fundamentally a protective and productive mechanism. In the presence of low alveolar oxygen concentrations (atelectasis, bronchitis), blood is shunted from poorly ventilated alveoli to areas of lung that are better oxygenated. Unfortunately, with generalized hypoxemia (high altitude, diffuse respiratory disease) generalized pulmonary vascular narrowing occurs. Such vasoconstriction probably involves both precapillary and postcapillary vessels. The increased pulmonary vascular resistance is reflected in elevated pulmonary artery systolic and diastolic pressures.

3. Hydrogen ion concentration—An increased hydrogen ion concentration of the blood perfusing the pulmonary arteries (acidemia) has a constrictor effect. Table 2–2 indicates the estimated relationship of mean pulmonary artery pressure to arterial blood oxygen saturation and pH.

TABLE 2–2. Estimated Relationship of Mean Pulmonary Artery Pressure to Arterial Blood Oxygen Saturation and pH

	Arterial Oxygen Saturation (%)	*pH*	*Estimated Mean Pulmonary Artery Pressure (mm Hg)*
NORMAL	97–99	7.35–7.45	15
	93	7.53–7.22	20
	90	7.40	24
	85	7.40	28
	85	7.22	50
	80	7.40	34
	80	7.22	64
	70	7.40	47
	70	7.30	70
	60	7.40	55

Adapted from Ferrer MI: Management of patients with cor pulmonale. Med Clin North Am (1979) 63:255.

4. Pharmacologic agents—Medications have varying effects on the pulmonary vasculature. *Pulmonary vasoconstrictors* include epinephrine (Adrenalin), norepinephrine (Levophed), and metaraminol (Aramine) and are associated with elevations in pulmonary artery systolic and diastolic pressures. *Pulmonary vasodilators* include isoproterenol (Isuprel), phentolamine (Regitine), nifedipine (Procardia), diltiazem (Cardizem), hydralazine (Apresoline), diazoxide (Hyperstat), and sodium nitroprusside (Nipride) and are associated with reductions in pulmonary artery systolic and diastolic pressures.

5. Blockage or destruction of part of the pulmonary circulation—Reduction in the cross-sectional area of the pulmonary circulation, as in pulmonary embolism, increases pulmonary vascular resistance, although such elevations are rare unless in the presence of a 30 to 50 percent or greater vascular obstruction.

6. Volume status of the pulmonary circulation—Volume overload results in an elevation of pulmonary arterial pressures; volume depletion produces pulmonary hypotension.

Overall, the low pressure pulmonary circulation may be converted to a high pressure circulation (pulmonary hypertension) by essentially three mechanisms: (1) an increase in pulmonary hydrostatic pressure due to pulmonary vascular volume loading as in left-sided heart failure; (2) a tremendous increase in blood flow as in ventricular septal defect; and (3) an increase in pulmonary vascular resistance due to pulmonary vasoconstriction or a decrease in the cross-sectional area of the pulmonary vascular bed.

Ventilation/Perfusion Ratios in the Lung. Normally, both lungs have an average alveolar ventilation of 4 liters per minute and a perfusion of 5 liters per minute; therefore, the ventilation/perfusion ratio (V/Q) is about 0.8 for the entire lung. The distribution of pulmonary ventilation and perfusion, however, shows variations dependent upon body position relating to gravitational forces. Both increase progressively downward from the apices to the bases when a person is in an upright position, although blood flow increases about three times more rapidly than does ventilation. Mean pulmonary artery pressure is about 13 to 15 mm Hg at heart level, and alveolar pressures are about equal throughout the lung, -3 to $+3$ cm H_2O with normal, quiet breathing. At the apex, mean pulmonary artery pressure is about 3 mm Hg; therefore, the V/Q ratio is higher at the apices (ventilation in excess of perfusion). At the bases, mean pulmonary artery pressure is about 21 mm Hg; therefore, blood flow is greater than at heart level and perfusion is greater than ventilation (V/Q ratios are lower). Clearly, ventilation is not perfectly matched to perfusion in all areas of the normal lung.

Three physical principles have major implications in caring for the critically ill.

(1) In patients assuming the lateral decubitus position, the upper lung experiences less ventilation and perfusion than do the apices normally, and the lower lung experiences increased ventilation and perfusion usually seen with the lower lobes in the upright position. Positioning the patient with the diseased lung side (diffuse atelectasis, pneumothorax) down increases blood flow through poorly ventilated areas and worsens hypoxemia.

(2) If pulmonary artery pressures are significantly decreased (hypovolemia) or alveolar pressures increased (positive end-expiratory pressure, or PEEP; continuous positive airway pressure, or CPAP), significant decreases in blood flow may occur to the least dependent segments of the lung. This would increase alveolar dead space ventilation (inspired air that does not interface with blood) and may contribute to hypoxemia.

(3) Interstitial and alveolar edema tends to accumulate in the dependent areas of the lung. This decreases ventilation in dependent areas through alveolar flooding, small airway obstruction, or atelectasis, whereas the dependent blood vessels continue to experience blood flow. This further increases the degree of perfusion in excess of ventilation normally seen at the bases and predisposes the patient to hypoxemia. The goal in therapy in this circumstance is to eliminate or reduce the degree of pulmonary edema.

TRANSPORT

Oxygen that diffuses from the alveoli to the pulmonary capillary blood is transported to the tissues in two forms.

Physically dissolved in plasma. Clinically, this is measured as the partial pressure of oxygen in arterial blood (PaO_2). Oxygen in physical solution accounts for less than 2 percent of the oxygen contained in a given volume of blood. The normal PaO_2 is 90 to 100 mm Hg at sea level when breathing environmental (ambient) air. At this value, the actual amount of oxygen in solution in plasma is 0.3 ml per 1 dl of plasma. Factors that influence the PaO_2 level include the volume of the lung, the adequacy of alveolar ventilation, the percent of oxygen in the inspired air (FIO_2), the physical characteristics of the lung tissue, age and the oxyhemoglobin dissociation curve.

Physically bound to hemoglobin. Oxygen is transported in reversible combination with the heme portion of the hemoglobin molecule and accounts for about 97 to 98 percent of the oxygen that reaches the tissues. The affinity of hemoglobin for oxygen varies with the PaO_2. When the PaO_2 is elevated, as in the pulmonary capillaries, oxygen binds readily with hemoglobin. When the PaO_2 is low, however, as in the systemic capillaries, oxygen becomes easily dissociated from the hemoglobin. *Oxygen saturation* (SO_2) is a percent measurement of the amount of hemoglobin bound with oxygen; normal arterial values are in the range of 96 to 98 percent. Each gram of hemoglobin can maximally (100 percent saturation) bind with 1.36 ml of oxygen.

The oxyhemoglobin dissociation curve relates the percent saturation of the hemoglobin molecule to the amount of oxygen dissolved in plasma (Fig. 2–3).

Illustrated in the *S* shape of the curve, one can see the progressive increase in oxygen saturation as the PaO_2 increases and decreases in saturation as the PaO_2 falls. Note the other characteristics of the curve. At a normal arterial PaO_2 of 90 to 100 mm Hg, the hemoglobin is about 96 to 98 percent saturated. Even if pulmonary disease causes the arterial PaO_2 to drop by more than one third to 60 mm Hg, because of continued affinity for oxygen hemoglobin saturation undergoes a very small decrease to a range of 91 to

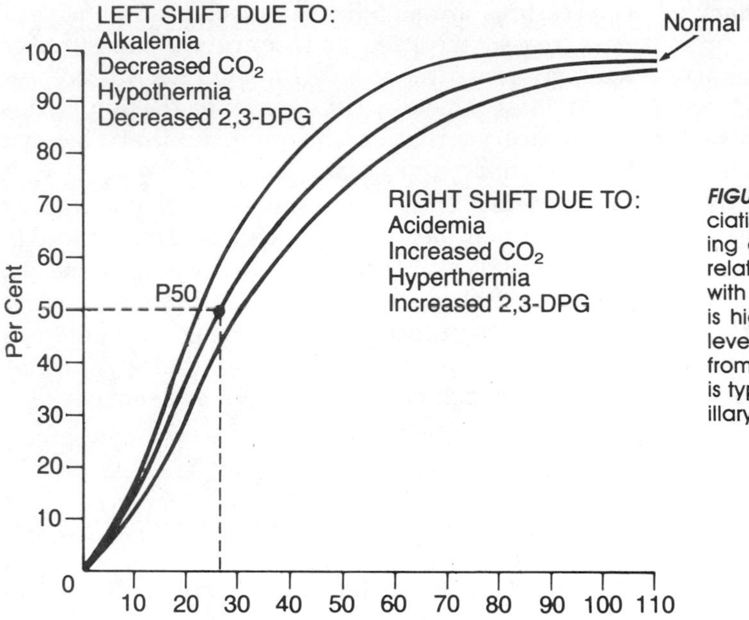

FIGURE 2–3. The oxyhemoglobin dissociation curve. Illustrated is the changing affinity of hemoglobin for oxygen, related to the Po_2 of plasma. Binding with oxygen is increased when the Po_2 is high, as at the pulmonary capillary level. Hemoglobin readily dissociates from its oxygen when the Po_2 is low, as is typically shown at the systemic capillary level.

92 percent. This protects the tissues from hypoxia. If the PaO_2 drops below 60 mm Hg, however, hemoglobin saturation changes dramatically as hemoglobin's affinity for oxygen progressively decreases. As illustrated in the descending limb of the curve (Fig. 2–3), smaller drops in PaO_2 produce greater decreases in oxygen saturation. Given a PO_2 of 40 mm Hg, a normal venous value, one can expect an oxygen saturation of 75 percent. The increased tendency for hemoglobin to release its oxygen and become desaturated at a lower PO_2 is important to facilitate tissue oxygen availability at the capillary level. Conversely, the tendency for hemoglobin to grab and bind oxygen at a high PO_2 facilitates uptake at the pulmonary capillary level and subsequent transport to tissues.

The *P50* is the estimated PO_2 level at an oxygen saturation of 50 percent. Given normal body temperature, normal blood pH, and normal levels of 2,3 diphosphoglycerate (2,3 DPG), at a hemoglobin oxygen saturation of 50 percent, the PO_2 is 26.6 mm Hg. The P50 may be changed, or, stated another way, the oxyhemoglobin dissociation curve may be shifted to the right or left, in the following circumstances:

Changes in body temperature—Increased body temperature increases the P50. That is, at an oxygen saturation of 50 percent, the PO_2 is greater than 26.6 mm Hg. Hyperthermia decreases the affinity of the hemoglobin molecule for oxygen, thus facilitating unloading for increased uptake and utilization by the cells. This is advantageous as increases in body temperature are met with proportionate increases in metabolic rate and oxygen demand. Decreases in body temperature, as occur when tissue metabolism is low, shift the curve to the left, as the hemoglobin molecule clings to its oxygen.

Changes in pH—If the blood is acidemic, as when around actively metabolizing tissue, the curve shifts to the right and the PO_2 is greater than 26.6 at an oxygen saturation of 50 percent. Alkalemia has the opposite effect; this has profound clinical implications, reducing oxygen availability at the tissue level.

Changes in the quantity of 2,3 DPG—A substance in the red blood cell, 2,3 DPG affects the affinity of the hemoglobin molecule for oxygen. Increased levels (as occurs at high altitude, during exercise, or during prolonged hypoxic conditions) shift the curve to the right. Decreased levels (as can occur following the administration of large quantities of banked blood, diabetic acidosis, or sepsis) shift the curve to the left.

To summarize, one can say that a rightward shift increases the P50 and decreases hemoglobin's affinity for oxygen. The PO_2 is greater than normal for any given oxygen saturation (SO_2). A leftward shift, on the other hand, decreases the P50, and increases hemoglobin's affinity for oxygen. The PO_2 is less than normal for any given oxygen saturation (SO_2).

The term *oxygen content (CaO_2)* defines the amount of oxygen in 100 ml of whole blood and is expressed in ml of oxygen in 100 ml of blood or "volume percent" (vol%). Because the PaO_2 only defines the partial pressure of oxygen physically dissolved in plasma and oxygen saturation only defines the percent of hemoglobin physically bound to oxygen, the CaO_2 value has important clinical application because it tells exactly how much oxygen is present in the blood. Because only a very small amount of oxygen in blood is physically dissolved in plasma, it is convenient and accurate to estimate oxygen content merely by multiplying the amount of hemoglobin by the known hemoglobin oxygen saturation by 1.36 (the amount of oxygen a fully saturated gram of hemoglobin can carry). For example, given a patient with a hemoglobin of 14 grams, a PaO_2 of 100 mm Hg and an oxygen saturation of 98 percent (the normal value when the PaO_2 is 100 mm Hg):

$$\text{Hgb} \times SO_2 \times 1.36 = CaO_2 \text{ expressed in vol\% (ml } O_2 \text{ in 100 ml blood)}$$
$$14 \text{ Gm} \times .98 \times 1.36 = CaO_2 \text{ 18.7 vol\%}$$

The CaO_2 can be decreased if the PaO_2 and, therefore, oxygen saturation fall or if the amount of hemoglobin is decreased. In the previous example, if the hemoglobin remains constant but the PaO_2 falls to 30 mm Hg with an oxygen saturation of 55 percent:

$$14 \text{ Gm} \times .55 \times 1.36 = CaO_2 \text{ 10.5 vol\%}$$

If the patient suffers a drop in hemoglobin due to hemorrhage but the PaO_2 and oxygen saturation remain constant:

$$7 \text{ Gm} \times .97 \times 1.36 = CaO_2 \text{ 9.2 vol\%}$$

It is also clinically significant to note that increasing the PaO_2 above 100 mm Hg through the administration of oxygen will have minimal effect on oxygen content because oxygen saturation cannot exceed 100 percent, which it nearly reaches at a PaO_2 of 90 to 100 mm Hg. In fact a PaO_2 greater than 100 mm Hg may place the patient at risk of developing oxygen toxicity.

Oxygen transport is an important calculation in the critical care setting. Remembering that the cardiopulmonary unit has as its end-point tissue oxygenation, oxygen transport defines how much oxygen is pumped out by the heart to the body tissues per minute. This value may be calculated by multiplying the cardiac output (in liters per minute) by 10 (the factor 10 converts Hgb from grams per 100 ml to grams per 1000 ml of blood) by arterial oxygen content in ml per 100 ml of blood. For example, given a patient with a cardiac output of 5 liters per minute and an oxygen content of 18.4 ml O_2 per 100 ml of blood:

$$\text{Cardiac output} \times 10 \times CaO_2 = \text{oxygen transport in ml } O_2/\text{min}$$
$$5 \text{ liters/minute} \times 10 \times 18.4 = 920 \text{ ml } O_2 \text{ transported to the tissues/min}$$

Oxygen consumption is the total amount of oxygen consumed by the body per minute. This value can be calculated with an arterial blood sample, a mixed venous blood sample, and a determination of cardiac output. By calculating arterial oxygen transport (total amount of oxygen carried *to* the tissues) and subtracting from it venous oxygen transport (total amount of oxygen carried *from* the tissues), one can determine the amount of oxygen consumed by the body in 1 minute. Oxygen consumption is calculated by multiplying cardiac output (in liters per minute) by 10, which converts Hgb from grams per 100 ml to grams per 1000 ml. This figure is multiplied by 1.36, the amount of oxygen a fully saturated gram of hemoglobin can carry. Finally, multiplying by the arteriovenous saturation difference yields the oxygen consumption. For example, given a cardiac output of 5 liters per minute, a hemoglobin of 14 grams, an arterial saturation of 99 percent, and a mixed venous saturation of 75 percent:

$$\text{Cardiac output} \times 10 \times \text{Hgb} \times 1.36 \times (SaO_2 - S\bar{v}O_2) = O_2 \text{ consumption in ml } O_2/\text{min}$$

$$5 \text{ liters/min} \times 10 \times 14 \times 1.36 \times (0.99 - 0.75) = 228.5 \text{ ml } O_2/\text{min consumed by the body/min}$$

The oxygen consumption for a normal resting adult is approximately 220 to 290 ml per minute. This value, however, does not indicate whether body oxygen demands have been met. Normal cell function requires that oxygen supply (blood oxygen content and cardiovascular transport) meets tissue oxygen demands. With a balanced supply/demand relationship, the amount of oxygen consumed by the tissues is equal to that demanded. When the body's oxygen delivery system fails, the amount consumed falls short of tissue demand, and cells are forced to metabolize anaerobically. This alternate metabolic pathway results in a 20 fold decrease in energy production and also in lactic acidosis. The metabolic acidosis evidenced on blood gas analysis predicts physiologic disaster because the acid environment further compromises cell and cardiovascular function and may ultimately result in death.

The following defects in the oxygen delivery system can threaten tissue oxygenation: (1) decrease in cardiac output; (2) a fall in hemoglobin saturation; (3) a decrease in the amount of hemoglobin (anemia); and (4) excessive tissue oxygen requirements (thyroid storm, hyperthermia) or an inability of the cells to utilize the oxygen brought to them (sepsis, cyanide or ethanol toxicity).

The body may attempt to compensate for these defects in three ways so that tissue oxygenation and metabolism remain normal. First, it may increase cardiac output. The healthy heart can increase cardiac output from 5 liters per minute to 15 to 25 liters per minute. Because of compromised cardiac function, however, many critically ill patients cannot respond in this way.

A second response of the body is to increase the arteriovenous saturation difference by extracting more oxygen from the capillary blood. Normally, hemoglobin in mixed venous blood has a saturation of 75 percent, which leaves considerable reserve for additional extraction. Under conditions of increased metabolic requirements, decreased amount of hemoglobin (anemia), decreased cardiac output, or decreased arterial saturation, venous saturation can be decreased to a level as low as 31 percent before anaerobic metabolism and lactacidemia occur. Since drawing on the venous oxygen reserve is a means of protecting the tissue from hypoxia, evaluation of mixed venous oxygen saturation can be an important parameter in evaluating the critically ill patient whose oxygen delivery system is frequently threatened (see Chapter 11). Although extracting more oxygen from the capillary blood is another major safety factor to protect the cell from hypoxic insult, many critically ill patients have serious arterial oxygenation deficits such as refractory hypoxemia, which may seriously reduce the reserve for additional oxygen extraction.

A final response is for the body to increase the amount of hemoglobin. This mechanism is not available on an acute basis. With chronic hypoxemia as is seen with COPD, however, hemoglobin and red cell mass increase to maintain oxygen transport and oxidative metabolism.

These measures illustrate that the body has excellent adaptive mechanisms designed to protect the cells from hypoxia. This is fundamental to preserving the specialized function of various body organs and life itself. Unfortunately, and not uncommonly, one or all coping mechanisms of the critically ill patient may be compromised. In addition, arterial desaturation (and, therefore, venous reserve) for each organ system varies depending on differences in functional metabolic need. For example, at rest, the myocardium extracts about 70 percent of the oxygen from its arterial blood, the brain 25 percent, the liver 20 percent, and the kidneys approximately 10 percent. The heart clearly has the least oxygen reserve, for at rest it nearly desaturates its perfusing blood. Increased myocardial oxygen demand can only be met by increases in coronary blood flow. The measured mixed venous hemoglobin saturation is representative of an average of all the systems' venous saturation.

Further, metabolic needs for oxygen may increase significantly if the specific organ is stressed. For example, seizure activity can adversely affect the brain's oxygen balance. At a time when brain oxygen requirements are four to five times greater than normal due to increased metabolic activity, the amount of oxygen in the arterial blood may be drastically reduced because of obstruction of the upper airway by the tongue and secretions and/or spastic or absent ventilatory movements.

Clearly, the critically ill patient walks an oxygenation tightrope. It is the responsibility of the care giver to vigilantly monitor all aspects of the oxygen supply/demand equation and make immediate corrections in defects as they occur.

REFERENCES

Burton GG: Respiratory gas exchange mechanisms. In Burton GG, Hodgkin JE (eds): *Respiratory Care: A Guide to Practice,* ed. 2. Philadelphia, JB Lippincott, 1985.

Cherniak RM, Cherniak L: *Respiration in Health and Disease*, ed. 3. Philadelphia, WB Saunders, 1983.

Guyton AC: *Textbook of Medical Physiology*, ed. 7. Philadelphia, WB Saunders, 1986.

Murray JF: Respiration. In Smith LH, Thier SO (eds): *Pathophysiology, The Biological Principles of Disease*. Philadelphia, WB Saunders, 1981.

Schweiss JF: *Continuous Measurements of Blood Oxygen Saturation in the High Risk Patient,* vol. 2. San Diego, Beach International, Inc., 1983.

White KM: Completing the hemodynamic picture: S_vO_2. *Heart and Lung* 1985; 14:272–280.

Wilson RF: *Principles and Techniques of Critical Care*, vol. 1. Kalamazoo, MI, Upjohn, 1979.

Physical Assessment of the Pulmonary System

3

Because this text relates to the acutely ill patient who is a candidate for or is receiving invasive hemodynamic monitoring, the chapters on physical assessment will be limited to the frequent and serial evaluations of the pulmonary and cardiovascular (Chapter 5) systems in the acute care setting.

Those who have been involved in critical care longer than 20 years can appreciate the tremendous technological advances in bedside care and increased use of invasive and noninvasive monitoring equipment. Nevertheless, their use must be kept in perspective. Although the monitors give "beat by beat" information of the patient's physiological status, which often can be observed at a distance from the patient, they must be considered an adjunct to patient evaluation and should never replace frequent bedside clinical assessment.

Complete objectivity is essential to accurate physical assessment. In the time-pressured, acute care setting, however, the human tendency to incorporate preconceived ideas and feelings into one's findings is especially prevalent: that is, we tend to perceive largely what we expect or want to perceive. This creates the potential for serious errors in judgment. A careful nonhurried attitude in assessment is important so that 1) we see and evaluate the patient realistically and not according to our own expectations; and 2) the approach is satisfactory to the patient. The individual who is acutely ill, apprehensive, and no doubt already feeling like an alien in a strange land, will become additionally disturbed if the examiner is indifferent, unsympathetic, and/or rushed. Such an approach may create barriers to effective communication and assessment as well as produce untoward physiologic alterations which may exacerbate the present illness. Because most people feel more comfortable and talk more freely if the examiner's eyes are at the patient's eye level or below, the examiner should sit at the bedside when questioning the patient.

During a crisis situation, the patient may be in too much distress to give a coherent or thorough account of the illness. On these occasions, the patient's family member or close friend may have to be consulted for information to establish what is "normal" or "usual."

Unfortunately, the critical care situation does not always allow for an optimum environment for examination. Nevertheless, every attempt should be made to provide a reassuring and comfortable milieu. This is especially important on admission to the unit as the patient's and family's first impression may strongly influence their attitude for the entire hospital stay.

Overall, errors in physical assessment may be minimized if we remain constantly aware of human and monitoring limitations. Conclusions should be tested against other findings and monitoring data to see if they fit into the total clinical mosaic.

CLINICAL EVALUATION OF SYMPTOMS AND SIGNS OF PULMONARY DISEASE

Symptoms

Symptoms are the patients' subjective account of changes in body function or indications of disease. Many of the following symptoms of primary pulmonary disease may be indicative of other conditions as well.

Cough. A sensation of irritation in the pulmonary system or cough is the most frequent symptom of pulmonary disease and may be caused by stimuli arising in any part of the airways from the pharynx to the terminal bronchi.

Because the character of the sputum, if present, may give important clues to the underlying disorder, it should be observed for volume, color, consistency, and odor. It is important that the specimen comes from the lungs and is not postnasal secretions or saliva which is clear, colorless, and watery. In the critical care setting, sputum is frequently collected via suctioning through an endotracheal tube or tracheostomy.

Copious, thick, mucoid, grayish-white, translucent sputum is commonly seen in cigarette smokers and in patients with COPD. Purulent looking and smelling yellow or green sputum is an indication of pulmonary infection. Rust-colored sputum is seen in lobar pneumonia.

Hemoptysis is sputum that is grossly bloody, blood streaked, pink, or contains small clots. Tumors of the lung or bronchus and chronic bronchitis are the most frequent causes of hemoptysis in the United States. Approximately one-third of patients with pulmonary embolism have blood-tinged sputum. Very high pulmonary vascular pressures may also result in bloody sputum. In acute cardiogenic pulmonary edema, the odorless, frothy, colorless or peachy-colored sputum may also be conspicuously blood streaked. Recurrent bloody sputum is also seen with pulmonary hypertension secondary to mitral stenosis. Trauma to the airways incurred during intubation or tracheostomy or during suctioning may be associated with bright red streaks in the aspirated secretions that resolve quickly unless trauma is recurrent. Hemoptysis may also indicate rupture of a pulmonary artery segment associated with flotation or wedging of the pulmonary artery catheter. (See Chapter 9, Complications of pulmonary artery catheterization.)

Dyspnea. The term dyspnea implies that the act of breathing has become a difficult, conscious effort. Most dyspneic patients also *appear* to have labored breathing, despite the lack of a consistent correlation of the apparent respiratory effort to the subjective sensation of breathing. Theories to explain dyspnea include: 1) excitation of intrapulmonary receptors by irritant substances or abnormalities within the structures of the lung such as bronchoconstriction, pulmonary edema, etc.; 2) abnormalities in blood gases such as hypoxemia or hypercarbia; 3) central nervous system mechanisms that relate to the perception of a disparity between work of breathing and adequacy of muscle contraction; 4) emotional factors such as hysterical hyperventilation; and 5) circumstances in which the patient's minute ventilation approaches his maximum breathing capacity. This may occur when minute ventilatory requirements are excessively high as in extreme exercise, or when the maximum breathing capacity is extremely low as in chronic obstructive pulmonary disease (COPD).

In patients with pulmonary disease, dyspnea is associated with: 1) airflow limitations due to obstructive lesions of the airways such as asthma; 2) conditions that reduce pulmonary compliance such as atelectasis, the adult respiratory distress syndrome; 3) conditions that resist lung expansion such as pneumothorax, pleural effusion, pleural thickening or inflammation; 4) increase in physiologic dead space as in massive pulmonary embolism; 5) severe hypoxemia or hypercarbia, both of which are associated with increases in pulmonary ventilation; and 6) respiratory muscle fatigue, which may occur either when the underlying disease increases the work of breathing beyond the work capacity of the normal ventilatory muscles, or when the ventilatory muscles become so weak that they cannot maintain even quiet, normal breathing.

The present level of dyspnea may be compared with that usually experienced and precipitating or alleviating factors explored.

Chest Pain. Pain of pulmonary origin includes: 1) upper retrosternal pain as seen in acute tracheitis; 2) retrosternal pain associated with lesions of the mediastinum; and 3) pleural pain due to pleurisy or pleuritic involvement secondary to pulmonary embolism. Pleuritic pain is typically sharp and stabbing in nature.

Signs

Signs are objective indicators of disease. Several signs are indicative of pulmonary disease but, as with symptoms, may also characterize other pathology.

The Level of Mentation. Several conditions can alter the patient's cerebral function. *Hypoxemia* (PaO_2 less than 55 mm Hg) and/or changes in $PaCO_2$ produce changes in affect, perception of reality, and level of consciousness. Accurate assessment may require detailed questioning as a patient may appear quite rational, but careful interrogation may unmask abnormalities in mental function.

HYPOXIA. There is no subjective recognition of hypoxia. The signs of *cerebral hypoxia* are nearly identical to those of ethanol intoxication. Just as drunkenness manifests differently among different people, cerebral hypoxia may be variably present with restlessness, agitation, an inappropriate sense of well being, euphoria, outbursts of hilarity, paranoia, combativeness, irritability, and/or uncooperativeness. There is also generally a loss of higher mental functioning (inability to perform complex mental tasks or think abstractly), confusion, as well as loss of muscular coordination and visual acuity. With progressive decreases in cerebral oxygenation, progressive descending central nervous system depression may ultimately end in stupor, seizure, or coma.

HYPERCARBIA. The symptoms of hypercarbia resemble depression due to anesthetic agents. The patient's behavior may be characterized by lethargy, confusion, slurred speech, poor coordination, mental depression progressing to somnolence, stupor, and coma. The patient may also complain of headache, a result of cerebral vasodilation and consequent increased cerebral blood flow and intracranial pressure that accompanies increases in arterial carbon dioxide tension.

Unless the patient is receiving supplemental oxygen, hypercarbia is always associated with some degree of hypoxemia. The clinical picture, therefore, may be a mixed bag of the effects of hypercarbia and hypoxemia. Severe mental aberrations such as hallucination, paranoid/combative behavior, or schizoid behavior may make it appear that the patient has a psychiatric disorder.

Both hypoxemia and hypercarbia (due to the associated acidemia) have a potent constrictor effect on the pulmonary vessels. This increases pulmonary vascular resistance (increased pulmonary artery systolic and diastolic pressures) and may lead to right ventricular failure.

Respirations. Patients with pulmonary disease will experience physiologic alterations that may produce changes in respiration. Patients should be observed for respiratory changes in:

FREQUENCY—The normal respiratory rate for a healthy, nonstressed resting adult is 8 to 12 breaths per minute. The respiratory rate increases with fever, septicemia, hypercarbia, hypoxemia, acidemia, strong emotional stimuli, pain, shock, pulmonary embolism, or any condition that produces a sudden increase in the work of breathing such as bronchospasm or pulmonary edema.

DEPTH—Depth of breathing is difficult to determine because chest and diaphragmatic movements cannot be accurately measured in the clinical setting; however, normal breathing is barely visible. When ventilatory movements are clearly noticeable, the minute volume has approximately doubled.

SYMMETRY—In health, the two sides of the chest move symmetrically with each breath. To assess symmetry the patient should be in the supine position with the chest exposed. From the foot of the bed, one can observe ventilatory movements in the infraclavicular regions, mid-chest, and lower ribs and abdomen.

In the obese patient, observations may be difficult and assessment may require palpation. Grasp the sides of the chest with the fingers. The outstretched thumbs should nearly approximate the area of the xiphoid process for anterior palpation and the tenth thoracic spine for posterior palpation. A loose fold of skin should be present between the thumbs as the patient takes a few deep breaths. The excursions of the thumbs are observed and the range and symmetry of ventilatory movements felt. Observe for any lag or absence or incomplete expansion. Asymmetry may be due to pleural effusion, obstruction of a major bronchus, or neuromuscular abnormalities. Patients with fractured ribs, pleurisy, or area surgery may splint one side of the chest to reduce pain.

CHEST/ABDOMINAL SYNCHRONY—With normal breathing, the chest and abdomen rise and fall smoothly and synchronously with inspiration and expiration. In the supine person, the movement of the abdomen normally is slightly greater than the rib cage. With the onset of respiratory muscle fatigue, the ventilatory movements become rapid and jerky. The abdomen is sucked in on inspiration and balloons out on expiration, producing a paradoxical movement of chest and abdomen which results in a rocking appearance to the ventilatory effort (Fig. 3–1).

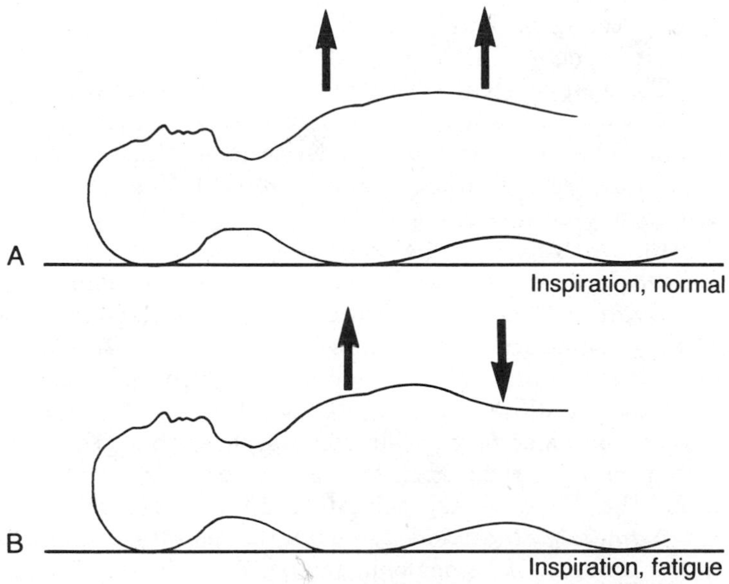

FIGURE 3–1. Respiratory paradox. *A,* With inspiration and descent of the diaphragm, the abdomen rises synchronously with the chest. Both fall smoothly on expiration as the diaphragm ascends. *B,* With respiratory muscle fatigue, as the chest rises during inspiration, the abdomen is sucked in. During expiration, the abdomen moves out as the chest falls. These rapid, uncoordinated respiratory movements may additionally be accompanied by CO_2 retention and hypoxemia.

The patient who is able to talk will also complain of dyspnea. Because this sign may herald acute respiratory failure, it is important to watch for it if a patient has any degree of ventilatory compromise or is being weaned from a ventilator.

CHARACTER OF BREATHING—With normal breathing, both intercostal and diaphragmatic muscles are utilized. Respiratory movements that are entirely thoracic may indicate that diaphragmatic movement is restricted by increased intra-abdominal pressure or pain. Respiratory movements that are entirely abdominal may be caused by paralytic involvement of the intercostal muscles. In bronchial asthma, emphysema, and diffuse pulmonary fibrosis, movements of the chest wall may be equally reduced bilaterally.

Labored inspiration occurs when adequate ventilation cannot be achieved with normal breathing. The accessory cervical muscles are used to lift the thoracic cage off the diaphragm. The increased negative intrathoracic pressure produces suprasternal, supraclavicular, intercostal and substernal retractions. The nares are also usually flared. This type of breathing occurs when the lung becomes stiff, as in severe fibrotic disease or pulmonary edema, where there is gross over-distention of the lung as in COPD; or from obstruction or narrowing of the bronchi, trachea, or larynx.

Labored expiration occurs when a disease process interferes with the free passive outflow of air. Use of the accessory muscles of the cervical area, intercostal area, back, and abdomen increase positive pressure in the thorax to expel air. Expiratory time is also prolonged. Patients usually prefer to sit upright and may purse their lips or grunt with expiration. These actions keep intra-airway pressures above that of the surrounding tissue and prevent small airway collapse. This type of breathing is seen in patients with asthma, chronic bronchitis, COPD, or ARDS.

The exaggerated intrathoracic pressure fluctuations associated with these types of breathing will be transmitted to the catheter tip in the pulmonary artery and pulmonary artery wedge tracing. This may make the determination of accurate values difficult. (See Chapter 9, Ventilatory effects on pulmonary artery measurements.)

REGULARITY OF BREATHING—Changes from regular, rhythmical breathing should be noted, e.g., Cheyne-Stokes respiration.

Cyanosis. As the amount of oxygen dissolved in plasma diminishes, the binding capacity of the hemoglobin molecule with oxygen decreases; this increases the amount of reduced (deoxygenated, desaturated) hemoglobin. Cyanosis—a diffuse, bluish discoloration of the skin and mucous membranes—becomes perceptible when greater than 5 gms per 100 ml of hemoglobin becomes reduced in the capillaries of the tissues. This usually occurs when the PaO_2 is approximately 50 mm Hg and arterial saturation is approximately 80 percent, although this point is variable and relates, in part, to the amount of hemoglobin in the blood. The higher the hemoglobin, the greater the likelihood of cyanosis because the amount of reduced hemoglobin in 100 milliliters of capillary blood will be greater for any given PaO_2. Therefore, cyanosis may occur before the actual oxygen-carrying capacity (blood oxygen content) is affected. For example, a polycythemic patient with a hemoglobin of 21 gm per 100 ml will appear cyanotic although the PaO_2 is in an acceptable range and there is no threat to tissue oxygenation. Conversely, anemic patients may suffer severe tissue hypoxia before cyanosis develops.

Cyanosis is most evident at the nail beds and mucous membranes and where skin is thin, such as the tip of the nose and earlobes. It is important to realize that cyanosis commonly occurs in the absence of disease when the arterioles of the skin, particularly in the hands and feet, narrow in response to cold or anxiety. Vasoconstriction slows blood in these superficial, peripheral capillaries so that more arterial desaturation occurs locally.

There are two types of cyanosis: In *central cyanosis*, blood leaving the left ventricle is poorly oxygenated. When associated with pulmonary disease, it occurs with tension pneumothorax, severe chronic bronchitis, or ARDS. Clinically, cyanosis is evident peripherally at the nail beds and earlobes as well as centrally in the conjunctiva or under the tongue.

In *peripheral cyanosis*, blood leaving the left ventricle is adequately oxygenated but becomes desaturated in the tissues due to poor blood flow. This typically occurs from narrowed peripheral arterioles due to a cold environment, or from excessive sympathetic nervous system stimulation due to anxiety or circulatory failure. Cyanosis is apparent peripherally; however, the conjunctiva and mucous membranes under the tongue remain pink because vasoconstriction never occurs in these areas. Peripheral cyanosis does not occur in isolated pulmonary disease.

Edema. Tissue swelling due to increased interstitial fluid is apparent in patients with COPD complicated by right ventricular failure. The increased venous pressure associated with right heart failure reflects back to the systemic capillaries resulting in increased capillary hydrostatic pressure and subsequent transudation of fluid into body tissue. Swelling will be most marked at the dependent parts of the body—the feet when upright and sacrum when supine. Associated venous distention reflects the increased venous pressure.

Subcutaneous Emphysema. Air in the subcutaneous tissue is indicative of a pulmonary air leak such as might occur from alveolar rupture in a patient receiving positive pressure ventilation. This is evidenced as swelling in various body parts and produces a characteristic crackling sensation on palpation. Although an intubated patient cannot complain, pain may be produced by palpating the areas of swelling as air dissects through the tissue under the pressure of the examiner's hand. Subcutaneous emphysema by itself does not pose a threat to the patient unless it is significant enough around the throat to compress and occlude the airway and blood vessels. It is, however, a warning that an air leak is present, and, therefore, the patient is at risk of developing a pneumothorax.

Posturing. The patient's position of comfort relates to the work of breathing. Patients with respiratory difficulty prefer to sit upright while grasping or resting their arms on a stationary object such as the back of a chair. This position enables the patient to stabilize the shoulders and enlist the assessory muscles to augment the respiratory effort. It also increases tidal volume because it allows for greater diaphragmatic descent. Moreover, the weight of the anterior chest wall, which can be very significant in the obese, does not have to be overcome with inspiration.

SPECIFIC TECHNIQUES OF PHYSICAL ASSESSMENT

In addition to symptoms and signs of pulmonary disease, the following specific assessment techniques may be utilized to detect distortion or abnormalities in the structures of the pulmonary system.

Percussion. Percussion is a technique to determine the density or consistency of the underlying lung by evaluating the sounds produced when the chest wall is tapped. Percussion should be performed with the patient sitting. The distal part of the middle finger is pressed firmly against the chest wall, palm side down, with the fingers slightly separated. The middle finger of the other hand, held at right angle, is used to tap the finger on the chest wall. The entire action must come from the wrist producing a sharp, hammer-like effect. Percussion begins at the apices and progresses downward. As each site is struck with equal force, symmetrical points on the thorax are compared. Percussion over the healthy lung produces a characteristic resonant tone, which varies depending on the amount of muscle and/or fat present. Table 3–1 lists the various pulmonary percussion sounds.

Tracheal Position. This assessment technique is utilized when shift of the mediastinal structures is suspected. The tip of the index finger is thrust gently into the suprasternal notch. The trachea is located and deviation of the trachea to either side can then be detected. An increase in volume/pressure on one side of the thorax (as in tension pneumothorax) shifts the trachea and

TABLE 3–1. Pulmonary Percussion Sounds

Sound	*Quality*	*Clinical Correlates*
Resonance	Loud, low in pitch	Sound heard over healthy, aerated lung
Hyperresonance	Very loud, lower in pitch than resonance	Occurs when the amount of air in the thorax is increased, as in emphysema or pneumothorax
Tympany	Musical, clear hollow tone; pitch is usually high	Tension pneumothorax; increased air under pressure
Dullness	Soft intensity, medium in pitch, short duration, damped quality	Occurs when lung is airless as in consolidation, collapse, fibrosis, tumor; or when lung is separated from the chest wall by pleural fluid or thickened pleura

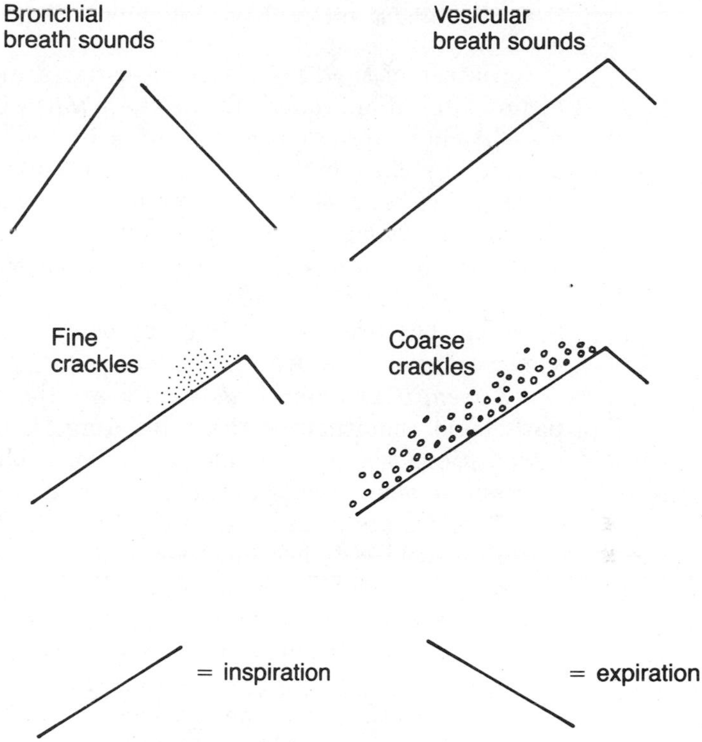

FIGURE 3–2. Breath sounds.

mediastinal structures to the opposite side. A decrease in volume (as in atelectasis) shifts the trachea and mediastinum to the affected side.

Auscultation (Breath Sounds). The bell of the stethoscope is used to auscultate the chest as most sounds reaching the chest wall from the airways and lungs are in the low frequency range. Alternate auscultation of both sides of the chest is essential for comparing the quality of breath sounds. The patient is asked to breath deeply with the mouth wide open. The patient should also be instructed to breath slowly with frequent pauses as prolonged hyperventilation may produce central nervous system excitability and cerebral and coronary vasoconstriction. Breath sounds are produced by turbulent air flow through airways and alveoli.

TYPES OF BREATH SOUNDS. *Bronchial sounds* are normally heard only over the trachea and main bronchi (upper anterior chest wall) (Fig. 3–2). They are high pitched and blowing; the expiratory sound is as long and as loud as the inspiratory sound, with a brief pause at peak inspiration. These characteristics are important to remember because bronchial breath sounds over lung tissue always indicate pulmonary disease characterized by consolidation or fibrosis.

Vesicular sounds are heard over normal lung and have a characteristic low pitched rustling quality (Fig. 3–2). The intensity of the sound increases steadily during inspiration and fades completely during the first third of expiration.

Disease of the lung alters vesicular sounds in several ways. If there is airflow limitation, sounds at the chest wall will be diminished or absent. This may be characteristic of severe bronchial asthma, atelectasis, obstruction of a large bronchus, or pneumothorax. Vesicular sounds are also diminished in emphysema because the abnormally large amount of air in the lungs damps the sound. Pleural thickening or effusion also interferes with the passage of sound to the chest wall. Should the lung tissue become consolidated as in pneumonia, tumor, or fibrotic pulmonary disease, the sounds picked up resemble but are quieter than bronchial sounds normally heard over the upper anterior chest wall.

Adventitious (abnormal) sounds are the result of vibrations produced by pathologic conditions within the lung. Unfortunately, terms to describe adventitious sounds are not consistent. The author suggests the use of descriptive adjectives to avoid confusion in nomenclature.

Crackles are sounds made by the sudden opening of small airways and alveoli previously stuck together by fluid or exudate and/or movement of air through secretions in the airways. They may be numerous or rare, loud or faint, coarse or bubbly, and gurgling or fine resembling the sound made by rubbing several strands of hair between the thumb and index finger in front of the ear. They may occur early or late in inspiration, expiration, or both phases of ventilation. Fine crackles are heard near the peak of inspiration and are due to the explosive reopening of the peripheral airways and alveoli that have been obstructed, during expiration, by exudate or edema. Coarse, inspiratory, or expiratory crackles are gurgling in quality and are produced by bubbling of air through secretions in the larger bronchi (Fig. 3–2). Crackles are associated with bronchitis, asthma, pneumonia, and/or pulmonary edema.

Wheezes are musical sounds with a wide range of pitch produced by the movement of air through narrowed bronchi. Since the bronchi normally become shortened and narrowed during expiration, wheezes are most frequently heard during expiration which also becomes prolonged and difficult. In cases of severe bronchial narrowing or when the airways become rigid and do not expand normally during inspiration, wheezing can occur both during inspiration and expiration. Wheezes are commonly associated with asthma, COPD, pulmonary edema, anaphylactic reactions, irritating inhalants, and pulmonary embolism.

Easily audible at a distance from the patient, *stridor* is a high-pitched, crowing inspiratory sound due to upper airway obstruction, which may quickly result in death. Retractions are visible over the sternal notch, above the clavicles, in the intercostal spaces, and below the sternum. Stridor may be due to laryngeal spasm or swelling, epiglottitis, tracheal stenosis, aspiration of a foreign object, or vocal cord edema. The presence of stridor is a medical emergency, indicating at least a 70 percent obstruction of the upper airway.

When the surface of the pleura is roughened by inflammation caused by pleurisy due to viral or bacterial infection or by pulmonary embolism, a creaking, leathery sound known as *pleural friction rub* occurs toward the peak of inspiration and early part of expiration. Since the greatest movement of the lungs occurs over the lower lobes, pleural rubs are most commonly heard over the lower thorax. The sound may vary in intensity and disappears when the patient holds the breath. In a healthy patient, no sound is produced because the pleura is smooth and moist.

SUGGESTED READINGS

Bates B: The thorax and lungs. In *A Guide to Physical Examination*, ed. 3. Philadelphia, JB Lippincott, 1983.

Carrieri VK, Janson-Bjerklie S, Jacobs S: The sensation of dyspnea: A review. *Heart and Lung* 1984; 3:436–447.

Cherniack RM, Cherniack L: Manifestations of respiratory disease and assessment of respiratory disease. In *Respiration in Health and Disease*. Philadelphia, WB Saunders, 1983.

Delp MH, Manning RT: Examination of the chest. In *Major's Physical Diagnosis; An Introduction to the Clinical Process*. Philadelphia, WB Saunders, 1981.

Weil JV: Dyspnea. In Horwitz LD, Groves BM: *Signs and Symptoms in Cardiology*. Philadelphia, JB Lippincott, 1985.

Ditchey RV: Cyanosis. In Horwitz LD, Groves BM: *Signs and Symptoms in Cardiology*. Philadelphia, JB Lippincott, 1985.

Henderson B, Ferguson GT: Concepts of physical assessment in critical care nursing. In Kinney MR, Dear CB, Packa DR, Voorman DMN: *AACN'S Clinical Reference for Critical Care Nursing*. New York, McGraw-Hill, 1981.

Cardiovascular Anatomy and Physiology

4

The respiratory and cardiovascular systems share an intimate relationship both anatomically and physiologically. The joint purpose of both systems is to sustain body cells by providing oxygen for metabolism and energy production and by removing metabolic waste products. The role of the respiratory system is the reciprocal exchange of gases between atmosphere and blood. The task of the cardiovascular system is to transport gases, nutrients, and other materials dissolved in blood to and from the cells. Abnormalities in one system, therefore, affect the successful function of the other.

The cardiovascular system is a continuous, closed, fluid-filled, elastic circuit equipped with a pump (Fig. 4–1). The constituent parts of the cardiovascular system include the following: the *heart*, the pump, which provides the force that drives blood through the vascular system; *arteries*, the delivery system, which distribute and regulate the amount of oxygenated blood flow to the various tissue beds; *capillaries*, the nutrient bed, where exchange of gases, nutrients and metabolites takes place; and *veins*, the return system, that brings deoxygenated blood back to the cardiopulmonary unit. Veins also act as a reservoir, accommodating about 70 percent of circulating blood volume.

With each beat of the heart, equal amounts of blood must move through all divisions of the cardiovascular circuit. Further, abnormalities or disturbances in flow in one division of the circuit must be reflected as abnormalities in all divisions of the circuit.

THE HEART

The heart is a four-chambered, muscular organ whose function is the forward propulsion of blood in an amount to meet the metabolic needs of the body. Structurally, the heart is formed of fibrous and muscular tissue.

The cardiac wall is composed of the pericardium, myo-

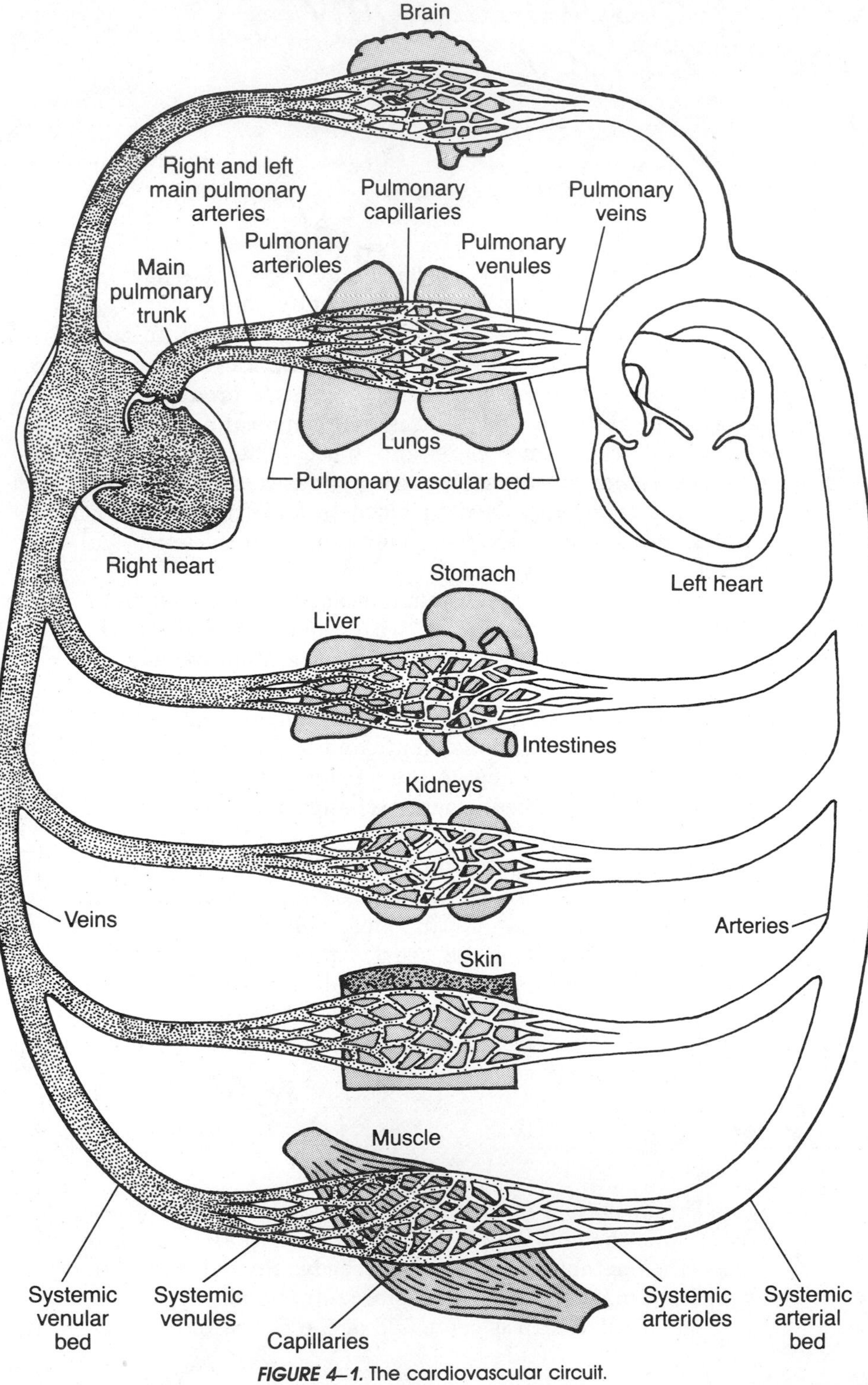

FIGURE 4–1. The cardiovascular circuit.

cardium, and endocardium. The *pericardium*, a fibroserous sac, attaches to the roots of the great vessels and encases the heart. The fibrous, nondistensible, parietal pericardium is the outermost layer. It is then reflected back to form the serous visceral pericardium, or epicardium, which is adherent to the myocardial surface. Between the parietal and visceral layers is a potential space containing 20 to 30 ml of pericardial fluid, which acts as a lubricant and provides a friction-free surface for the beating heart.

The *myocardium*, the muscular middle layer of the heart, is composed of interlacing specialized muscle fibers. Contraction of the cardiac muscle cell occurs when contractile elements within the cell slide over each other interdigitally, creating shortening and tension in the muscle fiber. The force of contraction relates to the amount of stretch provided by intrachamber volume applied to the muscle fiber just prior to systole, within physiologic limits. Increased stretch produces an increased force of contraction; decreased stretch results in decreased contractile dynamics. Myocardial cells connect in series at points called intercalated discs. These cell boundaries have tight junctions that offer low electrical impedance, allowing electrical stimuli to pass with ease from cell to cell. Stimulation of any muscle fiber, therefore, results in stimulation of the entire muscle mass.

The *endocardium* is a serous membrane that lines the inner surface of the heart and also extends out to form the heart valves.

Four heart valves normally permit only unidirectional blood flow. They

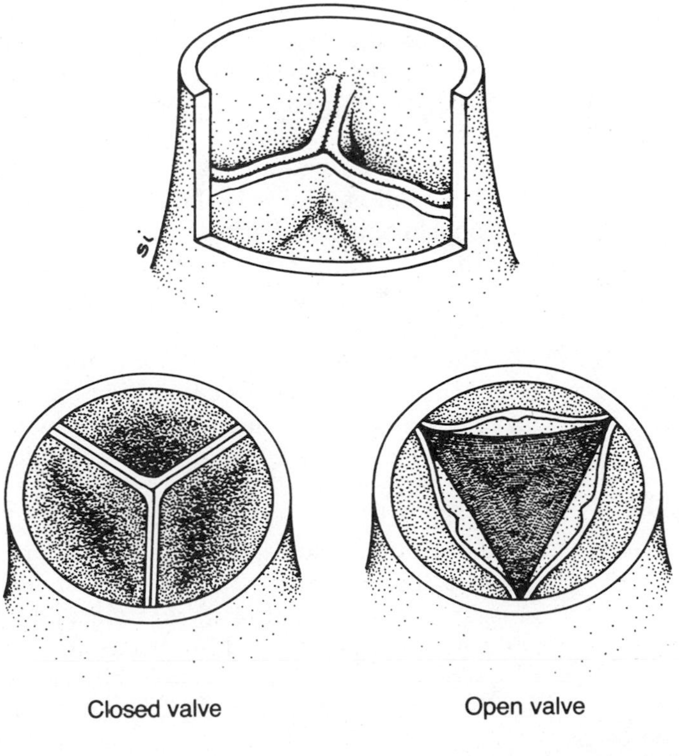

FIGURE 4–2. The semilunar valves. Though essentially the same in structure, the leaflets of the aortic valve are normally heavier than those of the pulmonic valve. This is because the aortic valve closing pressure (80 mm Hg) is greater than the pulmonic valve closing pressure (8–15 mm Hg). Thus, a structurally stronger valve leaflet is required for the root of the aorta.

are divided into two types according to their structure. *Semilunar valves* are located at the base of the aorta and pulmonary artery and consist of three delicate, half-moon-shaped leaflets attached to a fibrous ring or annulus (Fig. 4–2). Ventricular outflow forces the aortic and pulmonic valve leaflets open, and smoothed against the vessel walls. During ventricular diastole, reversal of blood flow fills the valve cusps, giving each valve the appearance of a small distended sac. The approximated valve edges seal off the roots of the great arteries and prevent backflow of blood into the ventricles.

The *atrioventricular (A-V) valves* are so named becaused they are located between the atria and ventricles (Fig. 4–3). The right A-V valve, or tricuspid valve, has three leaflets; the left, or mitral valve, has two. The leaflets open passively into the ventricles during diastole. During systole they are pushed upward by rising intraventricular pressure and ultimately approximate to occlude the valve orifice. Cordlike structures known as chordae tendineae connect the edges of the valve leaflets to muscular projections called papillary muscles that arise from the inner surface of the ventricles. Contraction of the papillary muscles during systole applies tension to the chordae tendineae, which in turn prevent prolapse of the valve leaflets into the atria and subsequent regurgitant flow. For normal function of the A-V valves to occur, all components of the valve apparatus—valve leaflets, chordae, papillary muscles, and adjacent myocardium—must be intact.

Blood Flow and Intrachamber Pressures

The factors responsible for the forward movement of blood through the heart are cyclic, transchamber pressure gradients—that is, a higher pressure in the delivering chamber and a lower pressure in the receiving chamber. The greater the pressure difference between chambers, the greater the rate of flow. As pressures approach equilibrium, flow rates slow.

Though anatomically the heart is one organ, each side serves a separate and physiologically distinct circulation. Normal blood flow is depicted schematically in Figure 4–4 with all four chambers visible to enhance conceptualization of circulation. For an anatomically correct view of the heart, refer to Figure 4–5.

The right heart (right atrium and right ventricle) receives venous blood from the systemic venous circulation and propels it through the low pressure, low resistance pulmonary circulation. Venous blood enters the thin-walled right atrium (RA) via the superior and inferior vena cava and coronary sinus. The pressure here is low, measuring 0 to 8 mm Hg. As blood enters the right ventricle (RV), the tricuspid valve (TV) is open, making the RA and RV openly communicating chambers, and pressures reach equilibrium at end-diastole. Therefore, RV end-diastolic or filling pressure is equal to mean RA pressure. At the onset of RV systole, right intraventricular pressure exceeds right atrial pressure, and the tricuspid valve closes.

When the RV pressure exceeds the diastolic pressure in the pulmonary artery (PA) (8 to 15 mm Hg), the pulmonic valve (PV) opens. As pressure

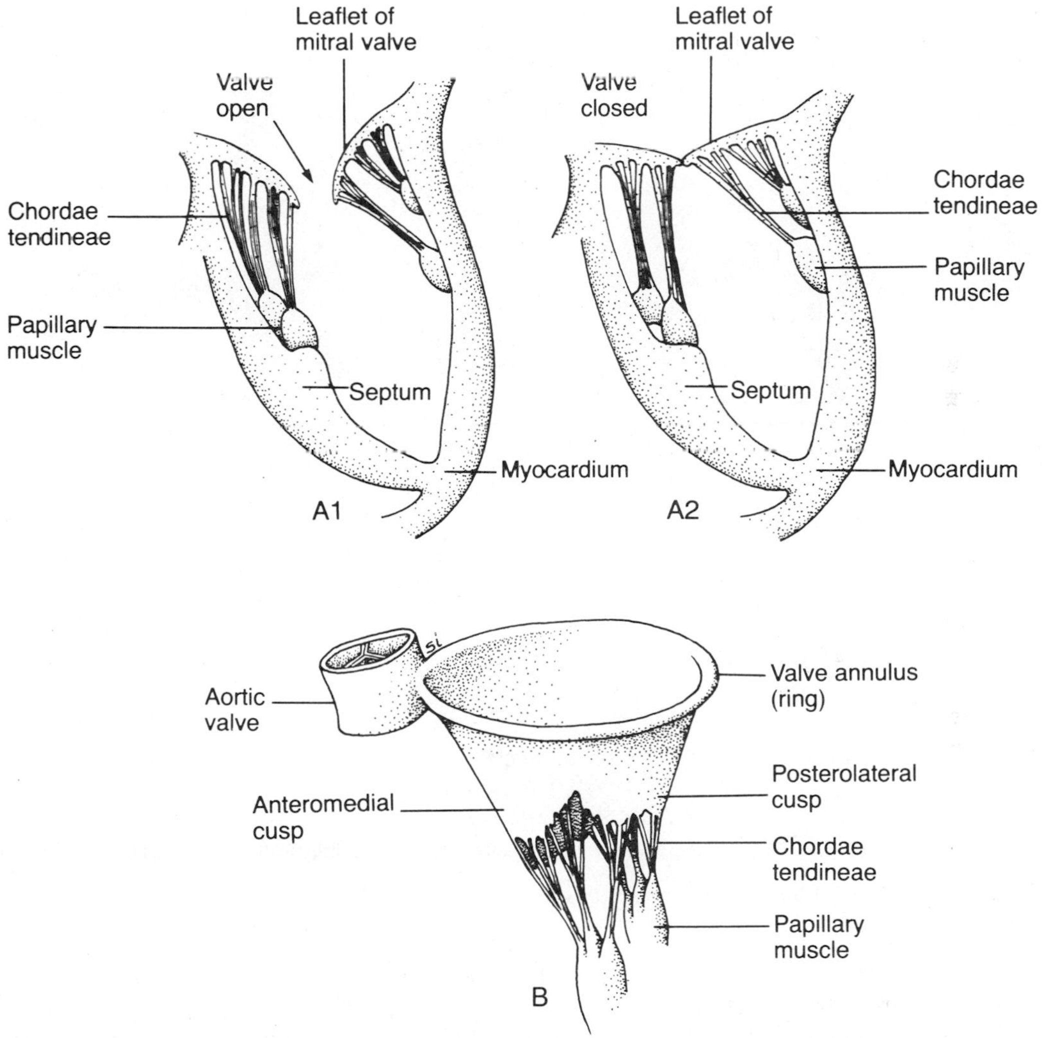

FIGURE 4–3. The atrioventricular valve structure (mitral valve). *A1,* The valve leaflets are widely open in ventricular diastole, thus allowing ventricular filling. *A2,* Closure of the valve leaflets in ventricular systole seals off the atria from the ventricles as ventricular contraction forces blood into the arterial circulation. *B,* The mitral valve annulus and the funnel-like structure of the valve apparatus.

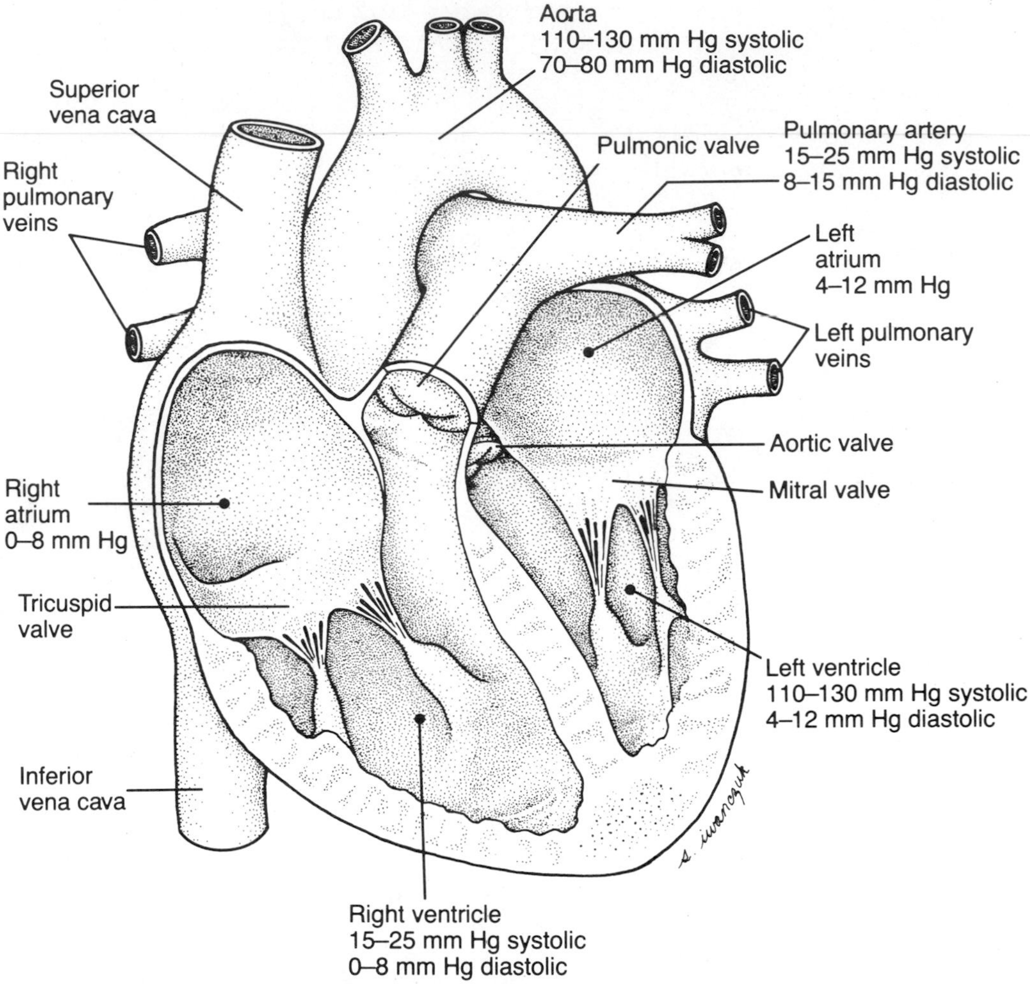

FIGURE 4–4. Normal blood flow through the heart and intrachamber pressures. A schematic representation of the heart showing all four chambers and valves visible in the anterior view to facilitate conceptualization of blood flow. Anatomically, this diagram is incorrect (see Fig. 4–5).

continues to increase to a systolic peak of 15 to 25 mm Hg, blood flows into the pulmonary circulation. At this time, the RV and PA are communicating chambers; therefore, RV and PA systolic pressures are equal. With ventricular relaxation, when RV pressure falls below PA diastolic pressure, 8 to 15 mm Hg, the pulmonic valve closes. Driven by a pressure gradient across the pulmonary circulation of approximately 4 mm Hg, blood flows through the capillaries of the lung where oxygenation of blood occurs and carbon dioxide is eliminated. The oxygenated blood then enters the left atrium (LA) via the four pulmonary veins.

The left heart (left atrium and left ventricle) pumps arterialized blood through the high resistance, high pressure systemic circulation. The thin-walled left atrium receives oxygenated blood from the pulmonary veins. The mean LA pressure is in the range of 4 to 12 mm Hg. As blood enters the left ventricle (LV) in diastole, the mitral valve is open, making the LA and LV openly communicating chambers where pressure then equilibrates at end-diastole. Thus, mean LA and LV end-diastolic pressures are equal at 4 to 12 mm Hg. The thick LV wall is less compliant than the thin RV wall; therefore, its end-diastolic (filling) pressure is normally higher than RV end-diastolic pressure, although ventricular end-diastolic volumes are normally equal—approximately 120 ml. With the onset of LV systole, the mitral valve (MV) closes and, as intraventricular pressure rises to exceed the pressure in the aortic root, 80 mm Hg, the aortic valve (AV) opens. Pressure continues to mount to approximately 110 to 130 mm Hg peak systolic pressure, which provides motive force for movement of blood through the large, high resistance systemic circulation. At this time, the left ventricle and aorta are communicating chambers. Therefore, LV systolic and arterial systolic pressures (as measured in the aortic root) are normally equal.

Table 4–1 lists normal intracardiac pressures and the factors affecting them, and also indicates means of obtaining bedside measurements.

Phases of the Cardiac Cycle

The thin-walled atria function primarily as entrance chambers for the ventricles, but they also contract to augment ventricular filling. The ventricles

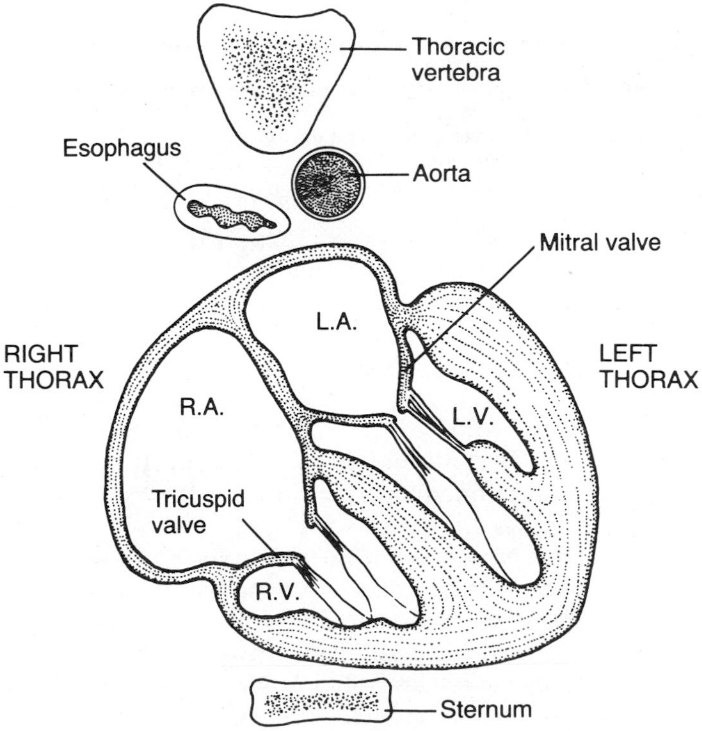

FIGURE 4–5. In situ, the heart is horizontally and asymmetrically positioned one third to the right and two thirds to the left of the sternum. The heart is suspended at the base by its great vessels; the apex is directed anteriorly, inferiorly, and to the left. The right ventricle is the most anterior structure of the heart and lies beneath the sternum. The right atrium lies superior and posterior to the right ventricle. The left ventricle is a posterior-lateral structure with only about one-fourth of the total mass visible in the anterior view. The left atrium is an entirely posterior structure lying in front of the aorta, esophagus, and thoracic vertebrae.

TABLE 4–1. Normal Intracardiac Pressure and Factors Affecting; Means of Bedside Measurement

	Normal Pressure Range (mm Hg)	Factors Affecting	Bedside Measurement
RA Pressure	0–8	Intravascular volume, directly reflects RVEDP in absence of tricuspid valve disease. Indirectly reflects pulmonary vascular resistance, left heart function, venous capacitance	CVP line placed in RA or preferably in SVC; proximal port of PA catheter
RV Systolic	15–25	Force of RV ejection, which relates to RV preload, afterload, and the contractile state of RV myocardium	PA systolic as measured with a pulmonary artery catheter
RV Diastolic	0–8	Intravascular volume; functional state of RV	CVP line; proximal port of PA catheter
PA Systolic	15–25	Pulmonary vascular volume; pulmonary vascular resistance (the resistance to flow through the pulmonary vascular channel)	Pulmonary artery catheter, distal port
PA Diastolic	8–15	Pulmonary intravascular volume; pulmonary vascular resistance	PA catheter, distal port
LA Pressure	4–12*	Intravascular volume, directly reflects LVEDP in the absence of mitral valve disease	LA line; PA catheter in wedge position
LV Systolic	100–130	Force of LV ejection, which relates to preload, afterload, and the contractile state of LV myocardium	Arterial line; arterial systolic pressure
LV Diastolic	4–12	Intravascular volume; functional state of LV	PWP correlates well in absence of mitral valve disease or PWP greater than 20 mm Hg

*Normally the measured PWP is 1–3 mm Hg less than the measured PA diastolic pressure (PAd-PWP gradient). (PAd = pulmonary artery diastolic pressure; PWP = pulmonary artery wedge pressure.)

Key:
CVP = Central venous pressure
LVEDP = Left ventricular end-diastolic pressure
RVEDP = Right ventricular end-diastolic pressure
SVC = Superior vena cava

supply the power that moves blood through the pulmonary and systemic circulations (Fig. 4–6).

Ventricular Diastole

Filling of the ventricles is accomplished in three phases:

Isovolumetric Relaxation. At the end of ventricular systole, the aortic and pulmonic valves close. At this point, ventricular pressures are still much higher than atrial pressure. In order to open the mitral and tricuspid valves, the pressure within the atria must exceed pressure within the ventricles. This means that for a period of time between closure of the aortic and pulmonic valves and opening of the A-V valves all four valves are closed and no blood is flowing. Intraventricular pressures, however, are decreasing as the ventricles relax. Blood flows into the atria from the systemic and pulmonary venous systems. (See Fig. *A*, p. 42.)

Passive Filling. When intraventricular pressures fall below atrial pressures, the A-V valves open followed by an onrush of blood—the period of rapid filling. As much as 60 percent of ventricular filling may occur during the rapid filling phase. Filling of the ventricles then becomes progressively slower in mid and late diastole as atrial and ventricular pressures approach equilibrium—the period of slowed filling. The duration of slowed filling depends on the heart rate; it becomes shorter with rapid heart rates and longer with slow heart rates. Overall, 70 to 90 percent of ventricular filling occurs during the passive filling phase. (See Fig. *B,* p. 42.)

Atrial Systole (Atrial Kick). The atrial contribution to ventricular filling is known as atrial systole or atrial kick. Because of active atrial contraction, blood flow into the ventricles again is increased. The additional volume pumped into the ventricles by the atria contributes approximately 10 to 30 percent to ventricular end-diastolic volume. (See Fig. *C,* p. 42.)

VENTRICULAR SYSTOLE

Ejection of the ventricles is also accomplished in three phases:

Isovolumetric Contraction. At the onset of systole, the ventricular walls press toward the center of the ventricular cavities, thus increasing

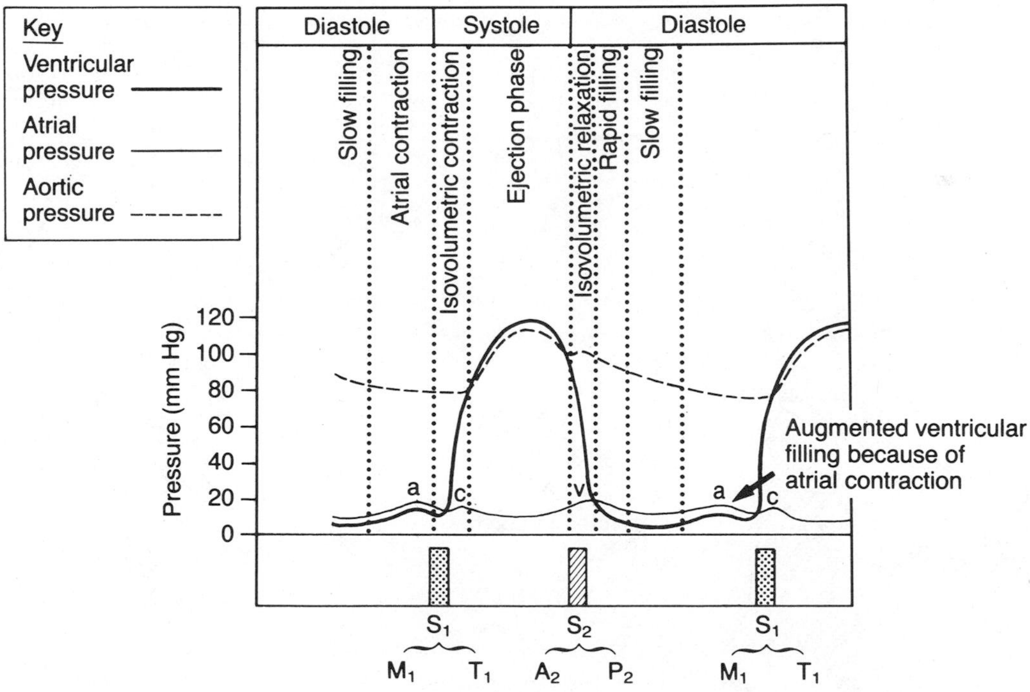

FIGURE 4–6. The cardiac cycle illustrating the pressure changes in the left atrium, left ventricle, and aorta as well as the relationship of these events to the production of heart sounds. S_1 = the first heart sound which occurs synchronously with closure of the mitral and tricuspid valves. S_2 = the second heart sound which occurs synchronously with closure of the aortic and pulmonic valves.

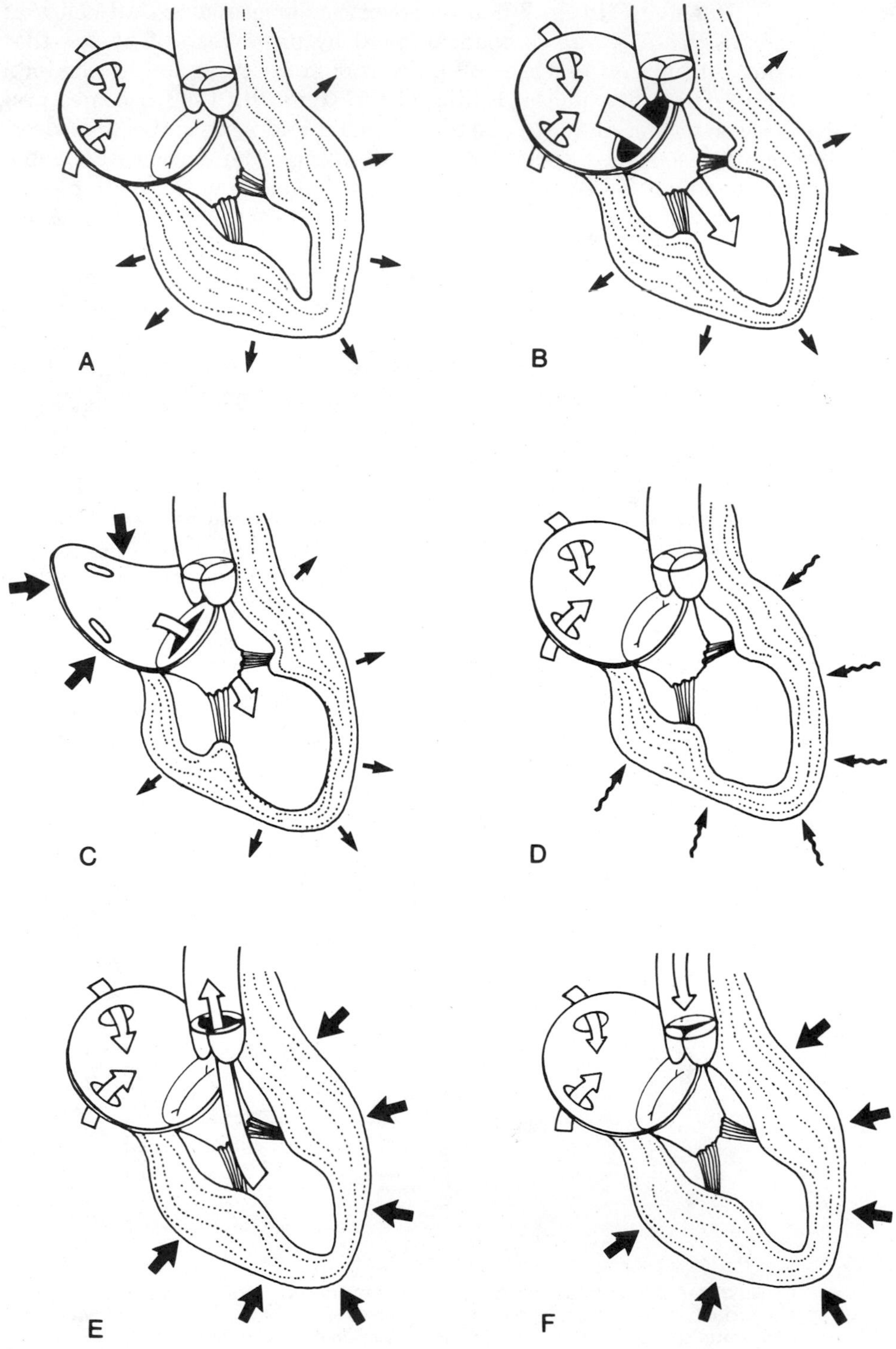
A
B
C
D
E
F

intraventricular pressure. When ventricular pressures exceed atrial pressure, the A-V valves snap shut. Intraventricular pressures continue to build to a level sufficient to push open the pulmonic and aortic valves against the diastolic pressures in the pulmonary artery and aorta; 8 mm Hg and 80 mm Hg respectively. During this phase of systole, myocardial tension increases, but there is no flow of blood. The greatest myocardial energy expenditure and oxygen consumption are associated with isovolumetric contraction. (See Fig. *D*, opposite.)

Rapid Ventricular Ejection. When LV and RV pressures exceed aortic and pulmonary artery pressures, the semilunar valves open and blood rushes out of the ventricles. Pressure continues to increase to 120 mm Hg in the LV and 20 to 25 mm Hg in the RV, forcing blood into the systemic and pulmonary circulations. This is followed by reduced rates of ejection during which the remaining 40 percent of ventricular emptying occurs. (See Fig. *E*, opposite.)

Protodiastole. This is the last phase of ventricular systole. During this brief period there is reversal of blood flow in the pulmonary artery and aorta as ventricular pressures fall below arterial pressures. This results in filling and closure of the pulmonic and aortic valves. (See Fig. *F*, opposite.)

Waveforms

Systolic and diastolic events can be correlated to specific components of the atrial, ventricular, and arterial waveforms.

The Atrial Pressure Waveform (Fig. 4–7). In sinus rhythm, two atrial

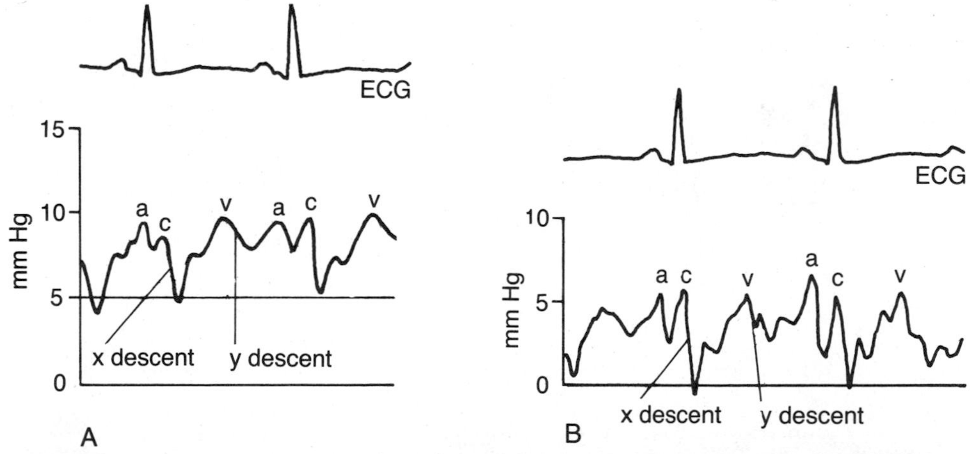

FIGURE 4–7. The atrial pressure waveform. *A*, Left; *B*, right. The mechanical events of the cardiac cycle as represented by the pressure waveforms follow the recorded electrical events represented by the ECG. In the recorded atrial pressure tracing, the *a* wave, which relates to atrial contraction, immediately follows atrial depolarization as represented by the P wave. Upward bulging of the A-V valves during early ventricular systole produces a *c* wave, which may be seen immediately following the QRS complex (ventricular depolarization). The *v* wave represents mechanical ventricular systole and follows electrical systole as represented by the QRS complex. The recorded relationship between the electrical and mechanical events may be prolonged if, for example, long tubing connects the transducer to the catheter sensing tip.

crests and troughs are associated with each heart beat. The pressure waveforms in the right atrium, left atrium, and pulmonary artery wedge position are fundamentally the same, except for minor differences in amplitude.

The first crest, the *a* wave, is produced by the small pressure rise accompanying atrial systole. The *x* descent immediately follows the *a* wave, reflecting the pressure fall occurring with atrial relaxation. Occasionally the *x* descent is distorted by a *c* wave, which relates to upward bulging of the A-V valves early in ventricular systole. The *c* wave is rarely seen in the pulmonary artery wedge waveform.

The second crest, or *v* wave, occurs with continuous vena caval and pulmonary venous inflow against closed, upward bulging A-V valves during ventricular systole. The *y* descent begins with atrial emptying and occurs with A-V valve opening and the passive filling phase of ventricular diastole.

The Ventricular Pressure Waveform (Fig. 4–8). The pressure waveforms for both ventricles have the same characteristics but have vastly different amplitudes. The smooth, nearly vertical upstroke coincides with isovolumetric contraction and intraventricular pressure rise. The semilunar valves open and pressure continues to mount to the systolic peak, which is approximately five times greater for the left ventricle than for the right. At the onset of the phase of rapid ventricular ejection, the pressure wave turns

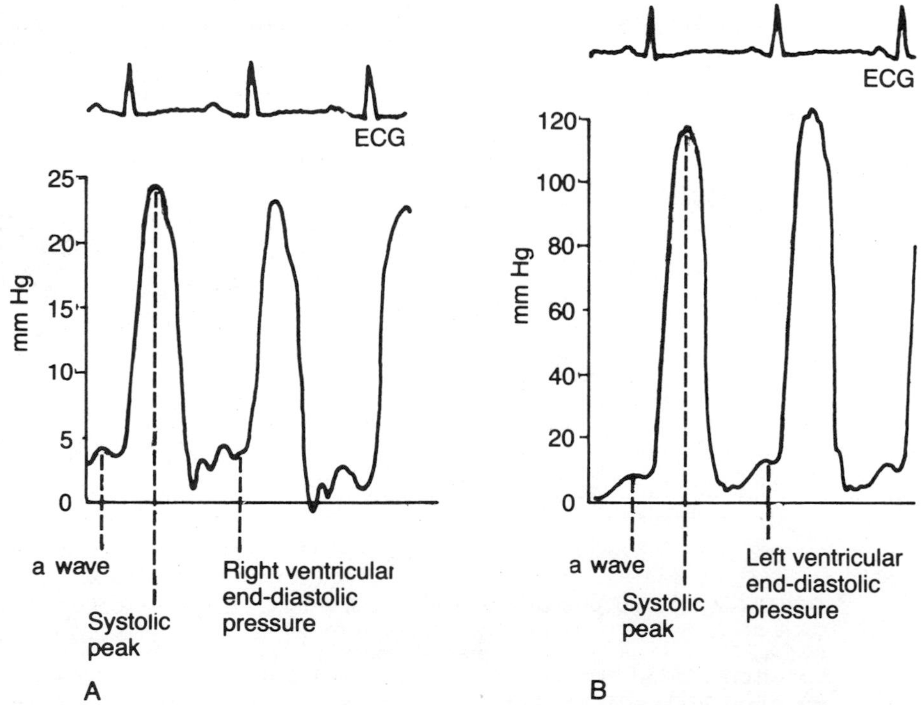

FIGURE 4–8. The ventricular pressure waveform. *A*, Right; *B*, left. Electrical systole precedes mechanical ventricular systole. The ventricular pressure waveform is usually seen in an area relating to the Q-T interval of the ECG. However, excessive tubing length may widen the recorded relationship.

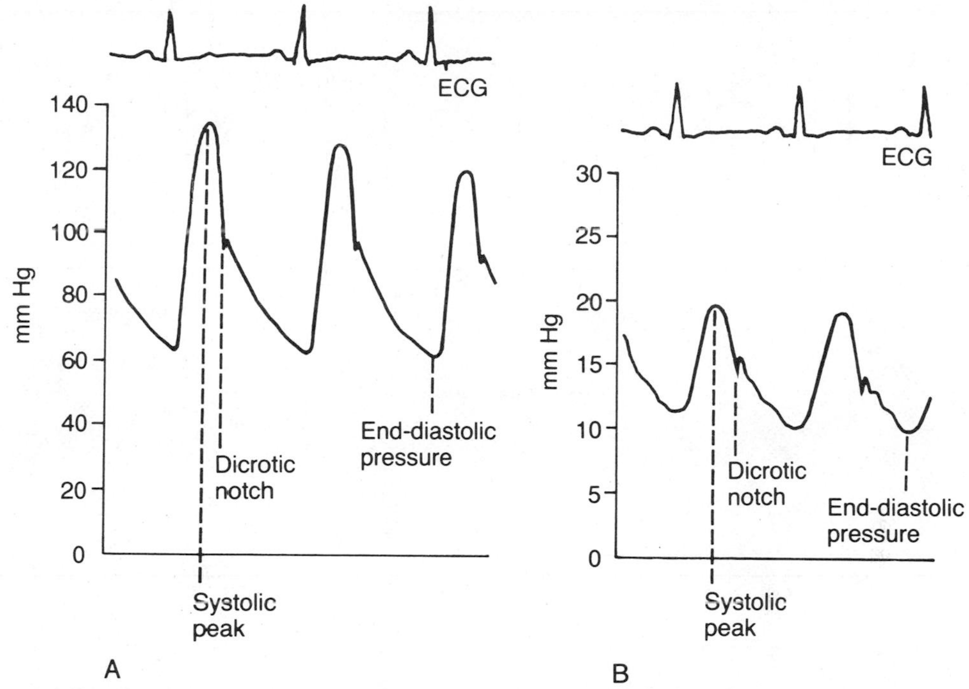

FIGURE 4–9. The arterial pressure waveform. The systolic rise in arterial pressure follows ventricular depolarization represented by the QRS complex. *A*, Aortic pressure; *B*, pulmonary artery pressure.

downward, forming a brief shelf. It then pursues a more vertical course relating to the phases of reduced rate of ejection and the isovolumetric relaxation phase of diastole. When ventricular pressures drop below atrial pressures, the A-V valves open and passive ventricular filling occurs. Early diastolic pressure is the lowest pressure recorded on the ventricular pressure waveform. The atrial kick or *a* wave produces a brief increase in pressure. The interval following the *a* wave is ventricular end-diastolic pressure.

The Arterial Pressure Waveform (Fig. 4–9). The phasic changes in pulmonary arterial and aortic waveforms are similar in contour except that the peak systolic pressure for the aorta is approximately five times that of the pulmonary artery.

The arterial pressure waveform begins with opening of the semilunar valves and ascends to the systolic peak. The slope of the upstroke, or rate of rise, relates to the velocity of blood ejected from the ventricle. The upstroke is more sharply vertical in people with hyperdynamic hearts (anemia, fever, hyperthyroidism, and excessive sympathetic nervous system stimulation) or increased peripheral run-off (aortic regurgitation). The upstroke is slowed with obstruction to outflow (aortic stenosis) or ventricular failure. Pressures in the pulmonary and systemic arterial circulations fall as blood runs off through the capillaries and veins. When intraventricular pressures fall below pressures in the great arteries, the semilunar valves snap shut, producing a

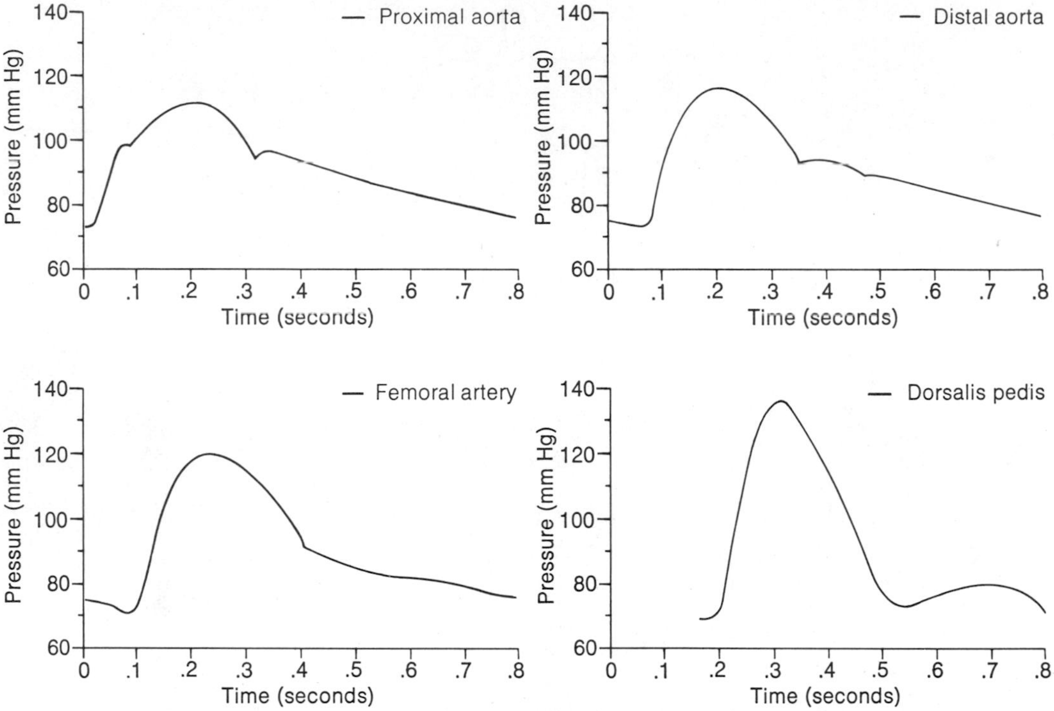

FIGURE 4–10. The contour of the arterial pressure waveform relative to the site used for pressure measurement. (From Wilson RF: Cardiovascular Physiology. In *Principles and Techniques of Critical Care,* Vol I. Kalamazoo, MI, The Upjohn Company, 1979, p 40; and Philadelphia, FA Davis.)

slight distortion in the waveform, the dicrotic notch. With continued run-off blood, pressures fall to end-diastole.

The form and numerical values of the systemic arterial pressure waves undergo changes relative to the site used for measurement. With arterial catheter placement in the more peripheral vessels, systolic pressures are higher, the waveform is narrower and has a steeper rise, and the dicrotic notch is delayed and lower (Fig. 4–10).

Factors Affecting Cardiac Output

Cardiac output is the amount of blood ejected by the heart measured in liters per minute. It is the product of stroke volume (the amount of blood ejected by the heart per beat) and heart rate. This is expressed in the following formula:

Cardiac output	=	Heart rate	×	Stroke volume
5–8 liters/minute		60–80 BPM		60–130 ml

Factors that determine stroke volume and cardiac output are shown in Figure 4–11.

Preload. Preload refers to the filling volume of the ventricle which stretches the relaxed ventricular wall at end-diastole. E. H. Starling, a physiologist, described the heart's ability to adapt its stroke volume to the volume of inflowing blood. The Starling law of the heart states that the greater the end-diastolic ventricular filling volume (the greater the amount of stretch on the myocardial muscle fibers) the greater the force of the subsequent contraction and stroke volume. Normally, there is a good correlation between ventricular end-diastolic volume (VEDV) and ventricular end-diastolic pressure (VEDP); therefore, for clinical purposes, a volume/pressure relationship is assumed. Right ventricular diastolic (filling) pressure is reflected in right atrial or central venous pressure measurements. Left ventricular diastolic (filling) pressure is reflected in the left atrial, pulmonary artery diastolic, or pulmonary artery wedge pressure measurements. The relationship between stroke volume and left ventricular end-diastolic pressure is demonstrated by the ventricular function curve depicted in Figure 4–12.

As preload increases, myocardial performance increases. The normal level of preload for the left ventricle ranges from 4 to 12 mm Hg; however, the preload level at which peak myocardial performance is achieved is variable among patients and is influenced by ventricular compliance (distensibility). Compliance is influenced by disease. For example, following acute myocardial infarction, the optimum preload for the stiff ischemic ventricle may be as high as 20 mm Hg, whereas in sepsis or hypovolemic shock the optimum level of preload may be between 10 and 15 mm Hg. Beyond the optimum level of preload for any given heart, performance levels off or declines. Pulmonary congestion and edema are likely beyond preload levels of 18 to 20 mm Hg.

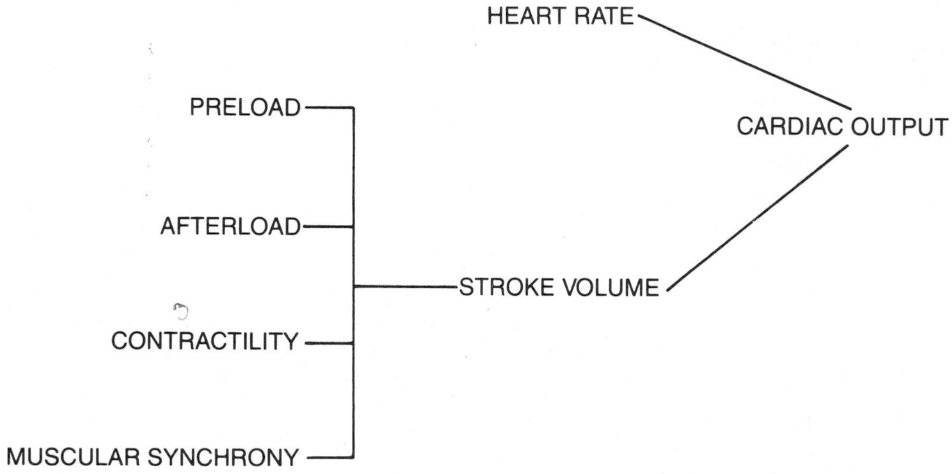

FIGURE 4–11. Determinants of stroke volume and cardiac output.

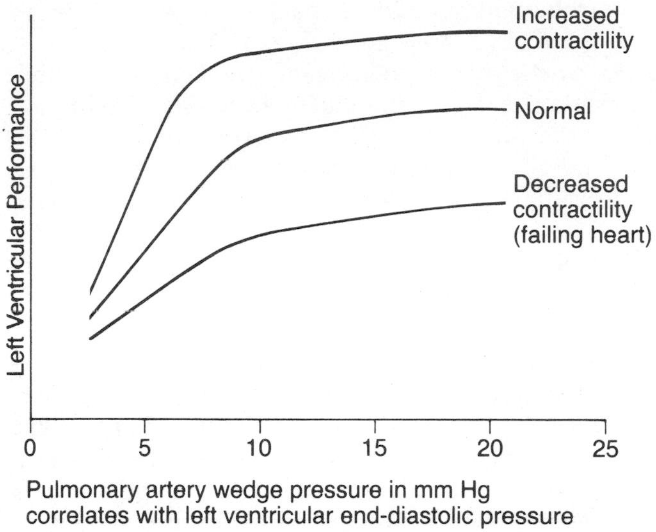

FIGURE 4–12. The ventricular function curve. Note that in the failing heart, increases in intraventricular volume, as reflected by increases in filling pressure, produce disproportionately smaller increases in performance compared with the normal ventricle. Conversely, with increased contractility due to catecholamine stimulation of the normal myocardium, more work is produced for any given filling pressure.

As previously stated, disease may alter the shape of the function curve and/or the pressure/volume relationship. For example, patients with myocardial dysfunction have only a small increase in stroke volume with increasing ventricular filling pressures and, therefore, have flatter, depressed function curves (Fig. 4–12, bottom curve). Furthermore, the ventricular end-diastolic pressure may be increased without a significant increase in end-diastolic volume when the ventricle is stiff and noncompliant as occurs in fibrotic or ischemic heart disease. Conversely, when the ventricle is abnormally compliant, as in dilated cardiomyopathies, there may be large increases in ventricular end-diastolic volume with minimal increases in end-diastolic pressure. The optimum filling pressure for any patient's left ventricle is that which produces an adequate cardiac output without producing pulmonary edema.

Afterload. Afterload refers to the resistance or impedance to right and left ventricular ejection. It is imposed by 1) pulmonary artery and aortic diastolic pressures which must be exceeded by intraventricular pressure during the isovolumetric phase of systole for pulmonic and aortic valve opening to occur; and 2) resistance to flood flow through the pulmonary and systemic circulations which is determined by vascular tone. If, for example, systemic vascular resistance is increased due to generalized arteriolar contriction (stress response, compensatory mechanism in heart failure, vasopressors), it becomes more difficult for blood to run out of the arterial circulation into the capillary bed in systole and, therefore, more difficult for the left ventricle, especially in a diseased state, to eject blood into the arterial circulation. As a result, stroke volume and cardiac output tend to fall as myocardial oxygen consumption increases proportional to the increase in heart work. Conversely, if afterload is decreased (vasodilator therapy, aortic regurgitation, hyperdynamic sepsis), the impedance to left ventricular ejection is decreased and stroke volume increases as myocardial oxygen consumption decreases. In other words, when changes in afterload occur, reciprocal changes in stroke volume and myocardial oxygen consumption result. Pathological conditions such as pulmonic or aortic stenosis or coarctation of the aorta also increase afterload. In these circumstances, afterload reduction requires surgical correction of the defect.

Afterload cannot be measured directly. Knowledge of aortic diastolic pressure and systemic vascular resistance (SVR) provides a guide. However, it is assumed that the ventricle is being unloaded if the patient is being treated with vasodilators and 1) cardiac output increases as systemic vascular resistance decreases; or 2) mean systemic blood pressure decreases or remains the same (the increase in stroke volume may compensate for the vasodilation and maintain mean arterial pressure).

Heart Rate. Changes in heart rate may profoundly affect myocardial performance. Rates beyond 170 beats per minute may be associated with cardiac decompensation because diastolic time is shortened, thus shortening coronary perfusion and ventricular filling time. Bradycardia may result in a severe drop in cardiac output if stroke volume is limited by myocardial disease or if venous return is reduced.

Coordinated Contraction of Individual Muscle Fibers. Coordinated contraction is necessary for efficient ventricular emptying. The organized contraction pattern may be impaired by regional ischemia or infarction, conduction defects, ventricular aneurysm, arrhythmias, or ventricular dilatation.

Myocardial Contractility (Inotropic State of the Myocardium). Contractility relates to the inherent capability of the myocardium to increase the extent and force of muscle fiber shortening independent of preload or afterload. A positive inotropic effect results in increased stroke volume if all other determinants of cardiac output—preload, afterload, heart rate, and muscular synchrony—are kept constant (Fig. 4–12, top curve). This results from stimulation of the sympathetic nervous system, the use of beta-stimulant drugs such as dopamine (Intropin), dobutamine (Dobutrex), or isoproterenol (Isuprel), or the administration of positive inotropic agents such as digitalis or amrinone (Inocor). A negative inotropic effect induced by beta or calcium blocking agents, most antiarrhythmic agents, acidemia, or ischemic heart disease reduces contractility and stroke volume (Fig. 4–12, bottom curve).

THE CORONARY CIRCULATION

Anatomy

The coronary circulation is depicted in Figure 4–13. The main coronary arteries extend over the epicardial surface of the heart and surround it like a crown. It is from these arteries and their small penetrating branches that the heart receives all of its blood supply. Only a tissue-paper thin area of the endocardium can obtain oxygen from blood in the heart's chambers. The two

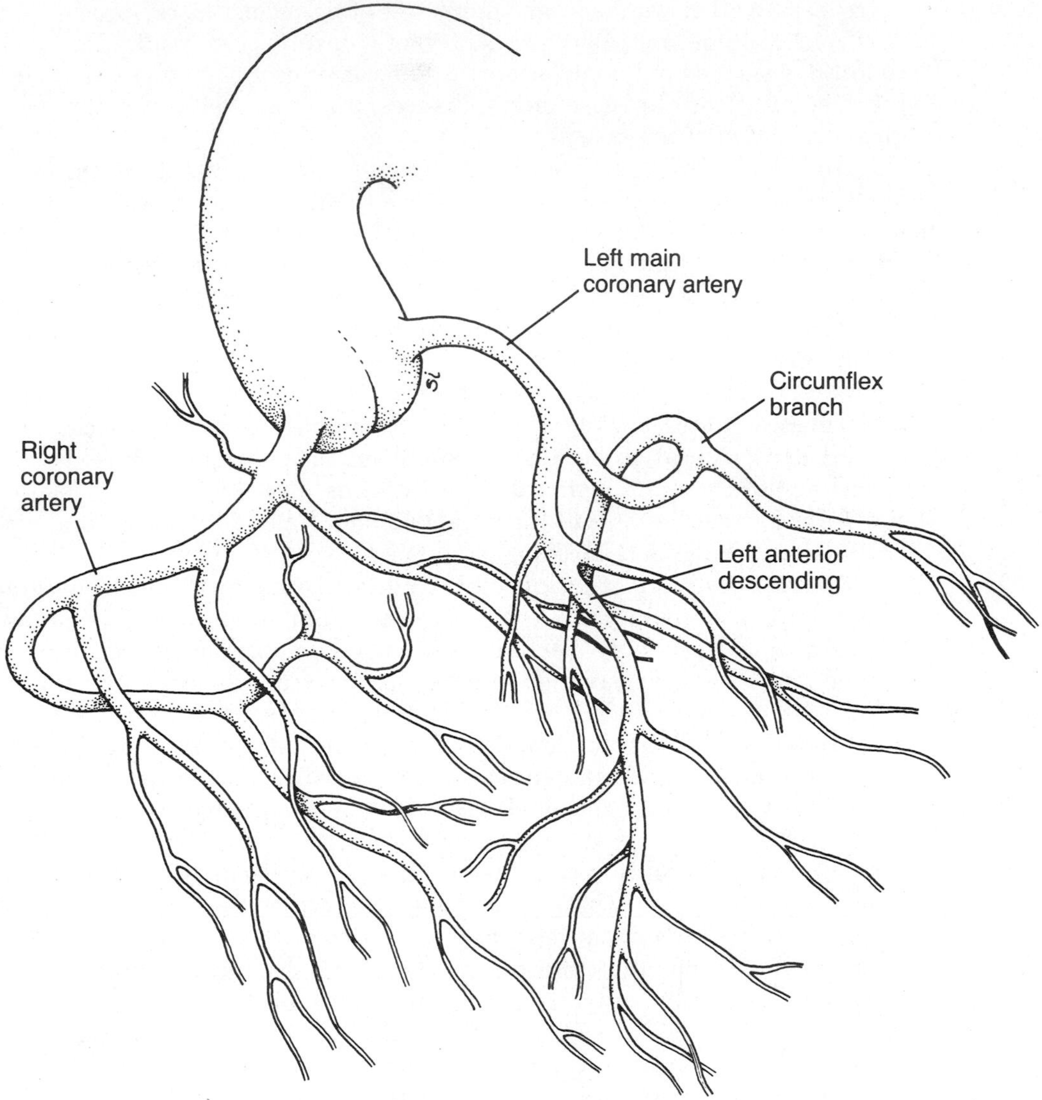

FIGURE 4–13. The coronary circulation.

coronary arteries arise from the region of the sinus of Valsalva at the level of the free edges of the aortic valve cusps.

The *right coronary artery (RCA)* originates behind the right aortic valve cusp and runs in a groove between the right atrium and ventricle until it reaches the crux (top of the ventricular septum posteriorly) where it becomes the posterior descending artery, which runs parallel to the ventricular septum. In 55 to 60 percent of persons, the RCA supplies blood to the sinus node and in 90 percent of persons it perfuses the AV node and the initial portion of the bundle of His. The penetrating branches of the posterior descending branch of the RCA provide nutrient flow to the posterior one-third of the ventricular septum.

The *left main coronary artery* originates as a single vessel in the small opening behind the left aortic valve cusp. It averages about 14 mm in length and usually divides into two main branches. The *left anterior descending (LAD)* artery runs anteriorly and downward, parallel to the ventricular septum, and, in its course, forms a reverse *S* curve. The first curve is around the base of the pulmonary artery; the second curve is around the apex where it then ascends 2 to 5 cm in the posterior intraventricular groove. The LAD sends some branches to the free wall of the right ventricle; some course over the free wall of the left ventricle, and about three to five branches penetrate into the septum to nourish the bundle of His, the bundle branches, and the anterior two-thirds of the septum.

The circumflex branch runs in a groove between the left atrium and ventricle and then descends on the posterior surface of the left ventricle to supply blood to the lateral and posterior portions of the left ventricle. In approximately 10 percent of the population, it reaches the crux and sends a penetrating branch to the AV node. A sinus nodal branch is provided by the circumflex in approximately 40 to 45 percent of the population.

Coronary anatomy varies considerably among individuals. For example, in some persons the left main coronary artery trifurcates, whereas in others it may send a lavish shower of vessels over the anterior surface of the heart.

The terms *right* or *left dominant circulation* are commonly used and do not imply which circulation supplies the most blood to the heart. The left circulation uniformly provides flow to the greatest portion of the myocardium. Right dominant circulation means the right coronary circulation reaches the crux and feeds the AV node. Left dominant circulation means the circumflex reaches the crux to vascularize the AV node. In other words, the coronary circulation perfusing the AV node is designed as the dominant circulation. In a small percentage of people in whom both the RCA and circumflex reach the crux, the term *balanced circulation* is used.

Coronary Blood Flow and Myocardial Oxygen Consumption

Blood flow through the coronary circulation, as in all circulations, is detemined by the pressure gradient across the vascular bed and the resistance to flow, which is determined by the caliber of the perfusing vessels.

Coronary perfusion for both ventricles is phasic because aortic pressure is phasic. Aortic diastolic pressure is the primary determinant of left ventricular blood flow, however, as almost all perfusion occurs during diastole. This is because systolic compression of the nutrient (penetrating) branches by the thick, strongly contractile, left ventricle increases resistance to flow progressively from epicardium to subendocardium. For this reason, the subendocardium (inner one-third to one-fourth of the myocardium) experiences no flow during systole whereas the epicardial layer enjoys some systolic perfusion.

The thinner-walled right ventricle develops less wall tension with systole; thus, penetrating branches undergo less compression, and phasic changes in coronary blood flow are less marked. The pressure head driving blood into both coronary circulations is approximately 80 mm Hg; outflow or coronary venous pressures are approximately 0 to 5 mm Hg. A decrease in aortic diastolic pressure or increase in venous pressure narrows the pressure gradient and has the potential to reduce coronary blood flow, especially in the presence of coronary artery disease.

The coronary circulation is unique because it supplies an organ whose energy expenditure and oxygen consumption are consistently extremely high. At rest, the left ventricle extracts approximately 70 percent of the oxygen from its arterial blood. This has two important physiologic implications:

- The left ventricle is very oxygen dependent for normal function.
- There is no reserve for additional extraction in times of increased need.

Increased myocardial oxygen needs can be met only by increased coronary blood flow; thus, the myocardium is also very flow dependent. In times of stress (exercise), the normal coronary circulation dilates to increase flow four to five times resting values. Decreased myocardial oxygen tensions seem to be the most potent stimulus to coronary vasodilation. Thus, coronary blood flow is determined by local metabolic need. The capacity of the coronary circulation to adapt its flow to myocardial need (autoregulation) is essential to maintain effective pump dynamics because contractility of the myocardium relates directly to oxygen availability and consumption.

The three primary determinants of myocardial oxygen consumption are wall tension, contractility, and heart rate. All can be manipulated pharmacologically in an attempt to keep myocardial oxygen supply and demand in balance. Two minor determinants are electrical depolarization and maintenance of cellular activity.

Wall Tension. Myocardial oxygen consumption increases proportionately with increases in wall tension. Wall tension is determined by two factors: 1) the pressure work of the heart; and 2) ventricular size. Increases in arterial pressure are met with linear increases in myocardial oxygen consumption. In addition, as the heart enlarges, greater wall tension is required to eject against a given pressure load. According to Laplace's law, the tension required to produce a given pressure increases proportionately with the diameter of the heart.

Contractility (The Inotropic State of the Myocardium). Positive inotropic agents such as epinephrine (Adrenalin), norepinephrine (Levophed), digitalis, dopamine (Intropin), amrinone (Inocor), or calcium ions increase contractility and the metabolic activity of the myocardium itself. This increases myocardial oxygen demand which, in the healthy heart, is met with a proportionate increase in coronary blood flow and oxygen consumption. Unfortunately, in the presence of coronary artery disease, this coronary autoregulation is not intact, predisposing the patient to ischemic events.

Heart Rate. The relationship of heart rate and oxygen consumption is very straightforward. Increases in heart rate are met with increases in oxygen demand and consumption; likewise, reduced heart rates result in decreased myocardial oxygen demand and consumption.

Activation. *Electrical depolarization* accounts for only 0.5 percent of total myocardial oxygen requirements.

Maintenance of Cellular Activity. Normal cellular metabolism accounts for only 10 to 15 percent of total myocardial oxygen consumption.

THE CIRCUIT (THE VASCULAR SYSTEM)

The vascular system is the conduit that carries blood to and from the cardiopulmonary unit and tissue and is composed of arteries, capillaries, and veins. Vascular flow rates in the resting adult are about 5 to 8 liters per minute. Blood flow through a vascular bed can occur only if there is a pressure gradient or difference between the two ends. For example, mean central aortic pressure is approximately 90 mm Hg whereas central venous pressure is approximately 0 mm Hg. This produces a pressure gradient of 90 mm Hg from the central arteries to the central veins. The rate of flow is determined by the pressure gradient at the beginning and end of the vascular bed, not by an absolute pressure (Fig. 4–14).

As blood flows through a vascular bed, several factors contribute to a resistance or opposition to flow.

Viscosity of the Blood. Thick fluid is more resistant to flow than thin fluid. Blood is a viscous fluid and its viscosity increases as the hematocrit (Hct) increases. For example, when the Hct exceeds 55 percent (polycythemia or overtransfusion) blood viscosity rises steeply, resulting in increased resistance to blood flow. Because the Hct normally remains constant and does not significantly affect viscosity, it is not taken into account when clinically calculating resistance to blood flow.

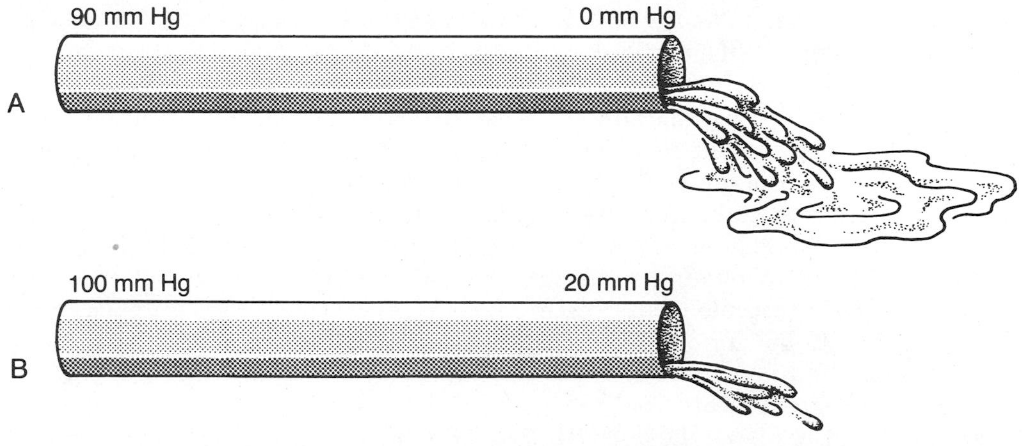

FIGURE 4–14. Rate of blood flow. *A,* A pressure gradient of 90 mm Hg drives fluid through the tube. *B,* Despite a 10 mm Hg increase in pressure at the beginning of the tube, fluid flow rates will be decreased because pressure at the end of the tube is increased to 20 mm Hg, thus decreasing the pressure gradient, or fluid driving force, to 80 mm Hg.

Length of the Vascular Bed. As the length of a tube increases, flow rates decrease because of the increased friction imposed by the increased length of the vessel wall. Blood vessel length does not change once adult growth has been reached; therefore, this factor is also not considered clinically when calculating vascular resistance (see Chapter 9, "Vascular Resistance").

Blood Vessel Diameter. The rate of blood flow through a vessel decreases in direct proportion to the fourth power of its diameter. If the diameter is decreased to one half by vasoconstriction, for example, resistance to blood flow is increased 16 times. The diameter of the vascular lumen, therefore, is the most important factor in determining vascular resistance. Because the arterioles and precapillary sphincters are the principal sites of changes in vessel diameter, they determine resistance and, therefore, distribution of blood flow.

Arteries

Arteries are vessels that carry blood away from the heart. Large arteries branch off the aorta and progressively divide, becoming smaller and smaller in diameter. The small arteries branch into arterioles that have a strong muscular wall and are the major area of resistance in the systemic circulation. Arteriolar tone is adjusted by local and systemic chemical, physical, and neural factors. Local tissue oxygen need is the primary determinant of arteriolar tone and profoundly affects capillary blood flow. For example, as oxygen availability at the tissue level decreases relative to need, vascular resistance decreases, bringing in additional blood flow. The arterioles divide into metarterioles before merging with the capillary bed. At the level of the metarterioles, a smooth muscle fiber known as the precapillary sphincter additionally regulates flow to tissues.

In summary, the arterial bed is a high pressure, low volume, high resistance system whose purpose is to deliver oxygenated blood in required amounts to the capillary bed.

Arterial pressure is a measure of the pressure, expressed in mm Hg, exerted by blood per unit area on the arterial wall. This pressure is the same at all points at the same level and is affected by the influence of gravity on hydrostatic pressure. Hydrostatic pressure results from the weight of blood within the column of the vascular structures; it progressively rises downward from heart level and progressively falls above heart level (Fig. 4–15). For this reason, to eliminate the influence of gravity on hydrostatic pressure and obtain accurate blood pressure measurement, the limb used for measurement should be supported at heart level. False high values will be recorded with the limb in a dependent position; false low values are obtained with the limb held above heart level.

Because of the pulsatile quality of blood flow through the arterial system, arterial pressure has two components: *Systolic pressure* represents the higher pressure and relates to contraction of the ventricles and ejection of a bolus of

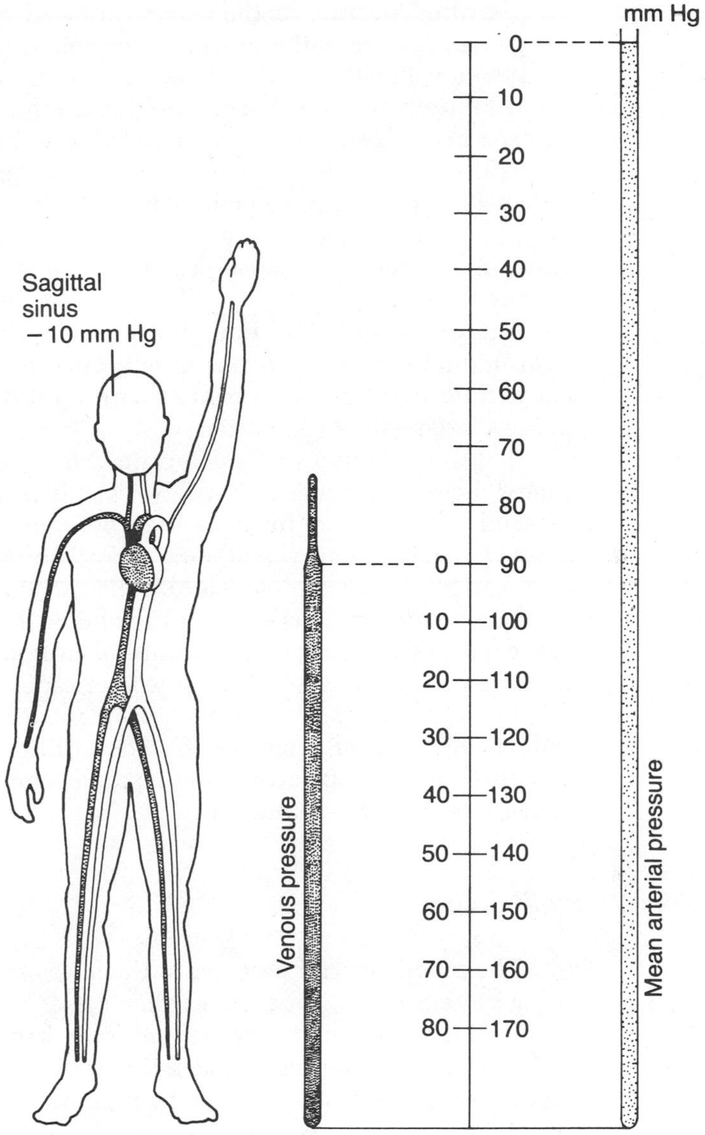

FIGURE 4–15. The effect of hydrostatic pressure on arterial and venous pressure. In the upright position, the mean arterial and venous pressures progressively increase from heart level to ankle. With the arm held vertically above the head, the arterial pressure progressively drops upward of heart level. The venous pressure is 0 mm Hg at heart level and becomes negative above that level.

blood into the arterial system. *Diastolic pressure* is the lower pressure and relates to relaxation of the ventricles and peripheral run-off of blood. Physiologic factors that influence systolic and diastolic pressure include:

Arteriolar Tone. The diastolic pressure is primarily determined by systemic vascular resistance. Arteriolar constriction, as seen with sympathetic nervous system stimulation, increases diastolic pressure. Decreased systemic vascular resistance, as seen with neurogenic shock, anaphylactic shock, or vasodilator therapy, decreases diastolic pressure.

Stroke Volume. As the volume of blood ejected with each beat increases, the pulse pressure (difference between systolic and diastolic pressures) widens. As stroke volume falls, the pulse pressure becomes narrower.

Elasticity of the Aorta and Its Large Tributaries. The walls of the arteries are far less distensible than those of the veins; however, they normally do yield somewhat to the bolus of blood delivered from the ventricle. The less distensible the system receiving pulsatile flow, the greater the pulse pressure. With increasing age the arterial system progressively loses compliance, resulting in the wide pulse pressure of systolic hypertension seen in some elderly persons.

Intravascular Volume. Since the systemic arteries are essentially noncompliant, volume increases will be met with pressure increases. Clinically, fluid overload is associated with hypertension whereas fluid depletion is associated with hypotension.

The systolic pressure is determined by a combination of all the aforementioned factors: peripheral vascular resistance, stroke volume, elasticity of the arterial system, and intravascular volume. All but elasticity can change acutely. These factors and how they interrelate have important clinical implications. For example, significant intravascular volume loss may occur without significant decreases in systolic or diastolic pressure. Compensatory vasoconstriction increases or maintains systolic and diastolic pressure within a "numerically acceptable" range when tissue perfusion may not be acceptable.

Pulse pressure is the most important assessment parameter because it reflects increases or decreases in stroke volume. If pulse pressure is narrowed by approximately 50 percent, for example, one can assume that stroke volume is decreased by about that much.

Mean Arterial Pressure

The mean arterial pressure is the average pressure within the cardiovascular system throughout one cardiac cycle. Some physicians prefer to assess perfusion status and/or titrate vasoactive drugs using mean arterial pressure rather than systolic and/or diastolic pressure. This is because mean arterial pressure represents the average pressure driving blood to the systemic circulation to the body tissue.

Because at normal heart rates diastole is approximately two-thirds of the cardiac cycle, the mean arterial pressure is closer to the diastolic value. The mean arterial pressure is calculated using the following formula:

$$\text{Mean arterial pressure (MAP)} = \frac{\text{Systolic} + (\text{Diastolic} \times 2)}{3}$$

For a blood pressure of 120/80:

$$\text{MAP 93 mm Hg} = \frac{120 + (80 \times 2)}{3}$$

Capillaries

Capillaries are microscopic vessels that branch off the arterioles to ultimately connect with venules. Capillaries might be conceptualized as a network of delicate vascular lace (Fig. 4–16). Capillaries are composed of a single layer of endothelial cells that are selectively permeable to water, sugars, electrolytes, and gases. They are the sole exchange stations that supply fuel to fire the life processes and also allow removal of metabolites from the tissues; no metabolic exchange occurs in the larger vessels; rather they only serve as conduits.

Diffusion is the most important means by which substances are transferred between intravascular and extravascular spaces. The rate of diffusion is determined by the concentration gradient on either side of the vascular membrane. Water diffuses back and forth freely; it is estimated that 3000 ml of water exits and enters the vascular space each minute in a 70 kg adult. Although tremendous two-way movement of fluid occurs across the capillary membrane, the fluid volumes on either side of the vascular membrane must be maintained in delicate balance.

Factors governing fluid movement across the capillary membrane, which determine intravascular and interstitial fluid volumes, include capillary permeability and the oppositely directed forces of hydrostatic and oncotic pressures.

The slitlike gaps between capillary endothelial cells and the diffusion capabilities of the endothelial cells themselves allow varying degrees of diffusion for different substances. For example, the capillary membrane is freely permeable to low molecular weight substances like urea, glucose, ions, and water but is relatively impermeable to high molecular weight substances like plasma proteins. The permeability of the capillaries can vary in different tissue beds, however. The capillaries of the liver and kidney are highly permeable; the capillaries of the lung are far less so. It is not possible to measure capillary permeability in the clinical setting.

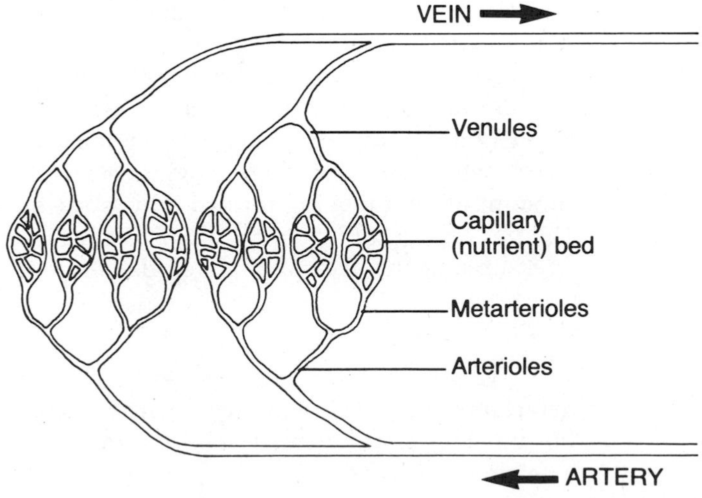

FIGURE 4–16. The capillary (nutrient) bed.

Hydrostatic Pressure. This is the pressure exerted by a volume of fluid within a given space. Capillary hydrostatic pressures are positive and tend to push fluid out of the vascular space into the interstitium. It is easily measured in the lung with a flow-directed pulmonary artery catheter while the catheter is in the wedge position (PWP). Measured left atrial pressure and pulmonary artery diastolic pressures also closely relate to pulmonary capillary hydrostatic pressure. Interstitial hydrostatic pressures are estimated to be subatmospheric and act as a vacuum, drawing fluid into the interstitial space. This pressure cannot be measured clinically; in fact, only assumptions have been made from laboratory work.

Oncotic Pressure or Colloid Osmotic Pressure (COP). This represents the pressure generated by the attraction of protein macromolecules for water across the semipermeable capillary membrane. Colloid osmotic pressure is proportional to the number of molecules in solution on two sides of the membrane. Fluid moves from an area of lower protein concentration to an area of higher protein concentration. Because capillaries are relatively impermeable to protein, plasma proteins are restricted to the vascular space. This results in a protein concentration gradient between the plasma and interstitium.

Plasma Oncotic Pressure. This tends to attract and hold fluid within the vascular space at a force of approximately 24 to 28 mm Hg in a healthy, ambulatory adult. Plasma oncotic pressure tends to decrease with illness or prolonged bedrest. Albumin contributes approximately 75 percent of the total plasma oncotic pressure; the remainder is contributed by the various globulin fractions and a very small amount by fibrinogen. Plasma oncotic pressure is easily measured with an oncometer. Since albumin contributes nearly three quarters to plasma oncotic pressure, the serum albumin also reflects the plasma oncotic state of the patient.

Interstitial Oncotic Pressure. This pressure tends to draw fluid out of the vascular space into the interstitium. This force is the result of the osmotic attraction for water imposed by the small amounts of protein that do escape from plasma across the capillary membrane into the interstitium. Interstitial oncotic pressure cannot be measured clinically, and only assumptions have been made from laboratory work.

Hydrostatic and oncotic forces differ in the systemic and pulmonary circulations because the systemic tissue and pulmonary tissue beds require slightly different fluid dynamics for normal function. In both systems, however, the amount of fluid moving outward is at near equilibrium to the amount of fluid moving inward. This state of near equilibrium is produced by the net effects of the oppositely directed forces of net hydrostatic and oncotic pressures at the arterial and venular ends of the capillary bed.

Systemic Capillary Fluid Dynamics

Hydrostatic forces differ at either end of the systemic capillary. At the arteriolar end of the capillary, hydrostatic pressures are approximately 25 to 30 mm Hg; at the venular end hydrostatic pressures are 10 to 15 mm Hg. The pressure gradient of 15 mm Hg across the capillary bed provides the impetus for blood flow. Because of the large cross-sectional area of the capillary bed, however, flow rates are slow, circumstances suitable for the reciprocal diffusion of substances from blood vessels to cells. Given a mean systemic capillary hydrostatic pressure of 17 mm Hg, the normal mean forces acting at the capillary membrane are as follows:

Average Forces Tending To Push Fluid *Out* Of The Systemic Vascular Space

Mean capillary hydrostatic pressure	17.0 mm Hg
Subatmospheric interstitial hydrostatic pressure (acting as a vacuum drawing fluid into the interstitium)	−6.0 mm Hg
Interstitial oncotic pressure	+ 5.3 mm Hg
Net Forces Directing Fluid Outward	28.3 mm Hg

Average Forces Tending To Pull Fluid *Into* The Systemic Vascular Space

Plasma oncotic pressure	28.0 mm Hg
Net Forces Directed Inward	28.0 mm Hg

Net forces:	Outward	28.3 mm Hg
	Inward	−28.0 mm Hg
Average Force Directing Fluid Into The Body Tissue		0.3 mm Hg

Pulmonary Capillary Fluid Dynamics

Hydrostatic forces at either end of the pulmonary capillary favor a driving pressure through the capillary bed of approximately 4 mm Hg. The normal mean forces acting at the pulmonary capillary membrane are as follows:

Average Forces Tending To Push Fluid *Out* Of The Pulmonary Vascular Space

Mean pulmonary capillary hydrostatic pressure	8.0 mm Hg
Subatmospheric pulmonary interstitial hydrostatic pressure (drawing fluid into the lung tissue)	−10.0 mm Hg
Interstitial oncotic pressure	+12.0 mm Hg
Net Force Directing Fluid Outward	30.0 mm Hg

Average Forces Tending To Pull Fluid *Into* The Pulmonary Vascular Space

Plasma oncotic pressure	28.0 mm Hg
Net Forces Directed Inward	28.0 mm Hg

Net forces:	Outward	30.0 mm Hg
	Inward	−28.0 mm Hg
Average Forces Directing Fluid Into The Pulmonary Tissue Space		2.0 mm Hg

Although the above values are not absolute and may vary within limits, neither systemic nor pulmonary capillary beds maintain perfect balance between outward and inward forces. In both systems there is slightly more fluid leaving than entering the vascular space. In the systemic circulation, this amounts to approximately 1.7 to 3.5 ml per minute. In the pulmonary circulation, this amounts to an estimated 20 ml per hour fluid leak into the lung tissue. This watery extract of plasma is ultimately returned to the venous circulation by the systemic and pulmonary lymphatics.

Veins

Veins are vessels that collect blood from the capillaries and return it to the heart. Venules, tiny veins that join with capillaries, merge into larger veins which ultimately merge into the large central veins (vena cavae). Because veins are subjected to lower pressures than arteries, they are thinner walled and more distensible, allowing them to expand and accommodate large volumes of fluids with very small changes in intravascular pressure.

At any time, approximately 70 percent of circulating volume is in the veins. Thus the venous system is also known as the capacitance bed. The veins are capable of changing capacitance in response to neural, chemical, and hormonal factors. Through increased venous tone, the collective volume of the veins shrinks and more blood is brought to the central circulation. Conditions that increase venous tone are hypovolemia, acidemia, hypoxemia, hypothermia, and severe pain. Venoconstriction may reduce venous capacity by 1 to 1.5 liters, thereby increasing preload and pulmonary capillary hydrostatic pressure. Venodilators may increase venous capacity by 1 to 2 liters or more, thus decreasing preload and pulmonary capillary hydrostatic pressure.

Venous pressures are low but, like arterial pressures, are influenced by gravity. That is, venous pressure is the same at all points of the same level but changes with changes in height. For example, venous pressures at the feet in a standing person may be as high as 90 mm Hg, but venous pressures in the dural sinuses of the head may be negative (see Fig. 4–14).

The pressure reading obtained at heart level from the superior vena cava or right atrium is termed central venous pressure and averages about 0 to 8 mm Hg. Central venous pressure is influenced by the heart's ability to pump out the blood returned to it; by the venous return, which relates to circulating volume; and by peripheral vascular tone. Pressure in the peripheral veins is usually 4 to 9 mm Hg higher than central venous pressure.

Venous return is augmented by the milking action of contracting skeletal muscles on veins as well as alterations in intrathoracic pressure associated with breathing (the intrathoracic pump). In summary, the systemic venous bed is a low pressure, high volume, low resistance system whose purpose is the return of deoxygenated blood from the tissues of the body back to the cardiopulmonary unit.

SUGGESTED READINGS

Ayres SM, Gianelli S, Mueller HS: *Care of the Critically Ill*, ed. 2. New York, Appleton-Century-Crofts, 1974, pp 50–71.

Cohn PF: *Clinical Cardiovascular Physiology*. Philadelphia, WB Saunders, 1985.

Daily EK, Schroeder JS: *Hemodynamic Waveforms: Exercises in Identification and Analysis*. St. Louis, CV Mosby, 1983.

Guyton AC: *Textbook of Medical Physiology*, ed. 7. Philadelphia, WB Saunders, 1986, pp 150–346.

Hurst JW: *The Heart*, ed. 5. New York, McGraw-Hill, 1982, pp 7–12.

Shapiro BA, Harrison RA, Trout CA: Cardiovascular anatomy and physiology. In *Clinical Application of Respiratory Care*. Chicago, Year Book Medical Publishers, 1985.

Underhill SL, Woods SL, Sivarajan ES, Halfpenny CJ: *Cardiac Nursing*. Philadelphia, JB Lippincott, 1982, pp 1–100.

Wilson RF: Cardiophysiology. In *Principles and Techniques of Critical Care*, vol. I. Kalamazoo, MI, Upjohn, 1979.

Physical Assessment of the Cardiovascular System

5

The only function of the cardiovascular system is to deliver oxygenated blood to the body at a rate equal to body need. In the critical care setting, a mere glance at the patient may reveal the present cardiovascular status. For example, an ashen, restless, confused or obtunded patient is characteristic of a low perfusion state. The patient's condition and the clinical setting should determine the frequency and rapidity of assessment as well as the sequence in which it should be done. For example, in the crisis situation, assessment is brief and focuses on parameters key to perfusion—presence and quality of pulses, capillary refill, color, and level of consciousness.

CLINICAL EVALUATION OF SYMPTOMS AND SIGNS OF CARDIOVASCULAR DISEASE

In assessing the symptoms and signs of cardiovascular disease, the influence of environmental or emotional factors or body position should be noted as such information may be pertinent in prevention and/or management.

Symptoms

Symptoms are the patient's subjective perception of changes in body function or indications of disease. The following are common symptoms of cardiovascular disease.

Chest Pain. Chest pain of cardiac origin is most commonly due to coronary artery disease. The areas of pain are quite variable and may involve the chest, back, neck, teeth, shoulder, arms (usually the left), and/or epigastrium. The pain is commonly described as a great pressure, burning, or crushing sensation. In some persons only a sensation of heaviness or tightness is perceived. Most patients sit or lie quietly during the painful episode; this may reduce the severity of pain by reducing heart work. Others become very restless and agitated.

In the postinfarction period or following heart surgery, chest pain may indicate pericarditis. The pain is sharp and stabbing and may radiate to the neck, back, and left shoulder. The severity of the pain is increased or appears abruptly from activities that have no effect on myocardial ischemic pain such as lying supine, deep inspiration, rotation of the trunk, or coughing as these activities stretch the inflamed pericardium.

Cultural and/or sexual differences as well as individual personality characteristics such as stoicism or the need to deny disease or pain may influence the pain threshold or may produce distorted information upon questioning. Therefore, an inclusive question such as "Are you having any pain, discomfort, pressure sensations, or unusual sensations in your chest, neck, face, teeth, arms, back or abdomen?" may facilitate communication that may then yield more pertinent information. If pain is acknowledged, a scale of 0 through 10 (10 being intolerable, 0 being complete freedom from pain) helps the clinician assess the severity of pain and the efficacy of analgesics. Precipitating or aggravating factors and/or measures that reduce the severity of pain should be determined.

Dyspnea. In the cardiac patient, dyspnea usually reflects pulmonary edema secondary to left heart failure. Generally, a pulmonary capillary wedge pressure (PWP) greater than 18 to 20 mm Hg is associated with the movement of fluid into the lung. Physiologic changes that may produce cardiac dyspnea include:

1. Increased venous return: A normal right ventricle easily transports an increased venous return through the pulmonary circulation. An impaired left ventricle functions on a depressed preload/stroke volume relationship so that a disproportionately high preload is required to generate the increased output for the left ventricle.

For example, given an end-diastolic volume that produces an end-diastolic pressure of 0 mm Hg, the right ventricle delivers 70 ml of blood into the pulmonary circulation (Fig. 5–1). An impaired left ventricle may match this output but requires an end-diastolic volume, producing a pressure of 15 mm Hg. This may be the patient's steady state when upright or at rest. At this time the lungs are clear and there is no complaint of dyspnea. Should venous return increase (volume loading, exercise, lying down), right ventricular end-diastolic volume increases to produce an end-diastolic pressure of 3 mm Hg. By the Starling mechanism, the small increased right ventricular preload raises the normal right ventricular stroke volume from 70 to 85 ml. An impaired left ventricle may be able to match this stroke volume to produce a new equilibrium only with an end-diastolic volume producing a pressure of 30 mm Hg. The increased pressure will be reflected back to the pulmonary capillary bed where the pulmonary capillary hydrostatic pressure of 30 mm Hg produces extravasation of fluid into the lung. Pulmonary edema and its clinical indicators, tachypnea and dyspnea, result.[1]

2. A sudden ischemic event: Acute ischemic cardiac events produce regional abnormalities in left ventricular wall motion that compromise pump

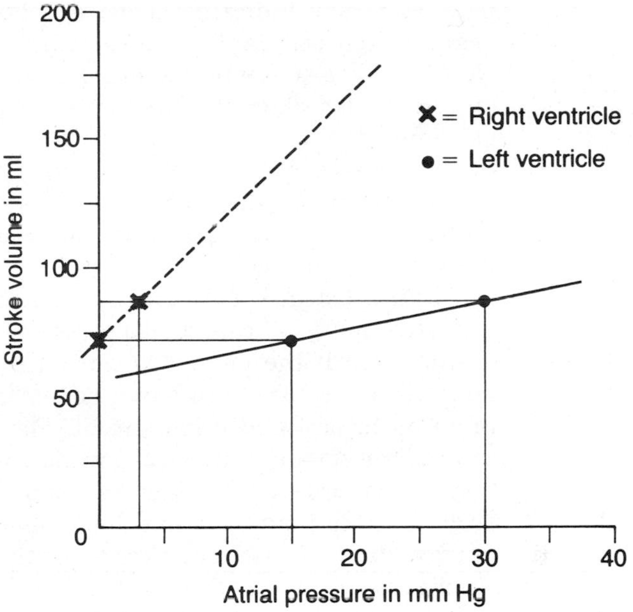

FIGURE 5–1. The relation between stroke volume and atrial pressure or ventricular filling pressure for the right heart is plotted by the broken line, and for the left heart by the solid line. The left ventricular filling volume required to establish the new dynamic equilibrium in stroke volume between the two ventricles may be associated with a left ventricular filling pressure sufficiently high to produce pulmonary edema. (Adapted from Bradley, RD: *Studies in Acute Heart Failure.* London, Edward Arnold Publishers, 1977, p. 3.)

function. Acute ischemic induced myocardial dysfunction leads to increased preload and the potential for pulmonary edema.

Weakness, Fatigue. The sudden onset of ventricular dysfunction precipitated by an acute ischemic event may produce sudden onset heart failure with its associated symptoms of weakness or fatigue. Chronic congestive heart failure is typically associated with feelings of weakness, tiredness, and varying degrees of exercise intolerance.

Signs

Signs represent objective indications of changes in body function or illness. The clinician caring for the acutely ill cardiovascular patient will observe for changes in the following:

Level of Mentation. Owing to its immediate need for steady state oxygenated blood flow, the brain is a sensitive indicator of the patient's perfusion status. Very early signs of cerebral underperfusion are the inability to think abstractly or perform complex mental tasks, restlessness, apprehension, uncooperativeness, and irritability. Short-term memory may also be impaired. A family member may need to be called upon for documentation of the patient's normal personality and intellectual status.

Skin Color and Temperature. During low perfusion states, blood is shunted from skin and muscle to central organs necessary for survival. Cool, pale skin may indicate perfusion failure. Color and temperature changes begin peripherally and move centrally with progressive cardiovascular deterioration. The anatomic site of color and temperature change should be noted (e.g., cool and clammy lower extremities; warm and dry trunk and upper extremities).

Cyanosis. Central cyanosis may be due to right-to-left intracardiac shunts as in tetralogy of Fallot. Peripheral cyanosis is apparent in low perfusion states such as cardiogenic shock. (See Chapter 3, Signs of pulmonary disease.)

Urine Output. Low urine output in a patient known to be adequately hydrated may indicate hypoperfusion secondary to acute left ventricular dysfunction. If the patient is not on a diuretic, the urine output is a very sensitive indicator of acute perfusion changes. As cardiac output falls so does renal blood flow and urine output. For example, a 10 to 20 percent drop in cardiac output may produce minimal blood pressure changes, but because renal vascular resistance increases immediately and disproportionately to the drop in cardiac output, renal blood flow and glomerular filtration rate may fall by 20 to 40 percent. Consequently, urine output may fall long before other signs of impaired tissue perfusion become clinically evident.[2] The scanty urine produced in sudden onset hypoperfusion states is typically concentrated (specific gravity greater than 1.025) and has a low urine sodium. Even if the perfusion deficit is slower in onset and urine output does not fall noticeably, the urine produced is more concentrated and urine sodium is low.[2]

SPECIFIC TECHNIQUES OF PHYSICAL ASSESSMENT

The following techniques are additionally utilized to obtain information about cardiovascular function.

Palpation of the Arterial Pulse

Several factors determine the quality of the arterial pulse. These include stroke volume and ejection velocity, peripheral vascular resistance, and the pressure waves that result from forward flow, which then are reflected back from the peripheral circulation. In the critical care setting, the arterial pulses are routinely checked for rate, rhythm, volume, and the equality of volume from limb to limb.

Rate. Tachycardia is defined as a pulse rate faster than 100 beats per minute (BPM) and bradycardia is a rate less than 60 BPM. In the clinical setting, the appropriateness of the heart rate and its hemodynamic consequences are far more significant than the absolute value.

Rhythm. A variety of circumstances may cause disturbances in pulse rhythm. If the pulse is irregular, the pattern of the irregularity should be noted.

Volume. Pulse volume reflects left ventricular stroke volume. The closer to the heart the vessel is palpated, the less influence the properties of the vessel wall will have on the quality of the pulse. Therefore, the carotid or brachial pulses are more reliable is assessing stroke volume than the radial or pedal pulses. Pulse volume is increased with hyperdynamic cardiovascular states as occur with fever, anemia, emotional excitement, or early sepsis. Pulse volume is decreased in tachyarrhythmias or in hypodynamic cardiovascular states as occur with left ventricular dysfunction or hypovolemia. Because pulse volume is variably affected peripherally, the heart rate is best counted by listening at the apex. However, palpating a peripheral pulse while auscultating at the apex discloses the number of "perfusing beats." For example, in ventricular bigeminy, a total of 76 beats (38 sinus and 38 ventricular premature beats) will be counted at the apex and visualized on the ECG oscilloscope. However, because of the shortened ventricular filling time, absence of the atrial kick, and distorted ventricular contractile dynamics, the ventricular beats may be so weak that they do not eject blood out of the semilunar valves and are, in essence, nonperfusing beats. Therefore, only the 38 sinus "perfusing" beats will be palpated at the wrist. Functionally, the patient has a significant bradycardia.

In hypoperfusion states, if the radial pulse can be palpated, the systolic pressure is at least 80 mm Hg. If the femoral pulse can be palpated, the systolic pressure is at least 70 mm Hg; and if the carotid pulse can be palpated, a systolic pressure of at least 60 mm Hg can be assured.

EQUALITY OF VOLUME. Alterations in cardiovascular function may produce characteristic changes in the arterial pulse. These include *pulsus alternans*, which manifests as a regular alternation in the force of beats so that a weak pulse regularly follows a strong pulse (Fig. 5–2). The underlying rhythm is regular. Stroke volume alters from beat to beat and, in some cases, is attributed to alterations in ventricular end-diastolic pressure (changing compliance). In other cases, there seems to be a primary alteration in contractility without changes in end-diastolic volume.

Pulsus alternans may be seen in patients with heart failure, particularly when there is increased resistance to left ventricular emptying as occurs in systemic hypertension or aortic stenosis. It may occur with heart failure due to cardiomyopathies and has also been noted in normal hearts following severe tachycardia.

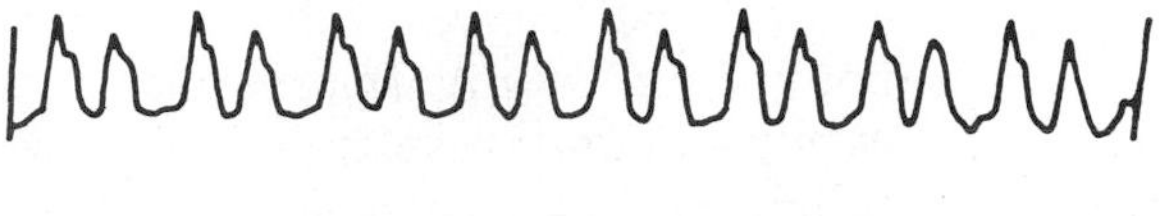

FIGURE 5–2. Pulsus alternans. Note the regular alternation in the amplitude of the radial pulse waveform.

Pulsus paradoxus is a decrease in pulse volume during inspiration and increase in pulse volume during exhalation. Normally, there is an approximate 3 to 4 mm Hg fall in systolic pressure with inspiration which produces no discernible change in the quality of the pulse. When detectable, a systolic pressure reduction greater than 20 mm Hg is usually present. Rarely, the weak pulse may be imperceptible. Pulsus paradoxus is commonly seen in cardiac tamponade, severe obstructive airway disease (asthma, COPD), hypovolemic shock, and pulmonary embolism. The cyclic changes in arterial systolic pressure may be visually appreciated on the arterial pressure waveform.

Extrasystolic beats, whether atrial, junctional, or ventricular, are weak beats because of the decreased ventricular filling time. If they occur early enough in diastole and are associated with altered systolic contractile dynamics, as in ventricular premature beats, they may not be palpable at all (nonperfusing beats). Usually the beat following the premature beat is stronger than normal because the compensatory pause allows more time for ventricular filling. As a general rule, a shorter cycle is associated with a weaker beat and a longer cycle is associated with a stronger beat.

Estimation of Venous Pressure

In the absence of a catheter for direct monitoring of right atrial pressure or central venous pressure, inspection of the external or internal jugular veins may give information relating to venous pressure, which is a reflection of the filling pressure and function of the right ventricle. However, certain clinical situations present pitfalls to neck vein examination, including (1) obstruction in the superior vena cava as seen in intrathoracic tumors; (2) increased intrathoracic pressures secondary to positive pressure mechanical ventilation (particularly with PEEP or CPAP) or pulmonary disease with obstruction to expiration as is common with COPD or asthma; (3) low perfusion states or hypovolemia due to the associated sympathetic nervous system–induced venoconstriction; (4) individuals with short, thick necks, which may make visualization of veins impossible; and (5) surgery, trauma, or dressings about the neck area.

The External Jugular Veins

The nonpulsatile external jugular veins are easily seen as they lie superficially in the neck. Normally, at a 30-degree angle, the crest of the vein column is just above the superior border of the mid-clavicle. Gentle compression of that site with the thumb or forefinger allows the vein to fill from above, become distended, and thus be identified. When the finger is removed and the vein column falls to its predistention level, the height of the crest is noted (Fig. 5–3 *A*, *B*). Normally, the full length of the partially distended external jugular vein is visible with the patient in the supine position; collapse suggests hypovolemia (Fig. 5–4).

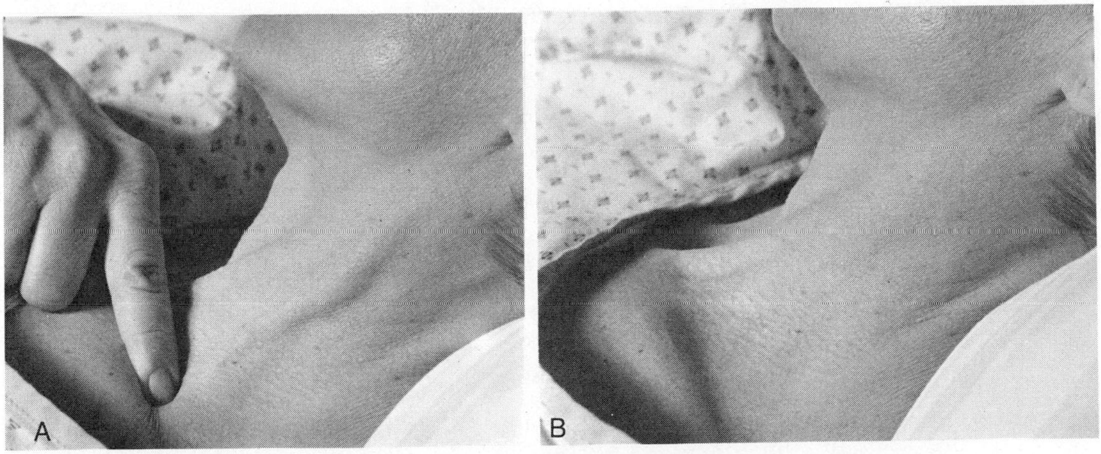

FIGURE 5–3. *A,* Compression of the superior border of the mid-clavicle allows filling and identification of the external jugular vein. *B,* Upon removal of compression, the vein column briskly collapses. The level of the crest of the fallen vein column is noted; normally it hovers just above the superior border of the mid-clavicle.

The Internal Jugular Veins

The right internal jugular vein most accurately reflects right atrial pressure because it lacks vein valves and extends in an almost straight line cephalad from the superior vena cava.

The internal jugular veins lie lateral to the carotid arteries deep in the neck. Therefore, the vein column itself is not visible; however, the crest of the vein column pulsates with each beat of the heart, thus forming *a* and *v* waves on the overlying skin.

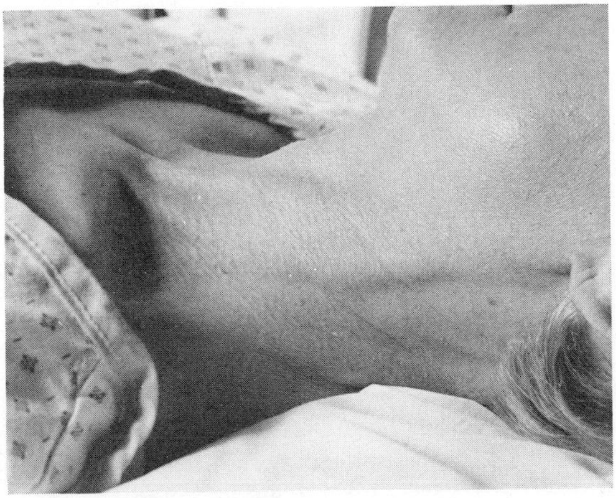

FIGURE 5–4. With the patient supine, note the normal slight distention of the full length of the external jugular vein column (clavicle to level of jaw).

TABLE 5–1. Characteristics of Carotid and Jugular Pulsations

Carotid Pulsations	Jugular Pulsations
Not clearly visible but clearly palpable	More visible but disappear on palpation
Do not change with position	Disappear when the patient is in the upright position
Compression above the clavicle has no influence	Pressure at the root of neck eliminates jugular pulse
Level of pulse not affected by respirations	Level of pulse descends with sharp inspiration

Carotid and jugular pulsations may be confused. The guidelines in Table 5–1 help distinguish them from each other.

For examination, the patient should be relaxed and breathing normally, with the head in a neutral position on a small pillow. Begin with 30 degree elevation of the head. An extremely high pressure may be missed if the pulsating crest is very high; visualization may be possible only if the patient is seated in an upright position. A low pressure may require a nearly supine position to visualize the pulse above the clavicle. The light source should strike the neck at an angle that casts shadows which enhance visualization of the veins and venous pulses. A pocket flashlight may be required. Normally, the sternal angle of Louis is 5 cm above the center of the right atrium regardless of the patient's position. It is easily located by running the forefinger centrally down the sternum. Very early a ridge will be noted. This angulation is formed by the junction of the manubrium and the body of the sternum and its union with the second ribs. A centimeter-ruler is placed on the sternal angle perpendicular to the top of the visualized vein column (Fig. 5–5). Central venous pressure is calculated to be the height of the blood column plus the 5 cm from the right atrium to the sternal angle. Thus, if the vertical height of the pulsation is 10 cm above the sternal angle, 10 cm + 5 cm = central venous pressure of 15 cm of H_2O. The normal vertical distance from the crest of the pulsating vein column to the level of the sternal angle is less than 6 cm, or a central venous pressure less than 11 cm of water.

Examination of the Veins at the Dorsum of the Hand

The patient is positioned with the trunk elevated 30 degrees or higher. The arm is initially placed in a dependent position, at which time the veins at the dorsum of the hand are normally distended. The extended arm is then slowly raised; when venous pressure is normal, the veins collapse when the dorsum of the hand reaches the level of the sternal angle. Early collapse suggests low venous pressure such as due to a fluid-depleted state; distention beyond that point suggests an elevated venous pressure.

Causes of elevated venous pressure include: (1) Right ventricular failure secondary to left heart failure (ischemic disease, mitral valve disease, etc.); (2) cor pulmonale; (3) pulmonic stenosis; (4) superior vena caval obstruction (thoracic tumors, scarring, etc.); (5) tricuspid stenosis; (6) cardiac tamponade; (7) constrictive pericarditis; and (8) increased blood volume.

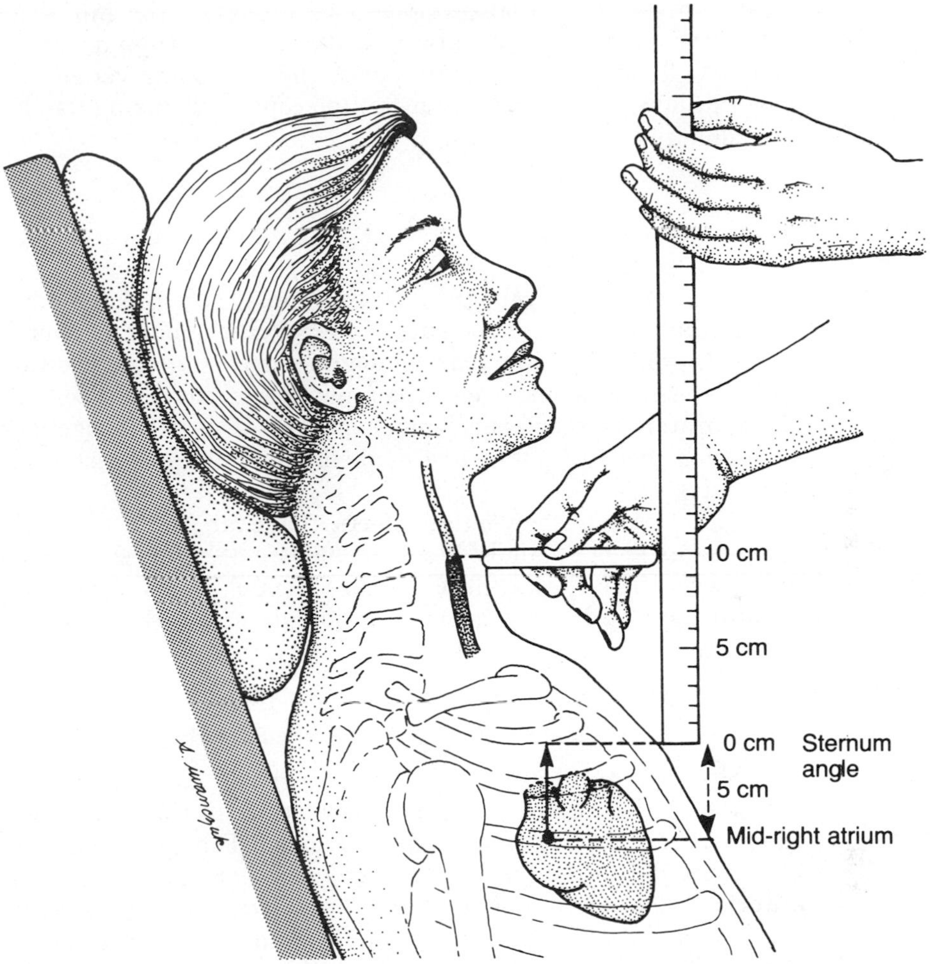

FIGURE 5–5. Estimation of central venous pressure using the vertical distance from the sternal angle to the pulsating crest of the internal jugular vein.

THE HEPATOJUGULAR REFLEX

In early right heart failure, the intravascular volume may be increased but the elastic, distensible venous system may initially be able to accommodate the increased volume without an increase in venous pressure. A more sensitive indicator of right heart failure is the hepatojugular reflex.

Firm, gentle pressure is applied over the mid-abdomen or right upper quadrant for 30 to 60 seconds while the jugular veins are observed. In individuals with normal cardiovascular function, the initial jugular venous distention is followed quickly by collapse of the jugular veins as the right ventricle quickly adjusts its output to the increasing venous return. In right heart failure, jugular venous distention continues during the 30 to 60 seconds of abdominal compression.

Palpation of the Anterior Chest

It is best to palpate the anterior chest with the patient supine. Some cardiac patients may not be able to tolerate the supine position, and elevation of the thorax to greater than 45 degrees may alter the position of the heart in the chest. However, it must be remembered that no assessment procedure, no laboratory test, or hemodynamic parameter justifies placing the patient in a position that will not be tolerated clinically and may usher in a physiologic disaster.

The person's body build affects the examiner's perception of cardiac movements and/or sounds. Weak or undetectable impulses or sounds occur in those with obese chests, muscular chests, emphysema, pericardial tamponade, or effusion. Cardiac movements or sounds may seem exaggerated in those with thin, small chest walls.

The Apex Beat

Also called *left ventricular thrust, apical impulse, point of maximum impulse* (PMI), the apex beat normally occurs in the area of the chest where the heart movement is maximally perceived. The apex beat is produced early in ventricular systole when the hardened, contracted left ventricle rotates anteriorly and to the right, thus tapping the anterior chest wall. It occurs synchronously with the carotid impulse and is sustained for the first half of systole. The apex beat is an excellent indicator of heart size and alterations or abnormalities in heart action. The apex impulse is examined for location, duration, and character.

Location. The normal apex beat is in the fifth left intercostal space at, or just medial to, the mid-clavicular line. In short, obese adults, or those with a distended abdomen, the apex beat of the horizontally displaced heart may be in the fourth left intercostal space. In tall thin people, the apex of the more vertical heart may be closer to the lower left sternal border. Therefore, *in the critically ill, changes are more important than absolute standards.*

As the heart enlarges with failure, the apex beat is displaced left of the mid-clavicular line and downward, for example at the anterior axillary line in the sixth intercostal space. With ventricular hypertrophy, as may be seen with systemic hypertension, the thickening myocardium tends to grow inward, encroaching on the ventricular cavity, and the apex beat occupies its usual position.

Duration. With ventricular enlargement, the apex beat extends into systole, sometimes lasting to the second heart sound. A prolonged impulse is also typical of pressure hypertrophy. The more severe the hypertrophy, the longer the impulse is perceptible.

Character. The normal apical beat is light and tapping. Any condition associated with a hyperdynamic cardiovascular state will produce a more forceful impulse which is not sustained. This may occur in anxiety states, catecholamine administration, fever, sepsis, anemia, or hyperthyroidism. Decreased force with increased duration and size occurs with ventricular dilatation from damage to the ventricle, such as ventricular failure due to ischemic heart disease.

The apical impulse may not normally be detectable in people over the age of 50 years while in the supine position. Turning the patient to the left lateral position brings the heart closer to the anterior chest wall and may make the apex beat palpable, especially at end-expiration. However, this maneuver shifts the heart leftward, and the apex will not occupy the usual position. In this circumstance, directional changes that occur with disease or therapy are noted.

The appearance of an ectopic impulse is important in the critical care setting. An acutely ischemic area of myocardium fails to contract in systole (ischemic paralysis) and may paradoxically bulge outward. Loss of a functional portion of the myocardial mass and paradoxical wall motion compromises function of the cardiac pump and may be associated with signs and symptoms of heart failure. The systolic bulge may be palpated or seen over the mid-precordial, apical, or epigastric areas. It will feel like a distinct, double impulse separated by a few centimeters. The extra impulse may occur in early, mid, or late systole. The double impulse may be present only during an anginal attack or may be persistent in myocardial infarction or ventricular aneurysm.

The Right Ventricular Impulse (Right Ventricular Lifts, Heaves, Thrusts)

Although the right ventricle lies closer to the anterior chest wall than does the left ventricle, a palpable right ventricular impulse is not a normal occurrence. Abnormal left parasternal activity may be associated with:

Increased Pulmonary Artery Pressures. With elevations in pulmonary artery systolic and diastolic pressures, right ventricular activity may be palpated at the left lower sternal border. Chronically, this may be associated with mitral stenosis or insufficiency, COPD, or cor pulmonale. Acutely, this may be seen with massive pulmonary embolism reflecting sudden pressure overload and dilatation of the right ventricle.

Right Ventricular Flow Overload. This is due to atrial septal defect or tricuspid regurgitation, both of which may be associated with a brisk, high-amplitude, left parasternal thrust.

Auscultation of the Heart

THE HEART SOUNDS

Opinions differ as to the precise mechanism producing heart sounds; ie, actual valve closure vs. acceleration/deceleration of blood associated with valve closure. As the issue is not yet resolved, it is expedient to state that the first heart sound occurs simultaneously with closure of the atrioventricular (mitral and tricuspid) valves, and the second heart sound occurs synchronously with semilunar (aortic and pulmonic) valve closure. Because most heart sounds are near the lower end of the range of human hearing, the clinician must optimize conditions for ausculation.

The environment should be as quiet as possible, requiring, for example, the silencing of a chest tube drainage system by discontinuing suction.

The stethoscope design should maximize transmission of heart sounds. The earpieces should fit sufficiently tight to produce slight discomfort when in place, and the total length of the stethoscope should not exceed 16 inches. The diaphragm chest piece is used for auscultating high frequency sounds, such as the sounds associated with pulmonic or aortic valve closure or the ejection sounds associated with full opening of the semilunar valves. The bell chest piece is used to detect low intensity sounds such as third and fourth heart sounds or the diastolic rumble of mitral stenosis. If the bell is applied with too much pressure, the underlying stretched skin acts as a diaphragm and filters out the low-pitched sounds. By altering pressure on the bell at one site, one may obtain bell or diaphragm effects on a given heart sound.

If capable of cooperation, the patient may assist with auscultation. This may involve breath holding to eliminate the noise of breath sounds, or a sustained hand grasp may bring out a sound by enhancing venous return to the heart.

Three concepts help one understand the principles of auscultation:

1. Heart sounds normally occur synchronously with valve closure. Normal valves do not generate sounds upon opening.

2. Heart sounds are heard best downstream from the source of the sound (Fig. 5–6).

3. The loudness of the sound depends partially upon the pressure at which the event occurs. (The aortic closure sound is louder than the pulmonic closure sound.)

The *first heart sound* (S_1) heralds the onset of ventricular systole. It has two components: M_1 is produced by mitral valve closure, and T_1 is the result of tricuspid valve closure (Fig. 5–7 *B*). However, these two events occur so close together that the human ear is usually unable to separate them. When tricuspid valve closure is delayed, as in right bundle branch block, both components may be heard. This splitting of the first heart sound is best heard over the left lower sternal border in the fifth intercostal space (tricuspid area).

The *second heart sound* (S_2) is produced by closure of the aortic (A_2) and pulmonic (P_2) valves and heralds the onset of ventricular diastole (Fig. 5–7 *D*).

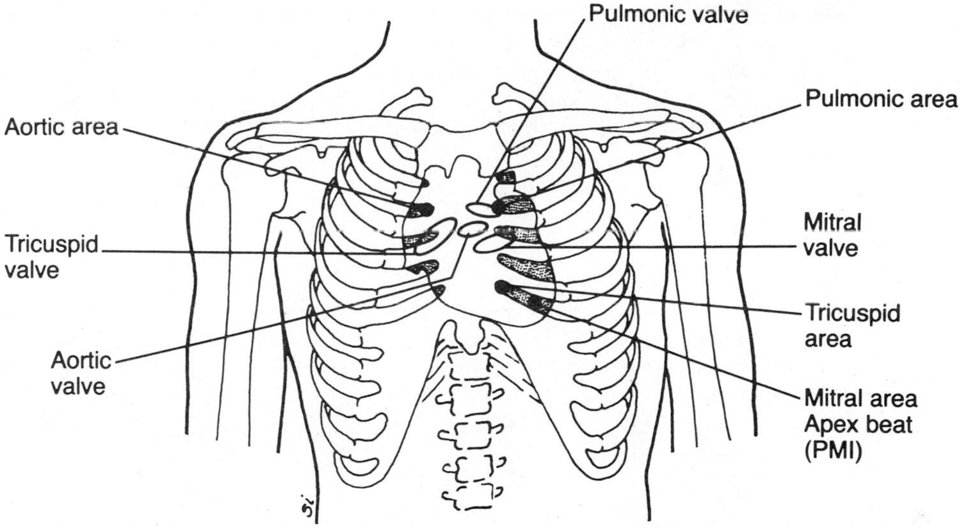

FIGURE 5–6. Areas of auscultation of heart valves. *Aortic area*—second intercostal space to the right of the sternum. *Pulmonic area*—second intercostal space to the left of the sternum. *Tricuspid area*—fifth intercostal space to the left of the sternum. *Mitral area*—over the apex beat (normally in the fifth intercostal space in the mid-clavicular line).

During expiration, the two components are nearly inseparable. However, during inspiration, P_2 tends to be delayed owing to slight prolongation of right ventricular systole secondary to increased venous return. This normal physiologic splitting of the second heart sound is best heard at the left sternal border in the second intercostal space (pulmonic area) with the diaphragm of the stethoscope. The intensity of the second heart sound depends on (1) aortic and pulmonic diastolic pressures—the loudness of A_2 or P_2 is increased in arterial or pulmonary hypertension; and (2) the mobility of the valve leaflets and their ability to close—the intensity of A_2 is decreased in aortic stenosis and/or regurgitation.

At heart rates less than 100 BPM, diastole is longer than systole. Therefore, it is easy to isolate and identify the first and second heart sounds. At faster rates they seem to run together, and it becomes very difficult to differentiate S_1 from S_2. A landmark may be identified by placing a finger over the carotid pulse or apical beat while listening to the heart. The pulsation felt will be synchronous with the first heart sound. In addition, S_1 is lower in pitch and more prolonged than S_2, which has a higher pitched, abrupt closing sound.

When the atrial kick is intact (sinus rhythm, atrial rhythms, high junctional rhythms), ventricular diastole is made up of three filling phases: rapid, slow, and active.

During the *rapid filling phase*, the mitral and tricuspid valves open followed by rapid flow of blood into the ventricle. If a third heart sound is present, it will occur at this point in the cardiac cycle (Fig. 5–7 *F*).

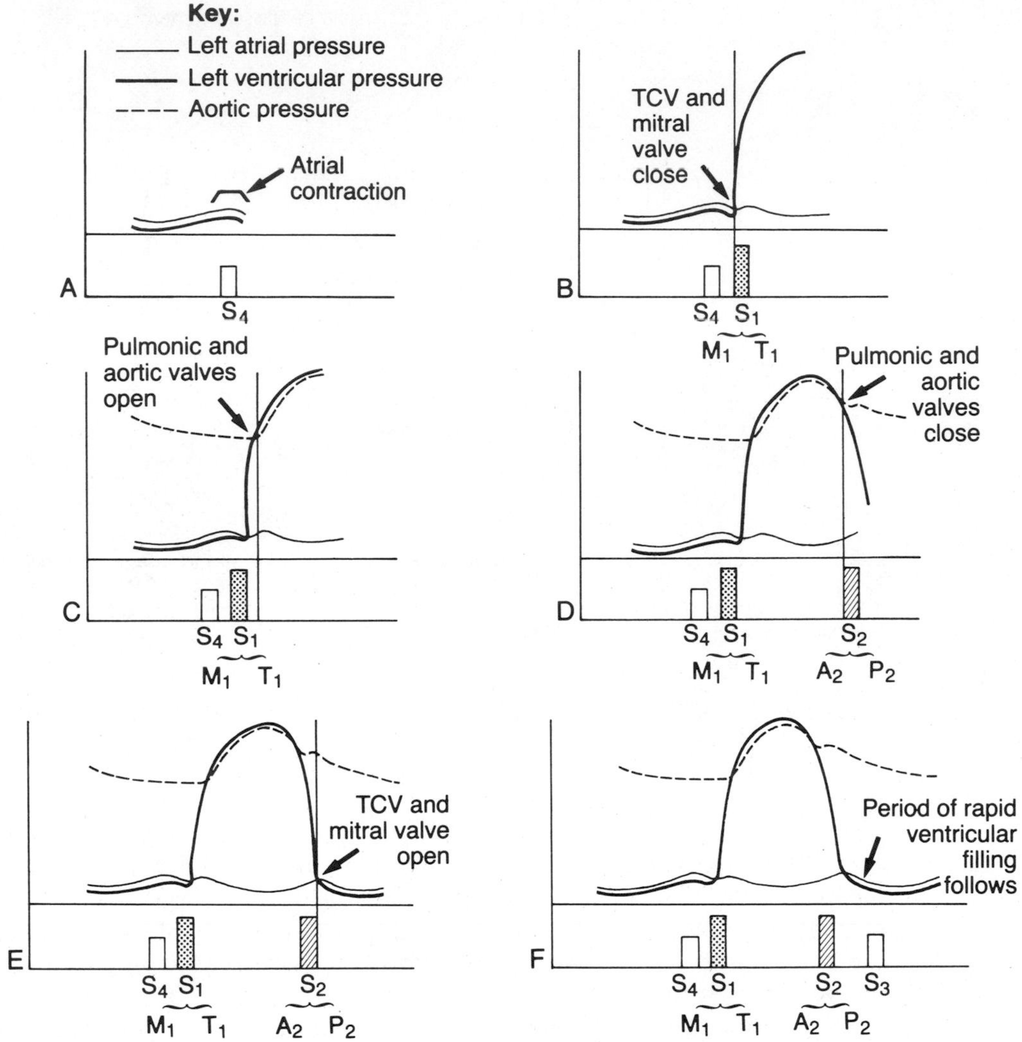

FIGURE 5–7. Relationship of cardiac events to the production of heart sounds. S_4 = fourth heart sound, S_1 = first heart sound, M_1 = mitral component of the first heart sound, T_1 = tricuspid component of the first heart sound, S_2 = second heart sound, A_2 = aortic component of the second heart sound, P_2 = pulmonic component of the second heart sound, S_3 = third heart sound.

At the end of the *slow filling phase*, ventricular diastolic pressures are normally low, and 70 to 90 percent of ventricular filling has occurred.

During *active filling* (atrial kick), the atrial contraction augments ventricular filling late in diastole. Through volume loading of the ventricle, this normally increases end-diastolic pressure a few mm Hg: If a fourth heart sound is present, it will occur at this point in the cardiac cycle, just before S_1 (Fig. 5–7 *A*).

Circumstances that produce large intraventricular diastolic pressure changes (ventricular failure), increased distending forces (a hyperdynamic cardiovascular state producing increased flow rates), or decreased compliance (myocardial ischemia) may result in accentuated or palpable third (S_3) or fourth (S_4) heart sounds.

Because third and fourth heart sounds are of very low intensity, the majority of them may go undetected, and the first subtle clue to the presence of heart disease may be missed. Therefore, conditions must be optimized to detect them. The patient's room should be as quiet as possible. S_3 or S_4 from the left ventricle is best heard with the patient in the left lateral position with the bell of the stethoscope lightly applied over the apical beat. S_3 or S_4 from the right ventricle is best heard with the bell of the stethoscope over the left lower sternal border with the patient recumbent. S_3 or S_4 may be augmented when intracardiac blood flows are increased. Having the patient cough a few times or a sustained hand grasp increases blood flow and may bring out the sound.

Third Heart Sound. This low-intensity sound, which is audible immediately after S_2, is produced by sudden distention of the ventricular wall by the onrush of blood during the initial part of the passive phase of ventricular filling. A distinct triple rhythm is produced: the first two components are the normal S_1 and S_2 sounds. The auscultated cardiac cycle sounds like "lup-dup-phaa," the softer "phaa" being the third heart sound. A third heart sound can

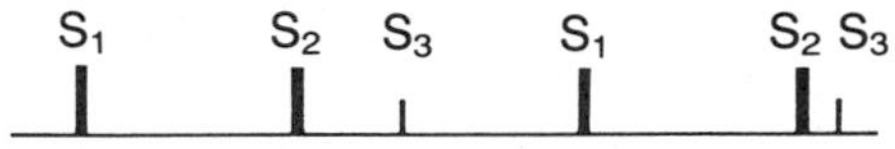

be heard in most children but gradually diminishes in adulthood to become inaudible. It may be a normal finding beyond the age of 30 years in thin-chested adults, particularly women. It becomes louder when cardiac output and flow rates are increased as in anemia, hyperthyroidism, exercise, anxiety, and so on. When present in a healthy heart, the term physiologic S_3 or third heart sound is used. With advancing age, only an accentuated third heart sound is audible. Its presence implies an enlarged failing ventricle with an elevated filling pressure. In this context, the term S_3 gallop or ventricular gallop is applied. The pathophysiologic S_3 sound is produced when atrial blood rushes into a ventricle incompletely emptied from the previous beat and unable to yield to the incoming blood. Its audibility becomes fainter with improvement or louder with deterioration. A ventricular gallop may also be palpable in patients with major elevations in left ventricular filling volume and pressure. Constrictive pericarditis may also produce a ventricular gallop because diastolic distention of the ventricles is limited by the constricting pericardium.

Fourth Heart Sound. The low intensity fourth heart sound occurs immediately before S_1. Because this sonic event is produced when ventricular filling is increased by atrial contraction, a fourth heart sound can be produced only when the atrial kick is present. The triple cadence, which sounds like "la-lup-dup," may occur in healthy hearts and is more frequently heard in the older patient. The term S_4 or fourth heart sound applies only to the

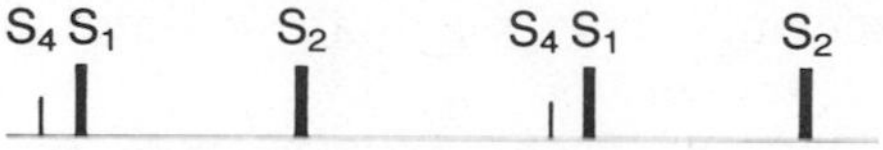

normal heart. In circumstances of disease, the terms atrial gallop or S_4 gallop are used. The fourth heart sound becomes particularly prominent and may also become palpable when there is decreased ventricular compliance. This helps distinguish it from a physiologic S_4, which is not associated with palpable precordial movement during systole. An atrial gallop is associated with an increased ventricular end-diastolic pressure, though pressure in early diastole may be normal. Clinically, this is seen with ventricular hypertrophy (particularly with outflow obstruction), ischemic heart disease, or acute mitral regurgitation. When present with ischemic heart disease, it may become more intense or audible only during an ischemic attack.

The auscultatory characteristics or cadence of sounds does not characterize normal from abnormal states. Rather, the setting in which the sounds appear helps distinguish normal from abnormal. For example, an S_3 sound in a teen-age victim of trauma is likely physiologic; however an S_3 sound in an elderly patient with ischemic disease is always a ventricular gallop.

Quadruple Rhythm

An atrial gallop in the presence of established ventricular failure produces two gallop sounds in addition to the two normal heart sounds. If the heart rate is sufficiently slow, all four sounds are separate and distinct, producing a quadruple rhythm that sounds like "la-lup-dup-phaa."

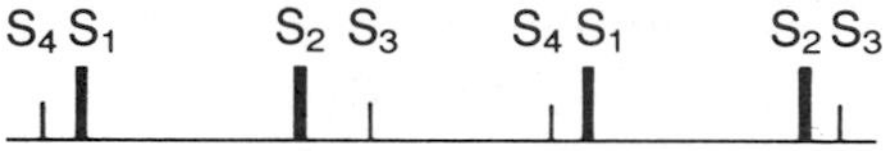

Summation Gallop

At rapid heart rates that typically accompany heart failure, the atrial and ventricular gallop sounds are merged or summated to produce a loud sound termed a summation gallop. The summation sound is typically louder than the first and second heart sounds.

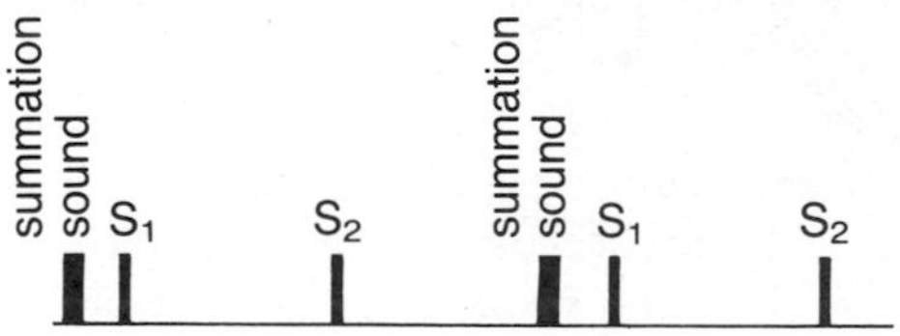

MURMURS

A cardiac murmur is an auscultatory sound that arises when: (1) the rate of flow increases across a normal structure, as in innocent heart murmurs; (2) flow occurs across a constricted area, as in aortic stenosis; (3) flow occurs across an abnormal structure without obstruction, as in the opening snap of mitral stenosis; (4) reverse or regurgitant flow occurs across an incompetent valve, as in mitral regurgitation; (5) flow occurs into a dilated structure such as the aortic root or pulmonary trunk in systemic or pulmonary hypertension, or (6) blood is shunted from a high to a low pressure area through an abnormal opening such as a ventricular septal defect.

Murmurs are described according to the following characteristics:

1. Pitch—high or low
2. Quality—musical, harsh, blowing, machine-like, etc.
3. Shape
    a. crescendo—increasing in intensity

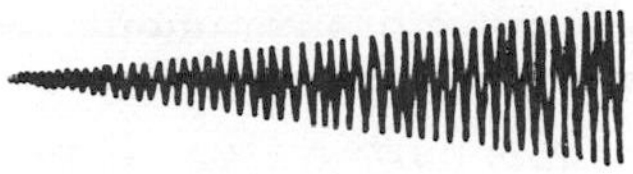

    b. decrescendo—decreasing in intensity

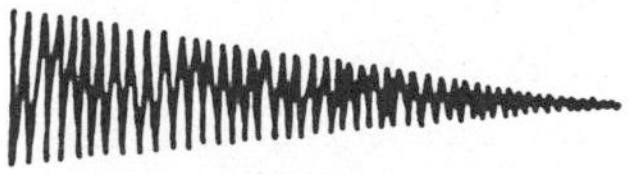

    c. crescendo-decrescendo, diamond-shaped—increasing in intensity to a peak then decreasing in intensity

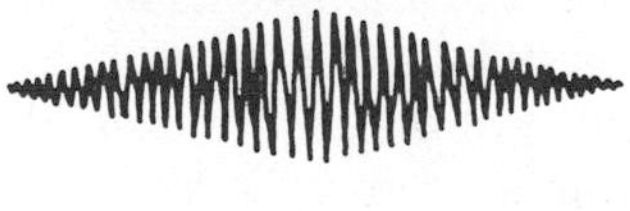

    d. plateau—consistent intensity throughout

    e. variable—intensity waxes and wanes variably

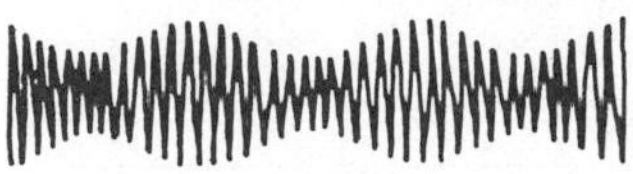

4. Location—where the murmur is maximally heard and its direction of radiation if applicable.
5. Timing—early, mid, or late systolic or diastolic. If the murmur occurs throughout systole, it is termed halo or pansystolic.
6. Intensity (loudness)—The intensity of a murmur may be graded from one to six.
   a. Grade I—The murmur is barely audible in a quiet room. For detection, it may require breath holding on the part of the patient as normal breath sounds may obscure the sound of the murmur.
   b. Grade II—The murmur is faint but clearly audible.
   c. Grade III—The murmur is conspicuous but not loud.
   d. Grade IV—The murmur is loud and may be accompanied by a thrill.
   e. Grade V—The murmur is very loud and is always accompanied by a thrill.
   f. Grade VI—The murmur may be heard with the stethoscope held just above the area of auscultation on the chest.

The presence of a murmur does not necessarily indicate heart disease. Innocent (functional) murmurs commonly occur that are systolic in timing, with no organic basis. These murmurs have numerous causes, such as episodic vibrations of the pulmonary valve leaflets at their attachments to the pulmonary trunk or an exaggeration of normal ejection vibrations within the pulmonary trunk.

Systolic murmurs are evident following S_1 since this sound heralds the onset of ventricular systole.

Aortic Stenosis. The murmur of aortic stenosis is usually loudest in the second intercostal space to the right of the sternum (aortic area) and radiates to the neck. It is harsh in quality, the sound being similar to that of a whispered "R." Beginning after S_1, it rises in crescendo to a systolic summit to fall in decrescendo and end before S_2. It therefore is a diamond-shaped murmur. The intensity of the murmur coincides with the rise and fall of blood flows in systole across the anomalous aortic valve. The more severe the aortic lesion, the later in systole is the summit. Patients with aortic stenosis develop concentric hypertrophy of the left ventricle; therefore, as an associated finding, the apex beat is prolonged and forceful.

Mitral Regurgitation. For normal valve function, all components of the mitral valve apparatus (valve leaflets, chordae tendineae, papillary muscles, and adjoining structures) must be normal and intact. The murmur of mitral regurgitation occurs when damage or distortion of the structures of the valve apparatus prevent valve leaflet closure, thus allowing backflow of blood into the left atrium during ventricular systole. The clinical, hemodynamic, and auscultatory findings differ with chronic and acute-onset mitral regurgitation.

CHRONIC MITRAL REGURGITATION. This type of murmur is usually associated with a dilated, thin-walled left atrium. The large compliant atrium accommodates the regurgitant flow throughout systole. Therefore, a pansystolic murmur ends with the aortic component of the second heart sound. The murmur, which is best heard over the apex, is typically high pitched and blowing in quality. Chronic mitral regurgitation may occur with rheumatic distortion of the mitral valve leaflets or chordae tendineae.

ACUTE-ONSET MITRAL REGURGITATION. This is frequently accompanied by sudden hemodynamic deterioration; early recognition, therefore, is of paramount importance in the critical care setting. The regurgitant blood streams into a normal, small left atrium, producing increases in left atrial pressure seen in the monitor as large "V" waves in the PWP tracing that may approach left ventricular pressures in late systole. This effect suppresses the regurgitant flow; therefore, the murmur is decrescendo and may end before the second heart sound. Mitral regurgitation may present acutely with ischemic damage or dysfunction of the papillary muscle or rupture of the chordae tendineae or valve leaflet. Also, severe left ventricular enlargement occurring with failure may sufficiently widen the valve annulus (ring) and distort the normal spatial relationship of valve structures, preventing approximation of the valve leaflets in systole.

Ventricular Septal Defect (VSD). In the acute care setting, septal rupture typically occurs within four days of infarction. The murmur is pansystolic because left ventricular pressures are higher than right ventricular pressures throughout systole, thus shunting ventricular blood from left to right. However, the murmur may occasionally occur only in mid-systole as the left ventricle reaches its peak pressure. The murmur itself is produced in the right ventricle by the turbulence of shunted blood. The murmur may cover a large area but is loudest at the left sternal border at the third, fourth, and fifth intercostal spaces. It is high pitched and harsh in quality, may be accompanied by a thrill, and is associated with hemodynamic deterioration.

Diastolic murmurs are evident following S_2 since this sound heralds the onset of ventricular diastole.

Mitral Stenosis. Blood attempting passage across a stenosed mitral valve produces a jet stream which impacts on the endocardial surface of the left ventricle at the apex producing the low rumbling murmur of mitral stenosis. It is best heard with the bell of the stethoscope lightly applied to the apical area with the patient in the left lateral position, which brings the heart closer to the chest wall. Other auscultatory findings coexist with the diastolic rumble or, in early disease, may stand alone. The full constellation of auscultatory findings of mitral stenosis is mimicked by the phrase "f-fout-ta-ta-roo," in which *f-fout* represents the accentuated first heart sound (S_1), the first *ta* represents the normal second heart sound (S_2), the second *ta* represents the snap produced on opening of the deformed mitral valve cusps, and *roo* represents the low-pitched rumbling diastolic murmur.

If right ventricular hypertrophy secondary to pulmonary hypertension has developed, the patient may also exhibit a right ventricular lift over the left lower sternal border.

Aortic Regurgitation. This murmur occurs when the aortic valve fails to close completely, thus allowing backward flow of blood into the left ventricle in diastole. The high-pitched, blowing murmur begins with the aortic component of the second heart sound and is decrescendo, reflecting the progressive reduction in rate of retrograde flow during diastole. Murmurs of aortic regurgitation may be all grades of intensity. When very soft, the murmur may be heard only when the patient leans forward and holds the breath at expiration. Firm pressure is applied to the diaphragm of the stethoscope at the mid-left sternal border.

Aortic regurgitation murmur may present acutely with infective endocarditis or proximal dissection of the aorta. With high levels of retrograde flow, the patient may develop severe heart failure or shock. Early detection and surgical correction (valve replacement) may be lifesaving.

Pericardial Friction Rub. Inflammation of the pericardium may be associated with noises concurrent with the beat of the heart. These noises are described as leathery, scratching, creaking, squeaky, and so on. They are most audible over the left sternal border with firm pressure applied to the diaphragm chest piece of the stethoscope during deep-held expiration. The sounds may have a to-and-fro cadence. In sinus rhythm, the rub may have three components: mid-systolic, mid-diastolic, and late diastolic. Pericardial rubs may be mistaken for murmurs; however, the relationship of a rub to a heart sound is less fixed than that of a murmur. A pericardial friction rub is not affected by respirations and may additionally be palpated over the precordium. The friction rub commonly disappears if a pericardial effusion develops.

REFERENCES

1. Bradley RD: *Studies in Acute Heart Failure.* London, Edward Arnold Press, 1977, pp 3–7.
2. Wilson RF: *Principles and Techniques of Critical Care*, vol. I. Kalamazoo, MI, The Upjohn Company, 1979, p 12.

SUGGESTED READINGS

Bates B: The heart, pressures and pulses. *In A Guide to Physical Examination*, ed. 3. Philadelphia, JB Lippincott, 1983.

Braunwald E: Part I: Examination of the Patient. *In Heart Disease: A Textbook of Cardiovascular Medicine*. Philadelphia, WB Saunders, 1984.

Delp MH, Manning RT: The cardiovascular system. *In Major's Physical Diagnosis*, ed. 9. Philadelphia, WB Saunders, 1981.

Henderson B, Ferguson GT: Concepts of physical assessment in critical care nursing. *In* Kinney MR: *AACN'S Clinical Reference for Critical Care Nursing*. New York, McGraw-Hill, 1981.

Horwitz LD, Groves BM: *Signs and Symptoms in Cardiology*. Philadelphia, JB Lippincott, 1985.

Hurst JW: Part II: Examination of the heart and blood vessels. *In The Heart*, ed. 5. New York, McGraw-Hill, 1982.

Perloff JK: *Physical Examination of the Heart and Circulation.* Philadelphia, WB Saunders, 1982.

6

Fluid-Filled Monitoring Systems

John VanRiper, BSN, RN
and Sharon VanRiper, MS, RN

From the time that Stephen Hales first cannulated the artery of an unanesthetized horse in 1733, various techniques for direct pressure monitoring have been available, although clinically cumbersome and impractical in most situations. It was not until the electronics revolution of the 1960s that equipment and techniques were developed which allowed the bedside practitioner to monitor patient hemodynamics in a relatively simple yet precise manner. Refinements continue today with the various components being reduced even further in size and made more reliable and less affected by external factors. These advancements have made hemodynamic monitoring a common element of the intensive care environment with some extension of these techniques into the special care areas of "ICU stepdown" units. As this deployment of technology continues, it becomes increasingly important for personnel involved in patient care to familiarize themselves with the function, use, and maintenance of the various components. This chapter focuses on these considerations, discussing first the pressure gradient effects on a fluid-filled system. The components, assembly, and calibration of the monitoring system are then presented.

PRESSURE GRADIENT EFFECTS ON A FLUID-FILLED SYSTEM

Fluid in motion exerts pressure which is referred to as hydrodynamic pressure while stationary fluid columns exert pressure known as hydrostatic pressure. Both must be considered when using clinical pressure monitoring systems. The electrical calibration controls of modern monitoring systems, in conjunction with proper set up and appropriate catheter size and location, will eliminate, or at least compensate for, most of the effects produced by these two forces. However, one factor known as the *dynamic pressure element* and another called the *static pressure head* are worthy of special mention.

The dynamic pressure element is the pressure exerted on the fluid within the monitoring system (eg, the fluid within the lumen of the indwelling arterial catheter) by the fluid outside the system (ie, blood flow) and is related to the orientation of the catheter with respect to the surrounding fluid medium. A catheter that is directed into the flow of the surrounding fluid will provide a more accurate representation of the dynamic pressure being generated than one that is directed away from the flow. In the case of arterial lines, a catheter that is too short or compliant may move around within the vessel (ie, not face directly into the blood flow) or become kinked, resulting in erroneous waveforms and pressure values. With pulmonary artery catheters, which involves cavity pressure measurement, this movement of the catheter tip, sometimes called *catheter whip*, can produce interference on the oscilloscope display in addition to inaccurate measurements.

The static pressure head is the pressure exerted on the transducer relative to its position to the monitored site. To put it another way, a transducer below the level of the tip of the catheter produces a positive static pressure head (gravity flow would be from the catheter tip to the transducer) while a position above the catheter tip results in a negative static pressure head (flow from the transducer to the catheter). On the electronic display, the former condition would produce a false high reading while the latter would produce a false low. For this reason, the transducer air fluid interface and catheter must be at the same level. This same principle applies when lowering the bag of IV solution to check its patency. With the bag lowered, the positive static pressure head means that the solution will flow from the patient to the solution bag (from high point to low point) and when the characteristic stain of blood backing up into the tubing is seen, IV patency is confirmed. When the IV solution is placed back on the IV pole, above the level of the IV catheter, the negative static pressure head assures that solution will flow into the patient.

To obtain accurate monitor readings, the effects of the dynamic pressure element and the static pressure head must be allowed for or corrected. This is accomplished through electrical calibration/zeroing, catheter orientation, and elimination of the static pressure head by assuring that the transducer and catheter tip are at the same level when obtaining readings. In the case of pulmonary artery catheters, this does not mean that the person must be completely horizontal. Research has shown that head elevations of up to 20 degrees will not greatly affect the accuracy of the readings as long as the transducer is adjusted to match the level of the tip of the catheter.

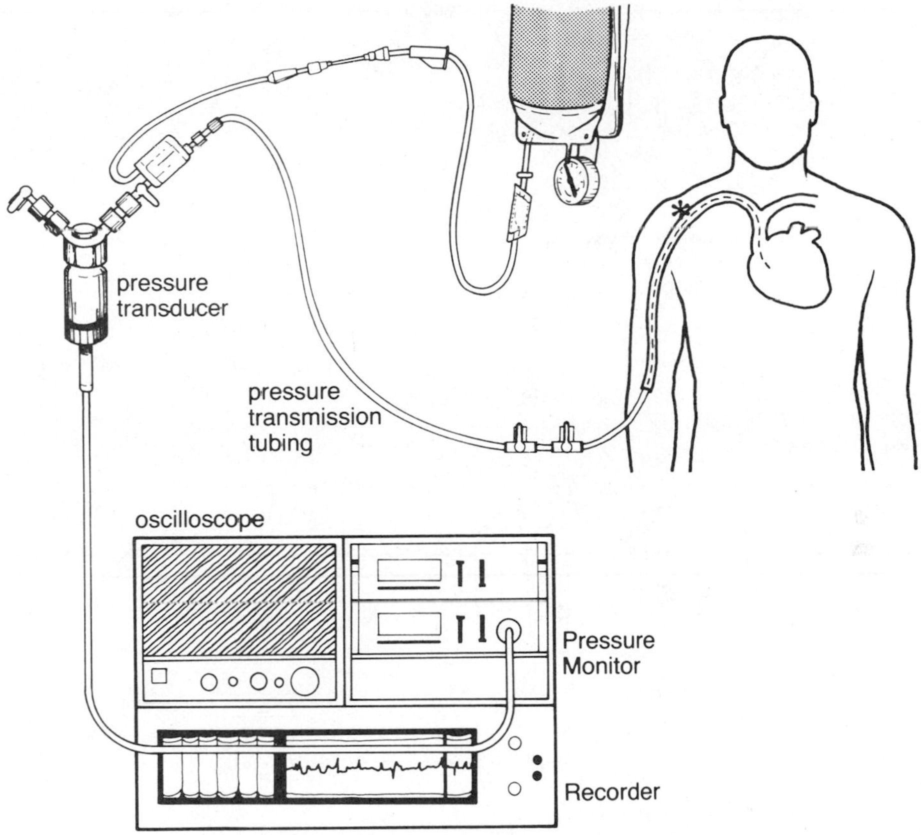

FIGURE 6–1. Set up for pulmonary artery monitoring.

COMPONENTS OF A PRESSURE MONITORING SYSTEM

The equipment required to do direct pressure monitoring consists of a transducer, transducer dome, amplifier, automatic flush device with pressure bag, some means of recording or displaying the collected information such as an oscilliscope or recorder, and assorted IV tubing and connectors. Various medical supply companies provide monitoring line set ups, and these are all quite similar in function if not in appearance. The following discussion can be applied to any of these commercial systems (Fig. 6–1 and 6–2).

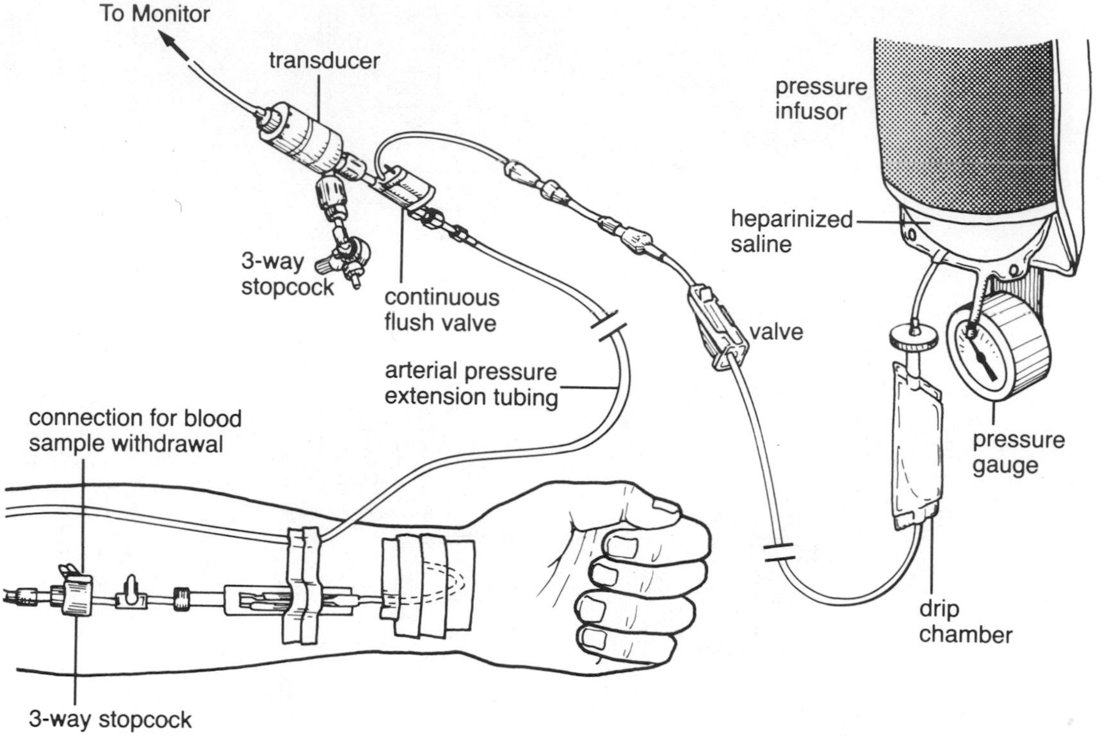

FIGURE 6–2. Arterial monitoring set up.

Transducer

The transducer is a device that converts one form of energy into another. In the case of arterial pressure monitoring, the mechanical energy created by the pressure wave strikes the transducer and is converted into electrical energy which can then be used by the rest of the monitoring system to display or record the information desired. The word transducer comes from the Latin *trans* which means across, and *ducere* which means to lead, calculate, or draw along. An alternative meaning of *ducere* is to charm, influence, or mislead and this secondary meaning should remind the practitioner that all information should be viewed within the context of the complete patient situation and not as separate from the clinical setting.

Most transducers are strain gauge devices. A strain gauge is an instrument that quantifies (gauges) the amount of pressure (strain) being applied to the system. Consisting of four wires attached to the inferior surface of the diaphragm of the transducer, it changes the electrical flow occurring through these wires in response to pressure changes. If the wires are stretched, they will become more resistant to electrical flow, and if they are compressed they will permit more electricity to pass through. Very simply put, when pressure (via the fluid column from the patient to the system) is applied to the top of the transducer diaphragm, the wires below are pushed downward or compressed and a greater amount of electrical flow occurs. This increased flow, if transmitted to an amplifier/monitor system, would be pictured on an oscilloscope as an upward deflection. If a blood pressure of 100 mmHg is applied to the transducer, the deflection will rise to the appropriate level and the digital display would read "100 mm Hg." If more pressure is applied, the value will rise even higher.

Quartz transducers are also available. These consist of two metallized discs separated from one another by a small air space. The reference voltage supplied by the monitoring equipment is then required to "jump" across the distance between the two discs. As pressure is applied to the transducer, the distance between these two points changes. Through electrical manipulation within the monitoring equipment, this change in distance is interpreted as being either positive or negative and is appropriately displayed on the monitor or readout. Quartz transducers appear to be more durable than their strain gauge counterparts and less affected by ambient conditions.

The latest development in transducer technology is the disposable or single use units. Most of these are strain gauge units or modifications of this prinicple and are thrown away after a single patient use. Although more convenient, it remains to be seen whether this is a cost-effective alternative in today's health care setting.

Transducer Dome

A dome covers the transducer and provides the connecting point between the transducer and the fluid-filled tubing (column), which terminates in a direct connection to the cannulated vessel. Unlike air, a fluid medium is not very compressible and allows for the accurate transmission of pressure or pressure waves from the patient to the transducer. The dome contains a very thin membrane that separates the fluid in the transmission column from the transducer surface. This membrane does not interfere with pressure wave transmission but does provide an interruption in the fluid column, thus decreasing the likelihood of contamination or electrical leakage back to the patient. Once assembled, the dome and transducer assembly should provide accurate readings within ± 5 percent or 1 mm Hg, whichever is the lesser. There should be no drift or variance in the output, and they should be electrically isolated from the patient.

Amplifier/Monitor

The purpose of the amplifier/monitor system is to take the very small electrical signal generated by the transducer, increase it to a level that can be used by the monitoring system, and then display that information for interpretation. It should be able to do this without adding distortion into the system or altering the frequency (occurrence rate) or morphology of the original waveform. An amplifier must also possess the quality of linear response. Linear response means that the amplitude of a 10 mv signal will be reproduced by the amplifier in such a way that it will be ten times greater than the amplitude of a 1 mv signal. This is an important requirement because it assures that, using arterial monitoring as an example, a systolic pressure of 120 mm Hg will be accurately represented by a waveform that is twice the height of one representing 60 mm Hg. Thus, visual trending (ie, observed changes in waveform height) and measurements obtained from strip chart recorders can be relied upon to be both accurate and reproducible.

Associated with this linear requirement is the ability to respond to changing parameters in a rapid and precise manner. For example, it would do no good to have a pressure monitoring system that takes a full minute to represent accurately a change in applied pressure from 0 mm Hg to 100 mm Hg. The shorter the amount of time it takes for the monitoring system to respond to changes, the greater the fidelity to the actual event. In actual practice, the monitoring systems used today are capable of responding to pressure changes in milliseconds. This quick response characteristic means that wide and rapid variations in pressure, such as occurs during arterial monitoring, will be received by the system and visually displayed as a rapid rise (systole) followed by a relatively rapid decline (diastole) rather than as slow and gradual elevations and depressions of the baseline. Another advantage of this nearly instantaneous response time is that it allows for accurate timing with other physiologic events (eg, the ECG).

Finally, the electrical damping of the system should be considered. An underdamped system will allow the rapid rise of the signal to extend beyond the actual upper limit of the pressure applied. Thus, a rapidly applied pressure representing 100 mm Hg may reach a level of 110 mm Hg in an underdamped system and result in inaccurate measurement. This phenomenon is called overshoot. A similar problem is found when the high pressure is suddenly removed and the rapid fall of the signal extends below the zero level or baseline, a phenomenon referred to as undershoot.

Nearly all systems have a calibration button which, when activated, feeds the known amplitude into the amplifier just as if that signal had come from the transducer. By observing the output display and the numerical readout on the monitor, one is able to tell if the signal rises to the proper level and then falls back to zero at the end of the test. Performing this function indicates only that the electronics of the system are functioning correctly but does not correct for any interference or inaccuracy in the rest of the system.

Flush System and Plumbing

The flush system consists of a heparinized solution of normal saline which is surrounded by a pressure bag and attached to the patient via assorted stopcocks and tubing. The pressure bag is pumped up to 300 mm Hg and clamped off to maintain that pressure. Housed within the tubing is a flush device that, under constant pressure, assures a continuous flow of 3 to 5 cc/hr of heparinized solution through the system. This prevents clotting and backflow through the vascular catheter. These flush devices also provide for manual flushing of the system if so indicated.

The plumbing consists of tubing that is as short as possible and nondistensible to maintain a low level of compliance or cushioning effect. To illustrate, banging a hammer against a noncompliant, underdamped surface such as a metal bell transmits energy from the hammer to the bell and converts it into sound. Placing a thick pillow over the bell and striking it again with the hammer produces a quite different result because the pillow absorbs much of the energy, producing very little sound. The same principle is true in a fluid-filled monitoring system. Factors that increase compliance adversely affect the transmission of the pressure wave by diminishing its intensity. This is particularly true in arterial monitoring where higher pressures are encountered. In this situation, distensible or "flabby" tubing would absorb some of the pressure being fed to the system, and inaccurate readings would result. Air bubbles are another source of error in these systems because they will increase compliance. While fluid is relatively noncompressible, air is highly compressible and will absorb a large amount of the pressure passing through the fluid column from the patient, resulting in a dampened waveform and false low readings. One should always be alert to the presence of air in the system and eliminate it when found. Tubing diameter and length have an effect on the compliance of the system as well, with long, small diameter, soft tubing being the most compliant. The optimal plumbing system then would be short in length, large in diameter, and as rigid as possible. Other sources or error in the plumbing are faulty connections—use Luer-lock connectors whenever possible and tape non-Luer-lock connections—kinking of the tubing, and cracks that sometimes occur at stopcock connections.

ASSEMBLY AND CALIBRATION OF THE SYSTEM

Although different institutions will have slightly different protocols to govern assembly, the procedure outlined below will apply to most of the commercially available monitoring kits. Aseptic technique should be employed at all times.

Assembly

To assemble the fluid-filled monitoring systems, complete the following steps.

- Collect the materials you will need for the set up, including a bag of sterile saline IV solution (not dextrose), a transducer and transducer dome, IV tubing with flush device, a pressure bag, IV pole, and transducer holder.

- Heparinize the saline IV bag with 1 to 2 units Heparin/cc of solution. (Different institutions have different Heparin concentration protocols.) Spike the IV bag and flush the tubing, taking special care not to allow even very small air bubbles to enter the system (Fig. 6–3*A*).
- Place the heparinized solution into the pressure bag, but do not pump it up to 300 mm Hg. To do so at this time may force the entrance of air into the system during the flushing and clearing of the transducer/dome assembly (Fig. 6–3*B*).
- Assemble the transducer and dome unit and affix it to the transducer holder (Fig. 6–3*C*). When recommended by the manufacturer put 2 to 3 drops of sterile saline solution on the transducer surface prior to placement of the transducer dome. During arterial monitoring, many institutions will tape this assembly to the patient's wrist to insure accurate monitoring placement at all times.
- Attach the IV tubing to the continuous flush device (Fig. 6–3*D*).
- Connect the flush device to one of the stopcocks attached to the transducer dome (Fig. 6–3*E*).
- Flush the entire system with solution, paying particular attention to the presence of any bubbles in the system. If any exist, they must be cleared from the line. This flushing is done with both of the stopcocks on the transducer dome in the open position (Fig. 6–3*F*).
- Attach nondistensible pressure tubing to the distal end of the flush device (the part that will attach to the patient) and, with the stopcock not attached to the flush device closed off to the dome, flush this line through (Figs. 6–3*G*, *H*).
- Pump the pressure bag up to 300 mm Hg and attach the nondistensible tubing coming from the flush device to the tubing connected to the indwelling catheter on the patient (Fig. 6–3*I*).
- Zero reference and calibrate the transducer/monitor assembly according to institutional and/or monitor system protocols. (*NOTE: It is a good idea to place two stopcocks at the catheter connecting point. This allows one to draw blood samples from the distal stopcock without breaking the sterile integrity of the proximal one. This "sample stopcock" can then be discarded when the tubing and dome are changed every 24 to 72 hours (depending upon institutional policy). (See Fig. 6–2.)*)
- Secure all non-Luer-lock connections with tape.

Calibration

Before beginning the calibration and zero-referencing procedure, the transducer assembly must be placed at the appropriate level to establish a zero reference point. In the case of pulmonary artery pressure or central venous pressure monitoring, the transducer should be placed level with a point known as the phlebostatic axis. (See Chapter 8, Fig. 8–5.) Although not standardized, the phlebostatic axis is defined as a point on the midaxillary

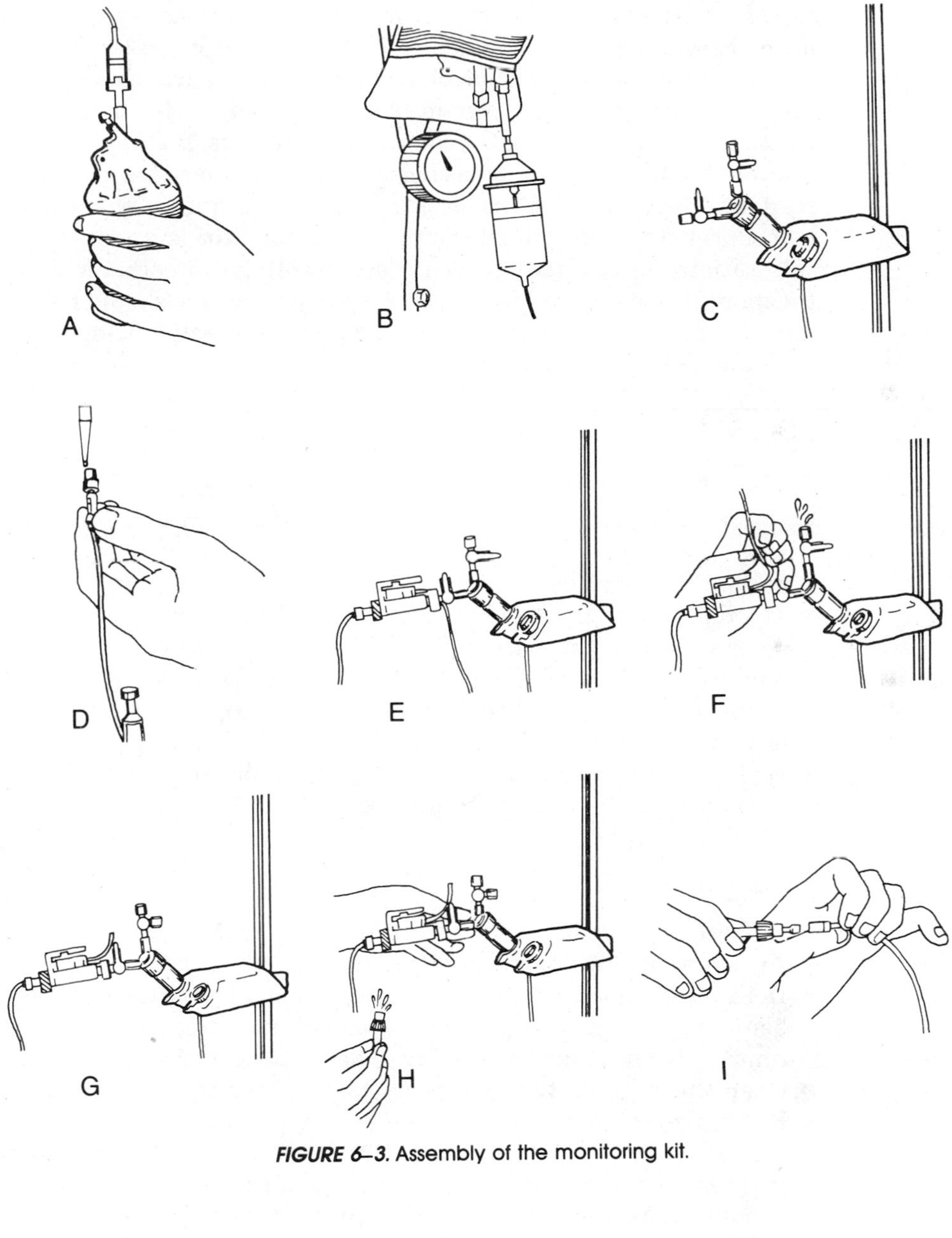

FIGURE 6–3. Assembly of the monitoring kit.

line at the level of the fourth intercostal space. Once this point is established, it should be marked so that all further measurements will be consistent and reliable. If the transducer is located above this point, the readings obtained will be falsely low and if located below this point, they will be falsely high. The degree of error is calculated at 1.86 mm Hg for each 1 cm deviation from the established axis. For arterial lines, the transducer should be at the level of the cannulated artery, which should also be at heart level.

Once the above conditions have been met, one can then proceed with the final adjustments in the system. Although frequently confused as one, zero referencing and transducer calibration are two distinct procedures. Zero referencing balances the transducer output to atmospheric pressure which is read as zero, while transducer calibration requires the exposure of the transducer to a known pressure. Some monitor systems have electronic calibration controls that send a present voltage to both the transducer and the monitor for calibration purposes. Both procedures should be done to insure monitor accuracy. It is recommended that zero referencing be done once a shift and calibration done once a day.

Zero Referencing

The following is the procedure for zero referencing.

- Having allowed the monitoring system and transducer sufficient time to warm up, adjust the stopcock on the dome so that it is turned off to the patient and open to air.
- The digital and oscilloscope displays should both read zero mm Hg. If they do not, follow the particular machine instructions and adjust the zero balance to achieve the desired value. (NOTE: *Some machines require calibration to a second value such as 40 mm Hg or 200 mm Hg in addition to zero*).
- When properly zeroed, close the stopcock that exposed the transducer to air and open the line to the patient.

Transducer Calibration

These steps should be followed to calibrate the transducer.

- Attach a mercury manometer to the transducer dome assembly.
- Determine the calibration pressure most appropriate to the parameter being measured. For pulmonary artery monitoring, 40 mm Hg is most commonly used and 200 mm Hg is used when measuring arterial pressure.
- Open the stopcock to the mercury manometer and close it to the patient.
- Pressurize the manometer to the selected pressure level. The monitor and digital display should reproduce this value. If there is a discrepancy of greater than 5 percent or 1 mm HG, replace the transducer. Replacement is not required for monitoring systems that have an adjustable gain control.

TABLE 6–1. Troubleshooting Pressure Monitoring Systems

Problem	Possible Causes/Solutions
NO WAVEFORM	☐ Check power supply. ☐ Check the pressure range setting on the monitoring equipment. ☐ Check balancing and calibration of the equipment. ☐ Check for loose connection in the IV pressure line. ☐ Check to be certain that stopcocks are not turned off to the patient. ☐ It is possible that the catheter is occluded or has moved out of the vessel. If this is suspected, try to aspirate blood from the line. NOTE: Fast-flushing the line may dislodge a clot. Never apply pressure to the irrigating syringe greater than that used for a standard IM injection.
ARTIFACT	☐ Check for electrical interference. ☐ Check for patient movement. ☐ Catheter whip may be the problem.
WAVEFORM DRIFTING	☐ Temperature change of IV solution (new flush bag hung) or environment. ☐ Be certain the electrical monitoring cable is not kinked or compressed.
UNABLE TO FLUSH LINE	☐ Check stopcocks and tubing for kinks. ☐ Check to see that the pressure bag is inflated to the appropriate level.
READING TOO HIGH	☐ Check balance and calibration. ☐ Check to see if the transducer is located at the appropriate level. ☐ Check stopcocks to make certain they are open to the patient. ☐ Suspect failure of the automatic flush device (flow too fast).
READING TOO LOW	☐ Check to see if the transducer is located at the appropriate level. ☐ Check for loose connections.
DAMPENED WAVEFORM	☐ Check for air bubbles in the system. ☐ Check for kinks in the tubing. ☐ Suspect possible occlusion at the catheter tip (ie, thrombus) or the catheter tip may be resting against the vessel wall. NOTE: A term sometimes used is "high pressure damping." This refers to a baseline that elevates and remains elevated—usually at the upper limit of the pressure monitoring range. This is invariably caused either by an electrical failure of the monitor/amplifier or by total occlusion at some point in the fluid-filled line. Check stopcocks, tubing, and catheter patency.

In this situation, follow the particular machine instructions and adjust the gain to achieve the desired value.

- Turn the stopcock off to the manometer and on to the patient to begin continuous monitoring.

COMMON PROBLEMS OF PRESSURE MONITORING SYSTEMS

Many common problems can occur with pressure monitoring systems. The caregiver must be able to recognize the signs, understand possible causes, and be able to take the measures necessary to correct the problems. Table 6–1 outlines some of the more common problems and suggests possible causes and remedies.

REFERENCES

Bartlett R, Whitehouse W Jr, Turcotte J: *Life Support Systems in Intensive Care*. Chicago, Yearbook Medical Publishers, 1984.

Bruner J: *Handbook of Blood Pressure Monitoring*. Littleton, MA, PSG Publishing Company, 1978.

Dechert R: *Hemodynamic monitoring*. UMMC-Towsley Presentation. May 6–8, 1985.

Kaye W: Invasive monitoring techniques: Arterial cannulation, bedside pulmonary artery catheterization, and arterial puncture. *Heart and Lung* (1983); *12*:395–424.

Kiyoshi M, Koepchen HP, Polosa C: *Mechanisms of Blood Pressure Waves*. Tokyo, Japan Scientific Societies Press, 1984.

Milnor W: *Hemodynamics*. Baltimore, Williams & Wilkins, 1982.

Nursing "81": *Using Monitors: Nursing Photobook*. Horsham, PA, Intermed Publications, 1981.

Pursley P: Arterial catheters: Nursing management to decrease complications. *Crit Care Nurse* July-Aug, 1981, pp 16–21.

Russell R Jr, Rackley C: *Hemodynamic Monitoring in a Coronary Intensive Care Unit*. New York, Futura Publishing Company, 1974.

Seifert P: Invasive hemodynamic monitoring. *AORN Journal*. (1983); *38*:416–425.

Stein J: Placing arterial lines. *Emergency Med.* May 15, 1983, pp 221–230.

7

Arterial Pressure Monitoring

Sharon VanRiper, MS, RN
and John VanRiper, BSN, RN

The ability to monitor blood pressure dates from the 18th century. Most methods, however, were unsuitable and impractical for use in the clinical setting. The advent of the electronics revolution in the 1960s ushered in a new era of technology that made possible sophisticated, accurate, and easily administered monitoring devices.

Arterial pressure can be monitored either by indirect or direct methods. This chapter outlines procedures for both. Indirect methods of monitoring include palpation, auscultation, automatic monitoring instruments, and Doppler ultrasonography. Direct methods include the monitored occlusion technique and the direct monitoring method via an intra-arterial catheter.

Also discussed in this chapter are the specific sites of arterial cannulation, including the radial, dorsalis pedis, femoral, and brachial and axillary arteries. The chapter concludes with presentations of how to interpret the arterial waveform and how to obtain blood samples from an arterial catheter.

INDIRECT METHODS OF DETERMINING ARTERIAL BLOOD PRESSURE

Palpation

This method is highly subjective and, as such, is of limited value as a consistent monitor of blood pressure. The method is quite simple and requires only a blood pressure cuff and the ability to palpate the brachial or radial pulse. The cuff is applied in the appropriate position, the radial (or brachial) artery is palpated, and the cuff is inflated 20 to 30 mm Hg above the point where the loss of the pulse is noted. The cuff is then slowly deflated and the point at which the pulse returns is the systolic pressure. This method is best reserved for acute situations when a "quick check" is all that is needed or as a baseline check for the systolic pressure when using the auscultatory method. The same technique can also be applied to the popliteal or posterior tibial arteries, though it may be somewhat more difficult to palpate these pulses.

Auscultation

The most common method of measuring blood pressure is the auscultatory (Riva-Rocci) method employing a sphygmomanometer and a stethoscope. An indirect method, it is dependent upon the production of certain sounds, called Korotkoff sounds, within the artery. These sounds are the result of turbulent flow within the vessel in response to some mechanical deformation (eg, a blood pressure cuff). With the stethoscope placed over the brachial artery (the most common site), the blood pressure cuff is inflated to an appropriate level and then slowly deflated. Korotkoff sounds signal the onset of systole and are produced by pulses of blood being pushed through the mechanically deformed vessel lumen, producing an audible turbulence. With further deflation of the cuff, the sounds generally disappear as the vessel lumen becomes large enough to permit unimpeded flow. The disappearance of these sounds marks the diastolic pressure. Many authorities interpret a change in character or intensity of the sound—not the disappearance of sounds—to be the diastolic pressure. When there is muffling of the sounds followed by their disappearance, the most accurate recording method may be the three-component format discussed later in this section.

It should also be remembered that the generation of the Korotkoff sound is totally dependent upon flow. Since flow may actually begin before audible sound is produced or since the sound may be absorbed by intervening tissue, the value obtained using auscultatory techniques may actually be lower than values obtained by direct monitoring. However, for most situations, this method is quite adequate as a tool for monitoring patient status.

Blood pressure is usually measured over the brachial artery but can be obtained from the radial, popliteal, or posterior tibial artery as well. To obtain a baseline measurement, the patient should be relaxed and pressure should be measured in both arms. A 15 mm Hg difference in systolic pressure between the right and left arms may indicate obstructive lesions in the aorta or subclavian arteries. The arm should be at the level of the heart during measurements. Despite the relative ease of this method, a number of technical errors can render the measurements inaccurate.

The first step to eliminate error in the measurement of blood pressure using the auscultatory method is the selection of the proper size of cuff. The cuff should fit snugly around the arm, be centered over the brachial artery, and be of proper bladder size. (The bladder is the part of the cuff that fills up with air when obtaining a measurement.) Bladder length should be at least 80 percent of arm circumference, and cuff width should be equal to 40 percent of arm circumference. If the cuff is too small or loosely applied, the reading will be falsely elevated. If the cuff is too large, a false low reading will be obtained. During measurement, the lower edge of the cuff should be about 1 inch above the antecubital space.

Next, palpate the brachial pulse and place the bell of the stethoscope over it. Although the diaphragm of the stethoscope is commonly used to obtain measurements, this practice should be avoided since the Korotkoff sounds are of *low frequency* and, as such, are better appreciated using the bell of the stethoscope. In addition, the "scratching" sounds associated with movement of the diaphragm on the skin surface are eliminated when the bell is used. Rapidly inflate the cuff to approximately 30 mm Hg above the expected systolic pressure. If the systolic blood pressure is unknown, palpate the radial artery as cuff inflation takes place. The disappearance of the radial pulse then becomes the estimated systolic blood pressure. Next, deflate the cuff at a rate not to exceed 3 mm Hg per second and listen for the appearance of the characteristic "tapping" (Korotkoff) sounds that mark the systolic blood pressure. Too rapid cuff deflation will produce false low systolic and false high diastolic readings because the onset of the Korotkoff sounds will be difficult to correlate with the level of a rapidly falling mercury column. The margin for error is increased with slower heart rates.

The diastolic pressure is that point at which the Korotkoff sounds either change in character or intensity or disappear entirely. If sounds muffle before they disappear, many authorities suggest that all three values be recorded. Thus, it is possible for a blood pressure to be recorded with three components (systolic/diastolic/cessation of sound) instead of the more familiar two-component format (systolic/diastolic).

Obese individuals or those with cone-shaped arms ("mutton arm") present difficulties in obtaining accurate auscultatory blood pressure measurements, with values usually being falsely low. In these individuals, accuracy may be increased if the examiner applies the cuff to the forearm and determines the point at which the palpated radial pulse returns during cuff deflation.

Another reason for false low readings is the failure to consider the possibility of an auscultatory gap. This phenomenon usually occurs in a small percentage of hypertensive individuals and is characterized by the appearance of Korotkoff sounds at some elevated systolic value followed by their disappearance and subsequent reappearance at a lower level. False low blood pressure values are prevented by simply being certain that cuff pressure is 30 mm Hg above the point at which the radial pulse is lost. An auscultatory gap should not be confused with another blood pressure phenomenon known as a paradoxical blood pressure.

A paradoxical blood pressure with a systolic gradient (difference) of less than 10 mm Hg is considered within normal limits for most individuals. Gradients of greater than this value may signal significant pulmonary or cardiac compromise, including cardiac tamponade. One checks for a paradoxical pressure by having the patient breathe normally while the cuff is slowly deflated. Note the appearance of the systolic sounds and determine whether

TABLE 7–1. Pitfalls in Measuring Blood Pressure

Problem	*Cause*	*Rationale*
FALSE HIGH READING	Cuff too small	Small cuff does not adequately disperse the pressure over the arterial surface
	Cuff not centered over the brachial artery	More external pressure is needed to compress the artery
	Cuff not applied snugly	Uneven and slow inflation results in varying tissue compression
	Arm below heart level	Hydrostatic pressure imposed by weight of blood column above site of auscultation additive to arterial pressure. Reposition arm to appropriate level
	Very obese arm	Cuff too small for large arm will cause too little compression of the artery at the suitable pressure level. Apply a large thigh cuff to the upper arm if necessary
	Cone-shaped arm	Uneven pressure with a circular cuff transmitted to the underlying artery within a conical arm. Employ forearm blood pressure measurements
FALSE LOW READING	Cuff too large	Pressure is spread over too large an area and produces a damping effect on the Korotkoff sounds
	Arm located above heart level	Hydrostatic pressure in the elevated arm causes resistance to pressure generated by the heart
	Failure to correctly determine the onset of the first Korotkoff sound	Difficult to correlate sounds with rapidly falling mercury column. Cuff deflation should not exceed 1 to 3 mm Hg/second

they occur only during *expiration*. If such is the case, continue to slowly deflate the cuff until the sounds are heard during both inspiration and expiration. The difference between first appearance and the point at which sounds are present throughout respiration is the systolic gradient.

Table 7–1 summarizes some of the common pitfalls in measuring blood pressure by auscultation.

Automatic Monitoring Instruments

Instruments that will take and record blood pressure without the aid of a stethoscope or the human ear are available for both home and hospital use. What appears to be a regular blood pressure cuff is applied to the arm over the brachial artery in the appropriate manner. In this case, however, a special type of microphone is housed within the cuff and is positioned over the artery. This microphone takes the place of the human ear and "listens" for the

Korotkoff sounds to appear and disappear during cuff deflation. The electronic equivalent of a manometer then displays the systolic and diastolic pressure as determined by the presence or absence of the Korotkoff sounds. In the hospital setting, these devices may be used on patients who require frequent blood pressure checks but who are not grossly unstable. Patients who have just undergone cardiac catheterization, who are undergoing exercise testing, or who have been given a drug that alters blood pressure are suitable candidates for this type of blood pressure monitoring. Many of these devices are adjustable, allowing the clinician to set the number of times the pressure will be checked within a predetermined period of time. For patients who require frequent blood pressure checks, the time-saving advantage is obvious.

Perhaps the most common of these automated bedside pressure monitors uses the principle of oscillometrics to obtain its readings. This is the same principle that causes the mercury column to pulsate up and down when the air is released from the bladder during a blood pressure determination. It results when the pressure produced by pulsations of the brachial artery are transmitted through the cuff and tubing onto the mercury column. In the case of the automated devices, these pulsations are transmitted to appropriate monitoring and recording devices which then display the results. These devices will tend to be less accurate than the Doppler or auscultatory methods in hypotensive individuals. However, the mean arterial pressure, as measured by this method, has been shown to be quite accurate. Additionally, these units can be quite expensive and may not be cost effective in today's health care setting.

Doppler Ultrasonography

Doppler ultrasonography is a term referring to two elements of sound generation that have been brought together and used as a means of determining blood pressure—the Doppler effect and ultrasonics of high-frequency sound waves. Most of us are familiar with the change in pitch that sound undergoes when a train approaches and then moves away from us. The pitch rises as the train gets nearer and then, suddenly, "downshifts" as the train goes by. Known as the Doppler effect, the phenomenon is dependent upon the speed (flow) of the object being measured. It provides information about the presence or absence of movement as well as the direction in which the object is traveling.

The principle of ultrasonics (high-frequency sound) is further refined in this setting into a technique known as "echo ranging." Echo ranging can best be thought of as an electronic yardstick and is easily visualized by using the analogy of a ball and string. Imagine that you are standing in front of a wall that is some unknown distance away from you. You throw the ball (with the string attached) at the wall and wait for it to bounce off the wall and return. While the ball is in motion toward the wall, the string is continually "reeled out" until the ball strikes the wall and this process ends. By retrieving the ball and measuring the amount of string that has been dispensed, one can obtain an accurate determination of the distance to the wall. Echo ranging uses sound waves in much the same way. By transmitting a high-frequency sound (which travels at a known and constant speed) and waiting for that sound wave to bounce off some object and return (echo), the distance (range) to the object can be determined.

The machinery that combines these principles to measure systolic and diastolic blood pressure uses a small transducer that serves as both a transmitter and a receiver and, as such, is called a transceiver. The transceiver is directed at the wall of a major arterial vessel, a high-frequency signal is emitted, and the transceiver then waits for that signal to bounce off the arterial wall and return. By taking a number of very rapid readings in this manner, not only the distance to the arterial wall but any changes in that distance—as occurs when arterial pressure waves pass through the vessel and cause it to pulsate—can be recorded. During a complete cardiac cycle, the rising arterial pressure that occurs during systole causes the vessel diameter to expand to some peak value which, under normal circumstances, is coincidental with systolic pressure. This same principle is then applied to the relaxation phase of the cardiac cycle (diastole) during which the vessel lumen becomes smaller. Depending upon how the information is processed, a determination of the systolic or diastolic pressure can be made. More sophisticated equipment uses these principles to observe vessel wall motion and then print out this information on paper. Machines used for echocardiography work on this same principle. By observing the change in diameter that the vessel lumen undergoes and correlating this information with an internal electric manometer connected to a blood pressure cuff, systolic and diastolic components can be obtained. In the less sophisticated or hand-held models, only systolic information is obtained because of the sole reliance on the Doppler effect (presence or absence of flow).

DIRECT METHODS

Monitored Occlusion Technique

This method requires a sphygmomanometer and the ability to observe the pressure pulse wave from an indwelling arterial catheter. The first observer inflates the cuff until the waveform disappears and then slowly deflates the cuff while watching the manometer. A second observer signals when the first deformation or "blip" appears in the flat line on the oscilloscope screen; the value noted on the manometer represents the systolic pressure. One might reasonably wonder why this method would be used if the patient was already attached to a monitoring system that, more than likely, provides continuous readout of both systolic and diastolic values. This method offers a quick check of the monitoring electronics of the system. If a wide variance exists between the value obtained and the displayed value, a check of the system should be done to determine the source of the problem.

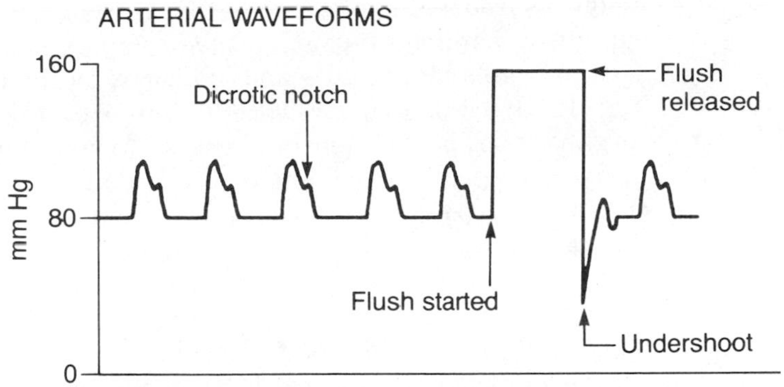

FIGURE 7–1. Waveform response created by activating the fast flush device. A rapid upward rise from the baseline, followed by an equally rapid return to a point below the baseline, confirms the integrity of the monitoring system.

Another rapid bedside check of the integrity of the monitoring system involves introducing a rapid pressure change within the system and observing the waveform response on the output display. This can be done by activating the fast flush device for 1 to 2 seconds and observing the waveform display for a rapid upward (straight line) rise from the baseline followed by an equally rapid return to a point located *below* the baseline. This last event is termed undershoot. Following the undershoot of the baseline the waveform will rapidly move (oscillate) above and below the baseline for a very short time before stabilizing at the zero or baseline level (Fig. 7–1). This observed response represents a "clean flush" and suggests a patent and functional monitoring system. If the return to the baseline is slow it may suggest an occlusion of some sort in the tubing or catheter. This possibility should then be examined and ruled out. An alternative method of performing the above procedure is to occlude the artery (in the brachial area, for example, if a radial site is being monitored) followed by quick removal of the occlusive force. The waveform is then observed for a similar response.

Direct Monitoring Method (Intra-Arterial Line)

This method involves an intra-arterial catheter, a complete monitoring system with continuous flush capability, and display of blood pressure information. It is the most reliable method of continuously monitoring systemic blood pressure and offers the advantage of providing pain-free, low-risk access for arterial blood sampling. The complete set-up required has been discussed in the preceding chapter.

CLINICAL APPLICATION OF THE INTRA-ARTERIAL CATHETER

The arterial catheter is usually placed in critically ill patients whose hemodynamic status is unstable or in patients whose cardiopulmonary status requires frequent sampling of arterial blood gases. Patients who need arterial pressure monitoring usually have complex health problems that necessitate critical assessment skills and judgment by the clinician.

In the critically ill patient, tissue perfusion and oxygenation of vital organs must be frequently assessed. Monitoring arterial blood pressure is a very important component of the bedside assessment. In the patient with profound hypotension (with its attendant decreased perfusion) due to shock or cardiovascular dysfunction, measurement of arterial pressure with a sphygmomanometer will most often be inaccurate or impossible. This is due to the absence of Korotkoff sounds as the arterial wall vasoconstricts (reducing its compliance) and becomes less likely to produce turbulent flow in response to mechanical deformation. In such a patient, the use of an arterial catheter will provide continuous information about the systolic, diastolic, and mean pressures. This rapid assessment of pressure is particularly valuable when vasopressors or dilator agents are used to help support the patient.

The oxygenation status of the patient can also be assessed through the analysis of arterial blood gases (sometimes in concert with venous blood gas analysis for determination of the arteriovenous oxygen difference). Patients who require invasive monitoring will usually be subjected to frequent arterial sampling. Providing this patient with indwelling arterial access reduces the risks associated with frequent arterial punctures, virtually eliminates the discomfort, and saves valuable time for critical care personnel.

PLACING AN ARTERIAL CATHETER

PLACEMENT

An arterial catheter is usually placed in either the radial, dorsalis pedis, femoral, axillary, or brachial artery. In choosing an appropriate site for cannulation, several factors must be considered. First, the artery must be large enough to accommodate the catheter without occlusion or thrombosis. Second, the site should be easily accessible for maintenance and free of contamination by body secretions. Finally, the artery and dependent limb should have adequate collateral circulation in the event that the cannulated artery is compromised or occluded.

A complete discussion of a fluid-filled system suitable for arterial pressure monitoring, its set-up, and factors that influence its operation can be found in Chapter 6.

CARE OF THE ARTERIAL LINE

The arterial catheter must be continuously assessed for perfusion to the involved extremity and for the signs and symptoms of other serious complications such as infection, hemorrhage, or embolus.

Scrupulous aseptic technique during insertion; routine dressing changes with replacement of tubing, stopcocks, and transducer domes; the use of an antiseptic ointment at the insertion site; and the removal of the catheter at the first sign of redness or drainage will all help prevent or limit the threat of infection.

REDUCING THE RISK/COMPLICATIONS

Although arterial monitoring is a relatively low-risk procedure, a number of potential complications are associated with its use. Those patients with peripheral vascular disease, arteriosclerosis, increased peripheral vasoconstriction, or marked alterations in blood pressure are particularly prone to the development of complications such as embolization and infection. In addition, individuals who have experienced multiple arterial punctures or those on anticoagulant therapy are also at increased risk. The use of 20-gauge Teflon catheters provides durability and availability while maintaining a sufficient degree of functional rigidity (ie, resistance to kinking or whipping).

Accidental disconnection of the arterial catheter from the connecting tubing may result in overt blood loss at a rate of 500 ml per min, depending on the size and location of the artery. So-called "hidden bleeding" may result from a puncture wound in the posterior wall of the artery or from catheter dislodgement. In such a situation, the bleeding will take the path of least resistance, which is all too often the surrounding tissue and the internal body cavities. Such bleeding can be difficult to detect and the individual may lose 2 to 3 units of blood before overt signs of hemorrhage become evident. Swelling or bruising at the insertion site may be the only clue to bleeding. In the case of femoral catheters, look for bruising or an increasing feeling of firmness in the lower right abdominal quadrant. Suturing the catheter in place at the time of insertion is the best way to guard against dislodgement.

Embolization in the peripheral arterial tree may result in ischemia or necrosis in the dependent area. The emboli are usually "seeded" from a primary thrombus that frequently forms at the end of the indwelling catheter. Air emboli may be introduced into the system through improper set-up of the system, as a result of blood sampling procedures or vigorous flushing of the catheter. Another source of embolization is particulate matter introduced during blood sampling. These pieces of dried blood or other elements result when the stopcock and connecting tube are cleared improperly following arterial sampling. The application of consistently good technique during catheter/system manipulation, the avoidance of vigorous flushing, and the use of a continuous infusion of heparinized saline with a pressure bag will help prevent embolization. One should remember that the pressure bag must be pumped up to a level higher than the systolic pressure to prevent reverse blood flow in the catheter. A pressure of 300 mm Hg, when used with an intraflow system, will ensure a continuous flow of 2 to 3 ml per hr of the heparinized solution. Patients experiencing hypercoagulation states (eg, from myocardial infarction, fever, cancer, or pregnancy) may require additional irrigation to keep the line patent.

Infection is another possible complication of indwelling arterial monitoring. Prevention of infection has been discussed previously and is also discussed in Chapter 12 on pathogenesis and prevention of line sepsis.

Finally, the portion of the extremity distal to the catheter site should be frequently assessed for adequacy of blood flow and neurologic integrity. The area should be checked for skin temperature and color, response to tactile stimulation, and motor response; the patient should be questioned to determine whether pain or altered sensation is present. Any changes should be promptly reported to the physician.

SPECIFIC SITES OF ARTERIAL CANNULATION

Radial Artery

The radial artery is the preferred site for placement of an arterial catheter. Once the adequacy of ulnar artery distribution has been assessed by the Allen test and determined to be sufficient, serious complications are rare. The radial artery is easily accessible and relatively free of neighboring structures that would preclude its use. A branch of the brachial artery, it extends along the radial aspect of the arm into the hand where it branches and connects to the ulnar artery to form a structure known as the deep palmar arch. It is interesting to note, however, that the majority of the blood supply to the hand is supplied by the ulnar artery and its branches. Thus, cannulation of the radial artery can be done safely when ulnar artery circulation is intact. To test for the adequacy of ulnar distribution and the patency of the deep palmar arch, the Allen test or Doppler plethysmography are done.

Performing the Allen Test

This test should be done before any radial artery puncture.

First, hold the patient's hand up and have the patient clench and unclench the hand several times to help drain blood from the hand. Compress both the radial and ulnar arteries while the patient is clenching and unclenching the fist. Lower the hand and have the patient relax the extremity to alleviate tension in the hand, which may give a false positive result. Release the ulnar artery while maintaining pressure on the radial artery. Observe for brisk return of color to the hand. If color returns within 5 to 7 seconds, the ulnar distribution is adequate. Should it take 7 to 15 seconds for color to return, then ulnar filling is impaired. If blanching persists for more than 15 seconds, then ulnar distribution is inadequate and radial artery cannulation should not be attempted.

Doppler Plethysmography

Although a Doppler study may provide more precise information than the Allen test, its cost and time factor cannot be justified for use as a general screening measure in arterial line placement and the Allen test is still preferable. The machinery used can be relatively large and expensive (such as that used for assessment of pedal pulses prior to vascular surgery) or a simple hand-held model common to most special care units. A special sensor detects blood flow and then translates that flow into an audible "whooshing" sound that the examiner can hear through a pair of headphones or a speaker on the unit itself. The simple Doppler assessment determines only the presence or absence of blood flow but does not address the question of flow adequacy. More expensive models can deliver a hard-copy printout for detailed analysis of the flow characteristics. It is noninvasive and requires only minimal patient involvement. For a more detailed discussion of this technique see the section on Doppler ultrasonics.

Care of the Radial Artery Catheter

After the catheter is inserted, fix the patient's hand in a neutral position to an armboard. Be careful not to hyperextend or dorsiflex the wrist as this can cause neuromuscular injury to the hand. It is common practice in many institutions to place the hand palm up on an armboard with a roll of dressing material or wash cloth lodged behind the wrist prior to securing the extremity to the board. This practice is not the preferred way since it can result in hyperextension of the wrist, but it is acceptable as long as care is taken to insure that the Kerlix roll offers support only. Some institutions use the Kerlix roll only during insertion and remove it afterward. Still others secure the armboard to the lateral instead of the dorsal aspect of the hand to further reduce the possibility of hyperextension. Cover the insertion site with an antiseptic ointment and a sterile dressing. Double check all connections and secure with tape those that are not Luer-locked. (It sometimes adds to one's peace of mind to tape even these connections.) Change the dressing routinely according to institutional protocol, and observe the insertion site for redness, drainage, bruising, or an increasing radial girth.

Complications of Radial Artery Cannulation

The most common complication of radial artery cannulation is thrombosis. This is particularly problematic in patients with inadequate ulnar circulation or those with Reynaud's disease. However, most patients with thrombosis show steady improvement if the catheter is removed before necrosis develops. Occasionally, spasm of the artery may impede circulation. This usually occurs shortly after insertion or removal of the catheter and is of short duration. Some clinicians use xylocaine (Lidocaine) or phentolamine (Regitine) to minimize the possibility of spasm. Air or particle embolism can enter the system through the catheter when large volumes of fluid are forced through it. The use of a continuous flush device and the observance of proper technique during set-up and sampling will virtually eliminate this complication.

Rarely, skin necrosis occurs around the insertion site. Observe for localized blanching of the skin during intermittent flushing. Should blanching occur, the catheter tip should be repositioned.

Radial nerve damage or irritation is another complication typified by numbness and tingling of the thumb and index finger.

Dorsalis Pedis Artery

The dorsalis pedis artery is an extension of the anterior tibial artery and can be palpated on the anterior (dorsal) part of the foot. It is usually positioned about halfway up the arch of the foot within a lateral range extending from the great toe to the third toe. If blood sampling is the primary reason for catheter placement, many practitioners regard this site as second in preference to the radial site. Blood pressure can be monitored from this site but is potentially subject to a variety of interfering factors. The physical distance from the heart is a consideration as is the possible existence of regional flow deficits or alterations in vascular tone. Any of these factors could produce an inaccurate or absent pressure wave.

Checking Regional Circulation

Just as the adequacy of ulnar blood flow is checked prior to radial cannulation, so too must the adequacy of collateral blood flow to the foot be assessed before cannulation is attempted. This collateral flow is supplied by the posterior tibial artery. To check for sufficient collateral flow, manually occlude both the posterior tibial and dorsalis pedis arteries with one hand while blanching the nail bed of the great toe with the other. Do this for about 15 seconds, then release the great toe and the posterior tibial artery at the same time and observe for the brisk return of color to the nail bed. The significance of the findings can be objectively evaluated by applying the same time frames as those used when performing the Allen test prior to radial artery cannulation.

Care of the Dorsalis Pedis Catheter

As with other arterial sites, one should apply antiseptic ointment and a sterile dressing, which is changed routinely. It may be more difficult to position the patient with a dorsalis pedis catheter as care must be taken to maintain the integrity of the catheter while avoiding abnormal positioning of the foot.

Complications of Cannulating the Dorsalis Pedis

The most common complication of a dorsalis pedis catheter is thrombosis. For this reason, catheters in this area are not recommended in patients with peripheral vascular disease. In addition, it is difficult for the patient with a dorsalis pedis catheter to walk. Thrombosis can be detected when prolonged blanching of the toe occurs. Prolonged ischemia may lead to necrosis and loss of tissue.

Femoral Artery

The femoral artery is quite large and easily cannulated. However, an indwelling arterial catheter at this site is much more prone to contamination, and the control of any oozing or bleeding is much more difficult to manage. More importantly, any serious compromise of the blood flow through this area exposes a much larger area of the patient to ischemic or necrotic complications. Despite these drawbacks, femoral artery cannulation may be necessary to obtain accurate pressures in patients with severe hypotension, peripheral vasoconstriction, or cardiac failure.

Care of the Femoral Artery Catheter

After the catheter is inserted and secured with suture material, apply antiseptic ointment and a sterile dressing. Maintain the patient in a straight leg position to prevent hip flexion. The use of soft restraints may be appropriate in some patients. Keep the area clean and observe for signs of bleeding into the leg or peritoneal cavity. Secure all connections with tape if appropriate. Assess the extremity frequently for adequacy of circulation.

Complications of Femoral Artery Cannulation

The most common complications are thrombus formation, embolization, and hemorrhage. Thrombosis occurs more often in patients with peripheral vascular disease or after prolonged, excessive manual pressure to the area following catheter removal. Emboli are generally fragments of the primary thrombus which forms around the tip of the catheter. These emboli then travel to the lower leg or foot and obstruct flow at that distal point. Frequent assessment of the pedal pulses and foot temperature are the best indicators of lower extremity vascular patency. Should pulses become absent, the catheter is removed and an embolectomy or thrombolytic therapy (eg, streptokinase) is instituted to restore circulation. Hemorrhage into the retroperitoneal space or leg can go undetected for quite some time, because of catheter dislodgement or posterior perforation of the artery during insertion. Firm pressure above the insertion site is usually required to stop the bleeding. This pressure should be maintained for 5 to 10 minutes. If left unchecked, bleeding from this site can occur at a rate of 300 to 500 ml per min.

Complications that occur less frequently following femoral cannulation are arterial dissection, aneurysm, and the development of an arteriovenous fistula. Dissection usually occurs during insertion, whereas fistulas and aneurysms are more likely to occur after catheterization involving large bore catheters such as those used in coronary angiography.

Brachial and Axillary Arteries

Both the brachial and axillary arteries are large and easy to cannulate. Since it is so close to the heart, the axillary artery also provides an accurate pressure recording that will remain accurate during profound hypotension or peripheral vasoconstriction. The axillary artery site has the additional advantage of having considerable collateral blood flow so that perfusion to the arm would not be impaired should thrombosis occur. However, if embolization occurs, an occlusion at the origin of the brachial artery would place the entire dependent limb at risk for ischemia and necrosis. In addition, cannulation of the axillary artery is technically difficult and requires prolonged extension, hyperabduction, and rotation of the arm at the level of the shoulder. This complicates patient movement and makes positioning the patient in bed more difficult.

Although cannulation of the brachial artery is relatively easy to do, prolonged use of this site may result in nerve damage and joint immobility from extended restriction of arm movement. The most common complication, thrombosis at the insertion site, compromises the entire limb.

The standard of care employed with all indwelling arterial catheter sites should be employed here as well. This includes aseptic manipulation, routine sterile dressing changes, and the application of an antimicrobial ointment to the insertion site.

Catheter Removal

The technique for removal of an arterial catheter is basically the same regardless of the site used. The sutures, if any, should be removed and an initial assessment of the site and surrounding tissue noted. The catheter is then rapidly withdrawn while firm pressure is applied with a sterile 4 × 4 gauze pad or other suitably sterile article. This pressure is maintained for 5 to 10 minutes or until bleeding ceases. In patients with radial lines, it sometimes is helpful to flex the arm at the elbow and elevate the hand 90° off the bed as the pressure is applied. Those patients with coagulopathies or increased bleeding tendencies may require the application of pressure for a greater length of time. In some situations a pressure dressing may have to be applied.

Following the removal, a note should be made in the record concerning the appearance of the arterial site, motor/sensory integrity of the involved limb, and any difficulties encountered during the removal process. The site should then be periodically assessed for any changes in the above parameters or for any signs of bruising or swelling (bleeding) or redness and drainage (infection).

INTERPRETING THE ARTERIAL WAVEFORM

The Normal Waveform

The normal arterial pulse pressure produces a characteristic waveform appearance (Fig. 7–2). This waveform is divided into the two components of blood pressure: systole and diastole. The initial sharp upstroke of the waveform (the anacrotic limb) represents the rapid ejection of blood from the ventricle through the open aortic valve, and its peak value is the systolic pressure. This peak is normally between 100 and 140 mm Hg. As blood flows into the periphery, pressure falls and the waveform begins a downward trend (the dicrotic limb). The pressure continues to fall until it reaches a point at which pressure in the ventricle is less than pressure in the aortic root. At this point the aortic valves close, producing a characteristic dicrotic notch in the descending waveform. Aortic valve closure signals the onset of diastole. As diastole progresses, aortic root pressure gradually falls to its lowest or resting (diastolic) level, which is normally between 60 and 90 mm Hg.

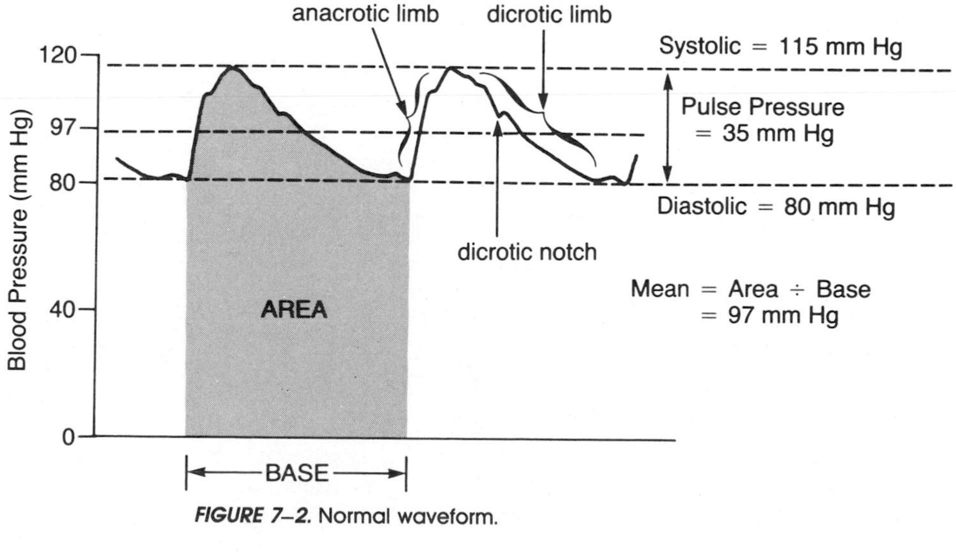

FIGURE 7–2. Normal waveform.

The configuration of the waveform and the actual pressure vary, depending on the anatomical site. For example, waveforms in the radial or dorsalis pedis arteries generally have a steeper upstroke and less obvious dicrotic notch. Femoral and dorsalis pedis pressures are usually 20 to 40 mm Hg higher than brachial or radial pressures.

Correlating the Waveform with the ECG

Electrical ventricular systole is represented on the ECG as the QRS whereas diastole occurs after the QRS and during the T-wave. The peak systolic pressure wave (mechanical systole) will appear just after the QRS, whereas the dicrotic notch is usually associated with the end of the T-wave.

Abnormal Waveforms

Ventricular premature beats (VPBs) cause a ventricular contraction to occur before the ventricle has completely filled with blood, resulting in a decreased stroke volume for that beat. The corresponding arterial pressure wave will show a diminished rate of anacrotic rise with a lower peak pressure. Multiple, consecutive extrasystoles will generally significantly lower systolic pressure. Single extrasystoles are usually compensated for by a greater stroke volume on the succeeding beat and will attain a greater peak systolic pressure on the arterial waveform (Fig. 7–3).

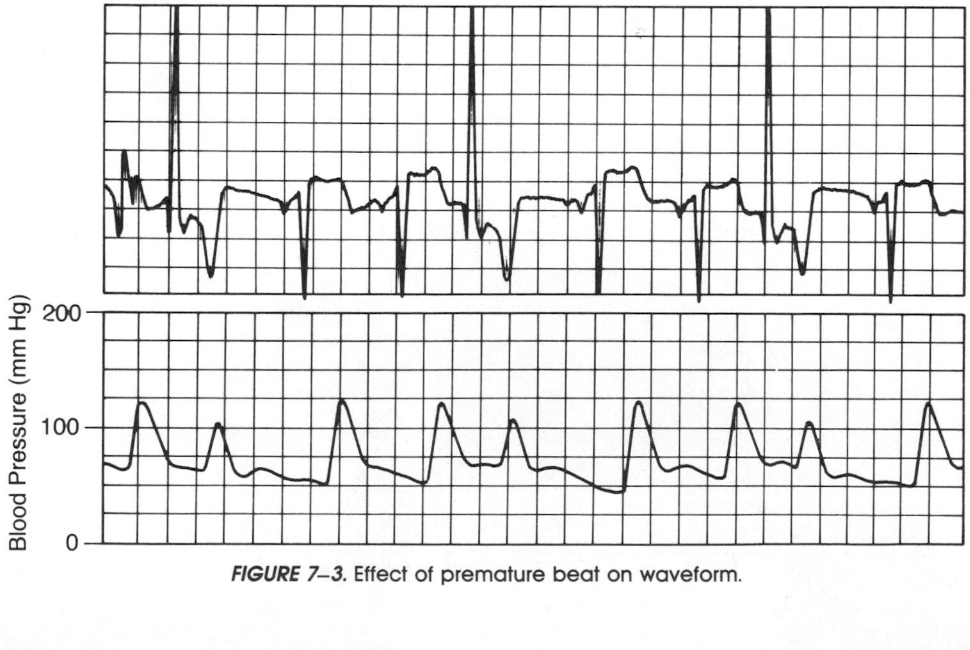

FIGURE 7–3. Effect of premature beat on waveform.

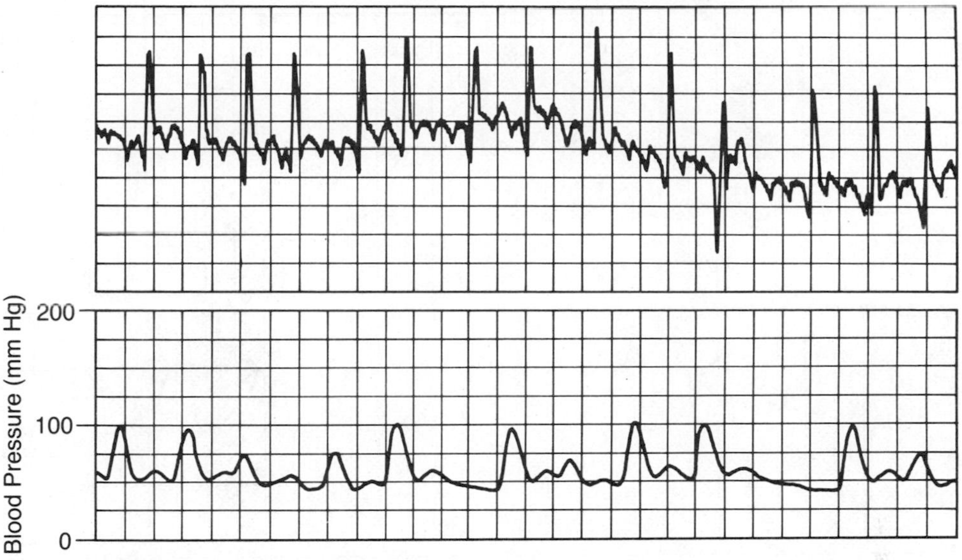

FIGURE 7–4. Effect of rapid, irregular supraventricular tachycardia on waveform.

Rapid atrial tachyarrhythmias may also diminish stroke volume and arterial pressure by limiting the amount of time for ventricular filling. In tachyarrhythmias where the R-to-R intervals are variable (eg, atrial fibrillation), the arterial waveform will show variable peak systolic pressures (Fig. 7–4).

Effects of Altered Physiologic/Anatomic States

Deviations from normal arterial pressures and pressure waveforms can also occur from a multitude of physiologic conditions, including systemic hypertension, shock, obstruction/coarctation of the aorta, and aortic valve disease. In hypertension, a rapid anacrotic rise reaches an initial peak pressure of greater than 140 mm Hg whereas the end-diastolic pressure may be 90 mm Hg or higher. Each phase of the waveform is clearly visible and may be significantly enlarged (Fig. 7–5). In shock or severe hypotension secondary to pump failure, quite the reverse is true. The waveform is small, with maximum peak systolic pressures of 90 mm Hg or less, and is associated with a significant reduction in the rate of anacrotic rise.

Patients with aortic stenosis will have a slower anacrotic rise time due to the delayed ejection of blood through a resistant aortic valve structure. The peak systolic pressure may also be less than 100 mm Hg because of this resistance. The dicrotic notch may be diminished or disappear altogether due to the stiffness of the valve leaflets during aortic closure. Aortic regurgitation or insufficiency, on the other hand, is commonly associated with a steep rate

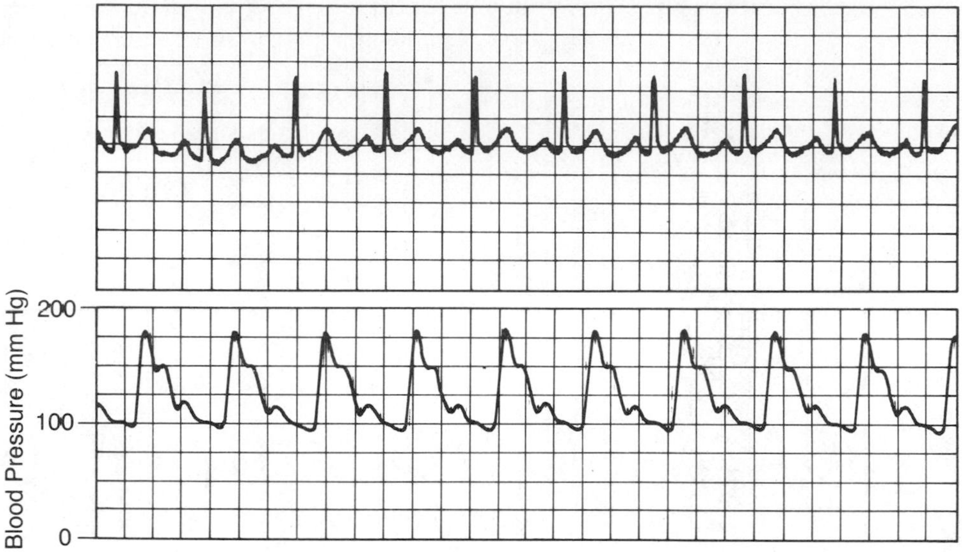

Figure 7–5. Effect of hypertension on waveform.

of rise, a high peak systolic pressure, a wide pulse pressure, and a poorly defined dicrotic notch.

Less common conditions such as cardiac tamponade or constrictive pericarditis may also influence the arterial waveform. In the case of cardiac tamponade, a paradoxical pressure may be observed.

Mechanical Factors That Influence the Arterial Waveform

Although a number of possible mechanical problems can affect the arterial waveform, the three most common problems are over-damping, catheter whip, and inaccurate monitor calibration/zeroing.

Over-damping may be caused by air bubbles in the monitoring system, thrombus formation at the tip of the catheter, or the lodging of the catheter tip against the vessel wall. The result is a small waveform with a slow anacrotic rise and a diminished or absent dicrotic notch. Air bubbles, if present, should be withdrawn from the system using aseptic technique. If a thrombus has formed and cannot be withdrawn from the system, a decision should be made regarding the benefits of leaving the catheter in place versus the possibility of embolization. A problem caused by the location of the catheter tip can be solved by repositioning and suturing of the catheter.

As the name implies, catheter whip is the spurious movement of the catheter tip within the vessel lumen, resulting in an erratic and "noisy" arterial waveform. The displayed values for systolic and diastolic pressures may also be significantly in error. Usually, repositioning or using a shorter length catheter will solve the problem. Catheter whip is not as much a problem with arterial monitoring systems as it is with pulmonary artery pressure monitoring systems.

Inaccurate calibration or zeroing of the monitor system may result from poor technique, infrequent calibration or zeroing, an electrical failure within the system itself, or thermal changes that affect the transducer. Calibration and zeroing should be done at least every shift by personnel who have been instructed in the proper method of performing this procedure. If variances continue, then the tubing or "plumbing" connecting the system together should be examined and the possibility of replacing the transducer considered. All new transducer set-ups should be given at least 30 minutes to 1 hour to adjust to ambient temperature conditions. If problems continue even after the transducer has been replaced, then a failure in the main electrical monitoring system may exist.

OBTAINING BLOOD SAMPLES FROM AN ARTERIAL CATHETER

Careful and aseptic technique when withdrawing blood samples from an arterial catheter can greatly reduce the chances of arterial trauma, embolus, and infection. Samples should be drawn from the *most proximal of the two in-line stopcocks attached to the short length of tubing at the insertion site* (Fig. 7–6). (See Chapter 6.)

When obtaining samples for blood gas analysis, the sterile cap covering the sample port is removed and a sterile syringe is attached in its place. The stopcock is then turned off to the flush system and 3 ml of blood is gently drawn off to clear the line of heparinized solution. The stopcock is then turned off to all three ports, the syringe is removed and discarded, and another sterile syringe that has been heparinized is attached in its place. The syringe has been heparinized by aseptically drawing up approximately 0.5 ml of 1:1000 sodium heparin, pulling back on the plunger to coat the inside of the syringe, and then expelling the excess heparin into a sink or other suitable

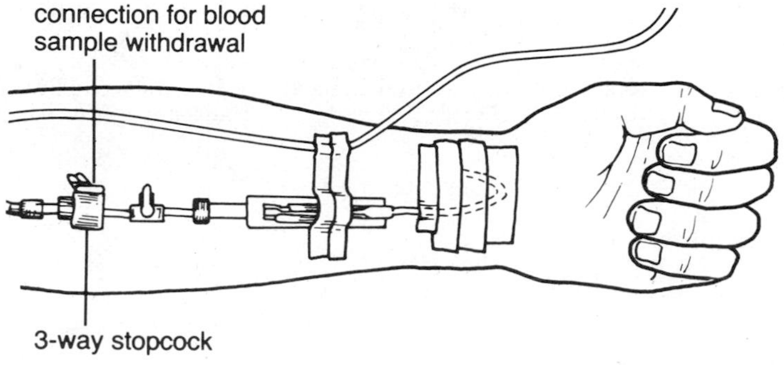

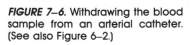

FIGURE 7–6. Withdrawing the blood sample from an arterial catheter. (See also Figure 6–2.)

receptacle. Once again the stopcock is turned off to the flush system and the desired amount of blood is drawn into the syringe. Next, the stopcock is turned off to the sample port, the syringe is removed and set aside, and the system is flushed for one to three seconds using the mechanism on the continuous flush device (pigtail or squeeze clamp) in order to rapidly infuse heparinized solution back into the catheter lumen.

The next step is the one most often forgotten but is, perhaps, the most important when it comes to preventing embolization and infection. The stopcock is turned off to the patient and the line is flushed (using the pressurized continuous flush system) with the heparinized solution to clear the sample port. It is most convenient to do this flush routine while holding a piece of sterile gauze over the port to collect the expelled solution. The stopcock is then turned off to the sample port, so that monitoring can continue, and a sterile cap is reapplied. When obtaining samples for tests other than blood gas analysis, the sampling syringe should not be heparinized.

Some institutions recommend rezeroing/calibrating the system following any sampling procedure. Depending upon the level of sophistication of the equipment as well as the age of the electronics/transducer combination, this may or may not be a necessary procedure. Be sure to check either with the manufacturer or the literature supplied to determine the needs of a particular monitoring system. As far as transducer technology is concerned, the modern quartz transducers tend to be very stable, as do the more recent strain gauge types.

REFERENCES

Bates B: *A Guide to Physical Examination, ed. 2*. Philadelphia, JB Lippincott, 1979.

Bruner John: *Handbook of Blood Pressure Monitoring*. Littleton, MA, PSG Publishing Company, 1978.

Braunwald E: *Heart Disease: A Textbook of Cardiovascular Medicine*. Philadelphia, WB Saunders, 1980.

Daily E, Schroeder J: *Hemodynamic Waveforms*. St. Louis, CV Mosby, 1983.

Kaye W: Invasive monitoring techniques: Arterial cannulation, bedside pulmonary artery catheterization, and arterial puncture. *Heart and Lung* (1983); 12:395–425.

Nelson W, Egbert A: How to measure blood pressure accurately. *Primary Cardiology* (1984); 10:14–26.

Pierson D, Hudson L: Monitoring hemodynamics in the critically ill. *Med Clin N Am* (1983); 67:1343–1358.

Pursley P: Arterial catheters: Nursing management to decrease complications. *Crit Care Nurse* (1981); 1:16–21.

Seifert P: Invasive hemodynamic monitoring. *AORN Journal* (1983); 37: 416–425.

Stein J: Placing arterial lines. *Emerg Med* (1983); 15:221–225, 230.

Underhill S, Woods S, Sivarajan E, Halfpenny C: *Cardiac Nursing*. Philadelphia, JB Lippincott, 1982.

Monitoring Central Venous Pressure

8

LINDA A. YACONE, RN, BS, CCRN

The introduction of central venous pressure (CVP) monitoring in 1962 was the first important step in invasive bedside assessment of cardiac function and intravascular volume status. A single or multiple lumen catheter is advanced from a peripheral or central vein until the catheter tip is in the proximal superior vena cava. Because the superior vena cava openly communicates with the right atrium, from this site central venous and right atrial pressure can be evaluated continuously via a pressure transducer or intermittently using a water manometer.

CLINICAL APPLICATION

The central venous catheter provides a means of assessing cardiac function and intravascular volume status. In addition, the catheter provides a central intravenous route which can be used to administer medications, fluids, and withdraw blood samples and may also serve as an emergency route for temporary pacemaker insertion.

Assessment of Cardiac Function

Right Ventricular Function. The right atrium is a thin-walled, low-pressure receiving chamber for venous blood. Mean pressure in the right atrium is normally 0 to 8 mm Hg. This value normally correlates well with the end-diastolic (filling) pressure of the right ventricle because when the tricuspid valve is open in diastole, the right atrium and right ventricle are openly communicating chambers and pressures equilibrate at end-diastole. If the compliance of the right ventricle remains constant, an elevated right atrial pressure suggests right ventricular failure. If the patient is showing signs of underperfusion, a low right atrial pressure suggests cardiac dysfunction from a fluid-depleted state.

Left Ventricular Function. Ordinarily, right ventricular end-diastolic pressure and left ventricular end-diastolic pressure correlate rather well in health.* Therefore, if the patient is young and without cardiopulmonary dysfunction, the CVP will accurately correlate with left ventricular end-diastolic pressure and may be used as a guide for fluid therapy. However, when there is a disparity between right and left ventricular function, the CVP may not accurately correlate with left ventricular end-diastolic pressure. This may occur with right heart dysfunction due to valve (tricuspid, pulmonic) defects, right ventricular dysfunction (infarction, contusion, cardiomyopathies), or right heart failure due to pulmonary disease (COPD, pulmonary embolism, primary pulmonary hypertension). If the left ventricle does fail in the absence of pulmonary or right heart disease, the CVP may still be within normal limits and not reflect pathological changes that are occurring or have occurred in the left ventricle for the following reason. As the left ventricle fails, stroke volume decreases and left ventricular end-diastolic volume and pressure increase. This volume/pressure overload is then reflected upstream of the failing left ventricular chamber as elevated left atrial, pulmonary venous, pulmonary capillary, and pulmonary arterial pressures. Right ventricular end-diastolic pressure may still be within normal limits at this point. By the time elevated pressures reflect back to the right atrium, pulmonary edema, the backward consequence of left heart failure, is well established (Fig. 8–1). The frequent disparity in right and left ventricular function in the critically ill makes hemodynamic monitoring with the CVP catheter alone a less common occurrence as it has largely been supplanted by the pulmonary artery catheter.

Assessment of Intravascular Volume Status

The central venous pressure measurement can be used to assess the patient's intravascular volume status. By measuring the mean pressure in the right atrium, it is possible to assess venous return to the heart as indicated by right ventricular end-diastolic pressure. As stated earlier, in the absence of cardiopulmonary disease, this value correlates rather well with left ventricular end-diastolic pressure (preload), which is a very important determinant of cardiac output. In hypovolemia, a reduced ventricular end-diastolic pressure compromises cardiac function and effective tissue perfusion. On the other hand, if the patient is volume overloaded, venous return and central venous pressure will be increased, as will cardiac output.

---

*In the normal heart, left ventricular end-diastolic pressure can be estimated to be twice that of right end-diastolic pressure + 2. For example, given a right ventricular end-diastolic pressure of 3 mm Hg, left ventricular end-diastolic pressure is 8 mm Hg (3 mm Hg × 2 + 2 = 8 mm Hg).

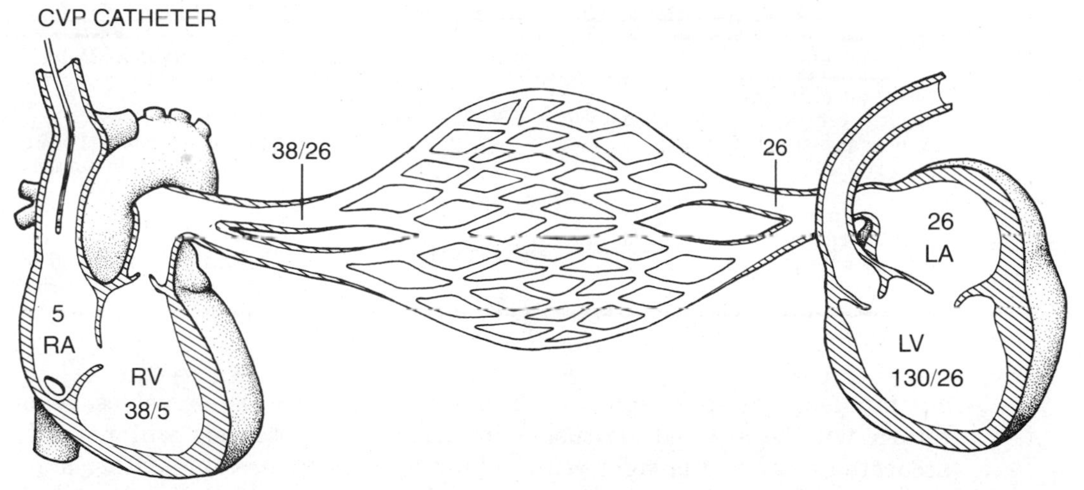

FIGURE 8–1. The left ventricle is failing and the elevated left ventricular end-diastolic pressure is reflected upstream of the left ventricular chamber to the level of the pulmonary arterial circulation. However, the right ventricle is still able to mount a systolic ejection pressure commensurate with its increased afterload and is not in failure. Therefore, right atrial or central venous pressure would not reflect the left ventricular disturbance.

Administration of Fluids or Drugs

Hypertonic or caustic fluids, such as potassium chloride at concentrations greater than 40 mEq/liter, cause vein irritation, pain, and phlebitis if administered via a peripheral vein, owing to slow peripheral venous flow and delayed wash-out of administered solutions. Blood flow in the great veins of the thorax is rapid, therby diluting the solution immediately upon entry into the circulation. In addition, peripheral venous sites may not be stable and subcutaneous infiltration of drugs such as norepinephrine (Levophed) causes local tissue necrosis. The stable central line is more suitable for administration of such medications.

Limitations

In several circumstances the central venous pressure may not be an accurate index of circulating volume or cardiac function. In hypovolemia, should venous tone be increased or coronary hypoperfusion compromise myocardial function, the CVP may not fall proportionate to the amount of fluid lost. If the patient is receiving ventilatory support, the central venous pressure value may be falsely elevated, reflecting the transmission of increased intrathoracic pressure on the cardiovascular structures. Additionally, the accuracy of the CVP measurement depends on the integrity and patency of the venous system. If there is tumor mass compressing the vena cava or

TABLE 8–1. Conversion Consideration in Value Interpretation

Scale	Method	Equivalent Value
mm Hg to cm H_2O (eg, the central venous pressure is 6 mm Hg)	6 mm Hg × 1.36 = 8.16 cm H_2O	8 cm H_2O (answer rounded off to nearest whole number)
cm H_2O to mm Hg (eg, the central venous pressure is 8 cm H_2O)	$\frac{8\ \text{cm H}_2\text{O}}{1.36} = 5.8$ mm Hg	6 mm Hg (answer rounded off to nearest whole number)

any problems with the patency of the veins or structure of vein valves, venous return will be affected. Tricuspid insufficiency or stenosis will not allow accurate assessment of right ventricular end-diastolic pressure. Other abnormalities such as left to right intracardiac shunts and restrictive or constrictive cardiomyopathies distort obtained values.

Conversion Considerations in Value Interpretation

When recording the central venous pressure in mm Hg using a transducer monitoring system, the normal range for venous pressure is 0 to 8 mm Hg. When the central venous pressure is read in centimeters of H_2O using a manometer, the accepted range is 3 to 11 cm H_2O. Since both methods are commonly used, the procedure for converting mm Hg to cm H_2O and vice versa must be understood. Mercury is heavier than water, therefore, a 1 mm

TABLE 8–2. Conversion of mm Hg to cm H_2O

mm Hg		cm H_2O
0	=	0*
1	=	1 (1.36)†
2	=	3 (2.72)
3	=	4 (4.08)
4	=	5 (5.44)
5	=	7 (6.80)
6	=	8 (8.16)
7	=	10 (9.52)
8	=	11 (10.88)
9	=	12 (12.24)
10	=	14 (13.60)
11	=	15 (14.96)
12	=	16 (16.32)
13	=	18 (17.68)
14	=	19 (19.04)
15	=	20 (20.40)

*cm H_2O reported in nearest whole number.
†actual equivalent value.

column of mercury would have the same weight as a 1.36 cm column of water (1 mm Hg = 1.36 cm H_2O). Conversion samples are illustrated in Table 8–1.

It is imperative that the same scale be used consistently for a particular patient when conveying values for interpretation. It should be reported in *cm H_2O* or *mm Hg*. A conversion chart is shown in Table 8–2.

Regardless of the scale used, serial trends are always clinically more important than isolated measurements. Whatever the central venous pressure value, it is imperative to continue to assess the patient physically, paying special attention to urine output, heart rate, blood pressure, lung sounds, and other signs or symptoms related to volume status and cardiopulmonary and cardiovascular function.

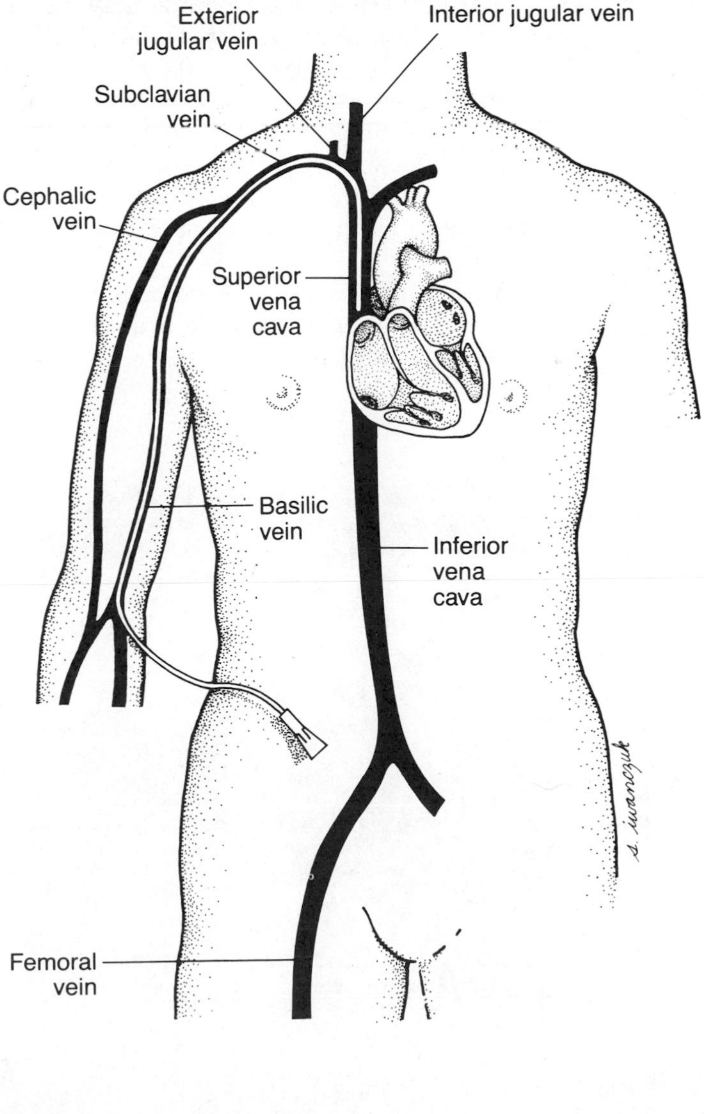

FIGURE 8–2. Sites for central venous or pulmonary artery catheter insertion. In the illustration, a CVP monitoring catheter is inserted at the antecubital fossa into the basilic vein. The monitoring tip rests in the superior vena cava.

Insertion Sites

Central venous pressure monitoring can be accomplished with the insertion of a catheter into either a central or a peripheral vein. There is no ideal site for insertion of a central venous catheter. Table 8–3 lists the advantages and disadvantages of the variously used sites, which are illustrated in Figure 8–2.

TYPES OF CATHETERS USED FOR CENTRAL VENOUS PRESSURE

Monitoring

Various types of catheters may be used to monitor central venous pressure. Pulmonary artery catheter utilization is discussed in detail in Chapter 7. When central venous pressure monitoring alone is desired, a single or multilumen catheter may be used. The multilumen catheter has three distinct infusion ports, 2.2 cm apart (Fig. 8–3). This catheter can also be used to: 1) withdraw venous blood samples; 2) administer different or incompatible drugs simultaneously; 3) administer hyperalimentation solutions; 4) administer blood, blood products or fluids; and 5) phlebotomize the patient as necessary.

When used with a percutaneous sheath introducer with a side-arm infusion port, four lumens are available for use. The multilumen catheter is not recommended for peripheral vein insertion because of its large outside diameter.

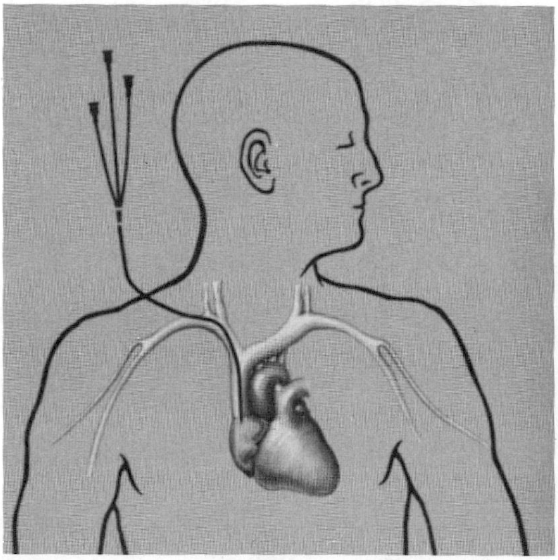

FIGURE 8–3. Anatomical positioning of the multilumen catheter. (Reproduced with permission from Arrow International, Inc., Reading, PA 19610.)

TABLE 8–3. Sites for Central Venous or Pulmonary Artery Catheter Insertion

Site	Advantages	Disadvantages
CENTRAL VENOUS ACCESS		
Subclavian Vein	easily accessible ease in maintaining a sterile, intact dressing unrestricted patient movements less likely displacement of catheter tip once in place reduced incidence of thrombotic complications because of rapid venous flow rates	possible puncture or laceration of subclavian artery possibility of a disastrous bleed (hemothorax, hemomediastinum) as pressure cannot be applied to bleeding site risk of pneumothorax risk of major complications increased in patients with prior surgery in the subclavian area, COPD, mechanical ventilation, especially with PEEP
Internal Jugular Vein	relatively short and direct pathway to right atrium reliable site for correct catheter placement patient movements not restricted; catheter displacement unlikely rapid venous flow rates decrease thrombotic complications lower incidence of arterial laceration or puncture and pneumothorax than with subclavian site	difficulty in maintaining an intact sterile dressing possible puncture of the common carotid artery possible puncture of the trachea or endotracheal tube balloon risk of pneumothorax
Femoral Vein	familiarity with site; used by clinicians for central venous access longer than other approaches greater ease in insertion in elderly patients with tortuous subclavian and jugular veins	possible increased risk of infection due to proximity to groin; contraindicated in patients with abdominal sepsis difficulty in maintaining an intact, sterile dressing difficult to locate in obese patients thrombosis of femoral vein is high risk factor to pulmonary embolism (risk is increased in low perfusion or hypercoagulable states) difficulty in immobilizing leg; increased risk of catheter displacement, particularly if patient is restless
PERIPHERAL VENOUS ACCESS		
External Jugular Vein	easily accessible, especially in children, because of superficial location of vein minimal risk of carotid artery puncture or pneumothorax	successful passage of catheter less likely than with internal jugular vein; J-tipped wire guide may be necessary to facilitate passage through junction to central veins risk of arterial puncture or laceration possibility of malposition into axillary or azygos vein venous flow rates less than central veins, thus increasing risk of thrombosis risk of pneumothorax difficulty in maintaining a sterile dressing, especially if patient has tracheostomy

Table continued on following page

TABLE 8–3. Sites for Central Venous or Pulmonary Artery Catheter Insertion (Continued)

Site	Advantages	Disadvantages
Antecubital Sites (Cephalic or Basilic Sites)	no risk of pneumothorax or of major hemorrhage bleeding from site more easily controlled in patients with coagulopathies	difficult to locate in obese or edematous patients cutdown is usually required because percutaneous insertion is more difficult stasis of blood in involved vein predisposes to thrombosis risk of septicemia may be higher advancement of catheter to central veins may be difficult vein may not be large enough to accept a large catheter involved arm must be immobilized to prevent catheter displacement access may be limited because of previous venous cutdown or venipucture venous spasm may prohibit catheter passage

Insertion Techniques

Catheter insertion for central venous pressure or pulmonary artery pressure monitoring can be accomplished via the percutaneous or cutdown technique. Most catheters are inserted utilizing one of the percutaneous approaches shown in Figure 8–4.

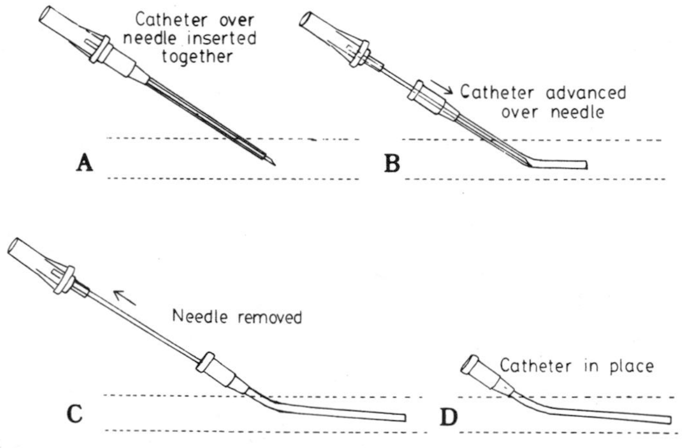

A — Insertion of catheter over needle.

FIGURE 8–4. Various techniques for catheter insertion. (Reproduced with permission from Textbook of Advanced Cardiac Life Support, American Heart Association, 1983.)

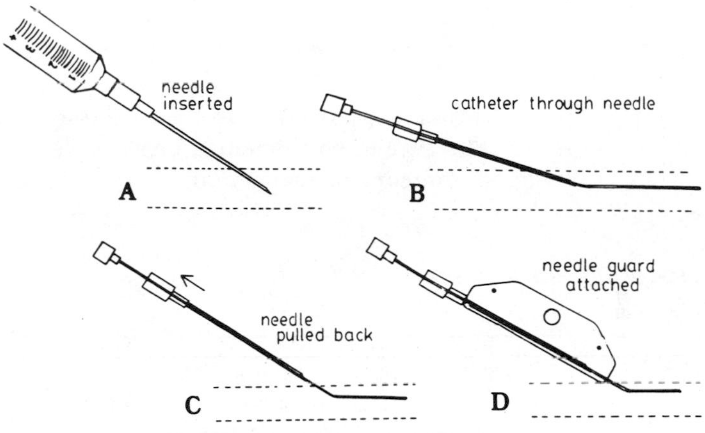

B — Insertion of catheter through needle.

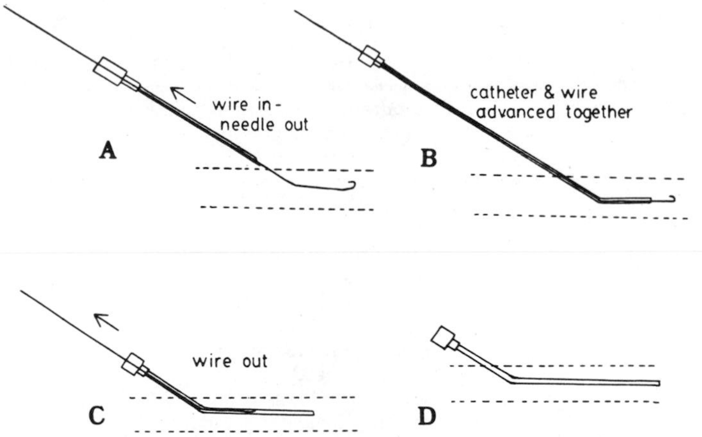

C — Insertion of catheter over guidewire (Seldinger technique).

FIGURE 8–4 Continued

To determine the length of the catheter to be inserted, the distance from the proposed insertion site to the suprasternal notch should be measured. Generally, a 12-inch catheter is used when performing a left subclavian vein insertion and an 8-inch catheter is used for a right subclavian vein insertion. A precise measurement before insertion insures that proper catheter placement can be achieved.

Special Equipment for Insertion of Monitoring CVP

In order to facilitate insertion, the appropriate equipment should be on hand. The type of equipment necessary depends on the kind of monitoring to be done, mercury or water manometer (Table 8–4).

Procedure for Insertion

As with all invasive procedures, aseptic technique must be observed during insertion to prevent both systemic and local infections. Proper positioning of the patient during insertion is necessary to prevent the occurrence of air embolism. The patient is asked to hold his or her breath at peak expiration at the moment of insertion and whenever the tubing is disconnected

TABLE 8–4. Equipment Necessary for Monitoring

Manometer Monitoring Technique
central venous pressure catheter
manometer
stopcock
suture material
sterile drapes
infusion solution with administration set
carpenter's level
sterile masks and gloves
local anesthetic agent with 10 ml syringe
21-gauge needle (5/8″)
25-gauge needle (1½″)
scalpel and blade (#15)—if cutdown technique used
nonLuer lock 10 ml syringe
4 × 4 gauze pads (10)
transparent surgical dressing (optional)
iodine antiseptic solution
nonallergic tape
arm board (if antecubital fossa used as insertion site)
extension tubing
Transducer Monitoring Technique
all equipment used with manometer technique except the manometer
transducer
pressure monitor

from the catheter hub. This maneuver increases intrathoracic pressure and prevents accidental entry of air into the patient's bloodstream. A head-down, supine (Trendelenburg) position of 15 to 30 degrees also promotes venous distention in the chest, head, and neck and makes cannulation easier. Another aid to insertion and safeguard against infection is to keep the patient's head turned in the direction opposite to the insertion site, with the chin pointed slightly upward. If the antecubital approach is used, it is not uncommon for the catheter to stop advancing smoothly. If this problem occurs, the arm can be extended and moved laterally 60 to 90 degrees to facilitate passage.

The skin should be cleansed with an iodine antiseptic solution. After the physician scrubs and dons the appropriate surgical attire, the patient is draped with the insertion site exposed. Local infiltration with the anesthetic agent should follow, first using the 5/8-inch needle and then the 1½-inch needle. An anesthetic agent such as xylocaine 2% or bupivacaine is best suited for this purpose. The skin puncture can then be made and the needle advanced in the appropriate direction. When the insertion of the catheter is done through a needle, a constant negative pressure is applied to the syringe as it advances. When cannulation occurs, dark blood will be seen in the syringe as the needle enters the vein. If bright red blood should appear in the syringe, however, it is indicative of arterial puncture and the needle must be withdrawn immediately. Pressure is then applied to the site for a minimum of 10 minutes. After successful cannulation has occurred, a free flow of intravenous solution indicates that the needle is in the vein. Until x-ray confirmation of venous position, the intravenous solution should be infused at a minimum rate (20 to 30 ml/hr). Other fluids such as TPN, lipids, blood, blood products or large volumes of fluids should not be infused until the correct position of the catheter is confirmed by chest radiograph.

Postinsertion Protocol and Site Maintenance

Once the catheter is in, it should be sutured in place and covered with a sterile dressing. An antibiotic/germicidal and transparent surgical dressing or sterile gauze may be used according to the individual hospital policy for central lines. Correct placement is then verified by a postinsertion chest radiograph. This can also rule out the presence of a pneumothorax, which is a common complication associated with insertion. The intravenous solution rate and type of fluid to be given may then be adjusted according to the needs of the patient after line placement confirmation. The dressing is changed according to hospital policy, usually every 48 hours and PRN.

MEASUREMENT OF CENTRAL VENOUS PRESSURE

Positioning of the patient is an important consideration when doing a central venous pressure measurement. Ideally, the patient should be supine

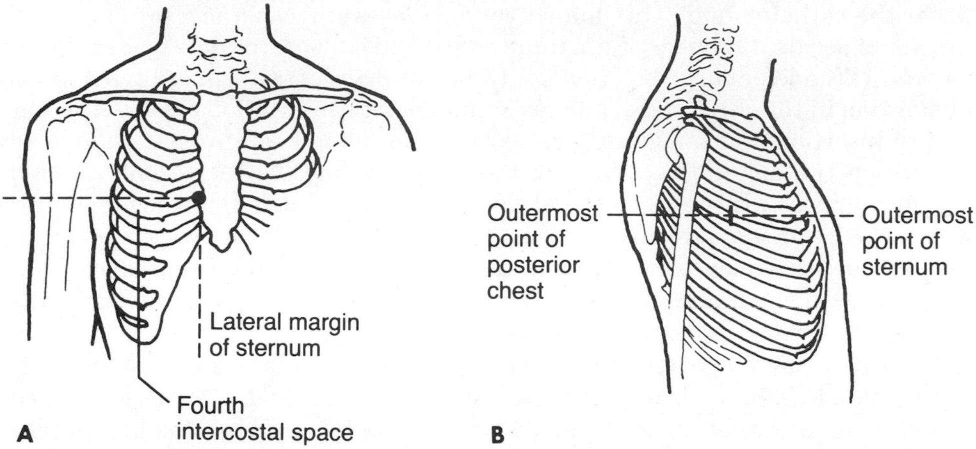

FIGURE 8–5. The phlebostatic axis. The crossing of two imaginary lines defines the assumed position of the monitoring catheter tip within the body, ie, right atrial level. *A,* A line that passes from the fourth intercostal space at the lateral margin of the sternum down the side of the body beneath the axilla. *B,* A line that runs horizontally at a point midway between the outermost portion of the anterior and posterior surfaces of the chest.

without a pillow. However, if the patient's condition does not permit this position, the reading may be performed with the head of the bed elevated to 20 degrees to obtain accurate data.[1] Any variation in the measurement procedure should be documented in the nurse's notes. The transducer or zero point of the manometer is leveled at the phlebostatic axis, regardless of patient position, to provide a zero reference point at the right atrium (Fig. 8–5).

Water Manometer Monitoring Technique

When setting up the initial intravenous infusion, it is best to have an extension tubing connected directly to the catheter and a stopcock between the extension tubing and the intravenous administration set. It is imperative that the stopcock port be covered with a completely closed protective cap to prevent infection. Either a rigid plastic water manometer or venous pressure manometer set with pliable tubing can be used. If pliable tubing is used, it must be attached to a precalibrated manometer stand in order to read the central venous pressure value (Fig. 8–6). The manometer stand is calibrated and the tubing set-up inserts into the stand at point 0. Hard plastic manometers are usually calibrated on the outside of the clear plastic itself and may also be stabilized by attaching the manometer to an intravenous pole. The zero reference point must be placed at the phlebostatic axis. If the manometer is secured to a point away from the patient, a carpenter's level can be used to confirm the accuracy of the imaginary line connecting the zero reference

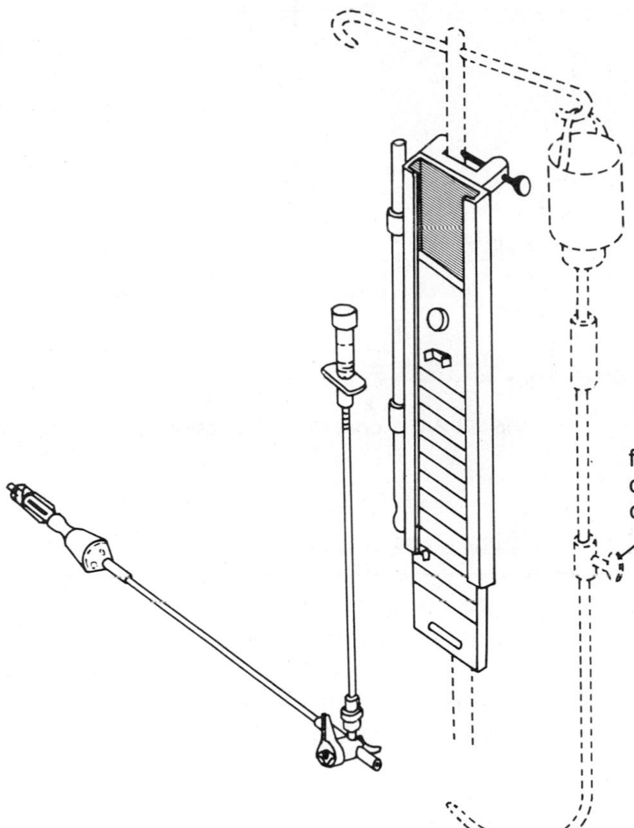

FIGURE 8–6. Venous pressure manometer set. (Redrawn, courtesy of Bard-Parker, Lincoln Park, NJ, a division of Becton Dickinson and Company.)

point to the patient's phlebostatic axis. The patency of the intravenous line should be checked before beginning measurements by opening it to free flow of solution (Fig. 8–7*A*).

The stopcock is turned off to the patient and opened to the manometer, allowing it to fill approximately 10 cm greater than the estimated central venous pressure reading (Fig. 8–7*B*). The manometer should not be filled to the point of overflow since this increases the chance for contamination of fluid. After the stopcock is turned off to the intravenous infusion (Fig. 8–7*C*), a drop in the fluid level should be observed. Fluctuation of the fluid level with respiration is expected. This is due to changes in intrathoracic pressure, which increases with expiration and decreases with inspiration. If the patient is on mechanical ventilatory support, true right atrial pressure may be altered, especially if PEEP or CPAP is applied. Removing a patient from the ventilator to perform readings is generally not advocated. However, all

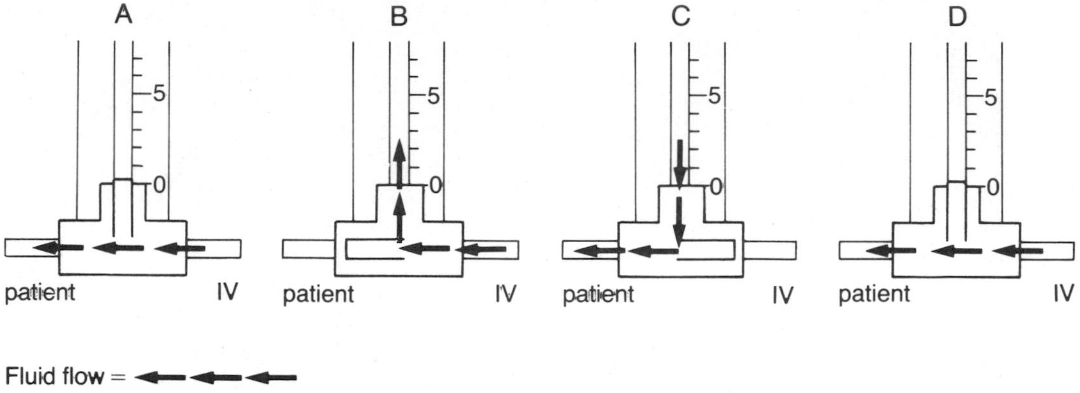

FIGURE 8–7. Proper stopcock positioning in a venous pressure manometer.

readings must be performed consistently. The fluid level in the manometer eventually stabilizes and a reading at eye level is taken at end-expiration. After the measurement has been made, the stopcock should be turned off to the manometer so that intravenous flow can resume (Fig. 8–7*D*).

Interpretation of an isolated reading is of limited value. The serial trends of the measurement correlated with the patient's clinical status offer the optimal benefit of monitoring central venous pressure.

Transducer Monitoring Technique

For frequent or continuous monitoring of central venous (right atrial) pressure, particularly when using the RA port of the pulmonary artery catheter, the transducer setup is the method used. Central venous pressure monitoring can be accomplished using a single or multilumen catheter and transducer or a pulmonary artery catheter and a single transducer to monitor both right atrial and pulmonary artery pressure. A right atrial waveform and pressure measurement can be obtained with a simple turn of two stopcocks (Fig. 8–8).

Several possible set-ups may be used, many of which involve custom-designed kits. In this way, adaptations are possible, and exactly the right type of equipment best suited to an individual unit's needs can be chosen. One possible setup utilizes an extra bridge tubing (Fig. 8–9). In this setup, the end of the pulmonary artery catheter with its infusion ports is secured to a short covered armboard with clear, nonallergic tape. This provides ideal stabilization and easy identification of the ports. When a transducer is used for this purpose, a central venous pressure reading may be obtained with greater accuracy and frequency. The reading obtained with the transducer technique will be in mm Hg. When this method is employed, the monitor should record the pulmonary artery pressures continuously rather than right

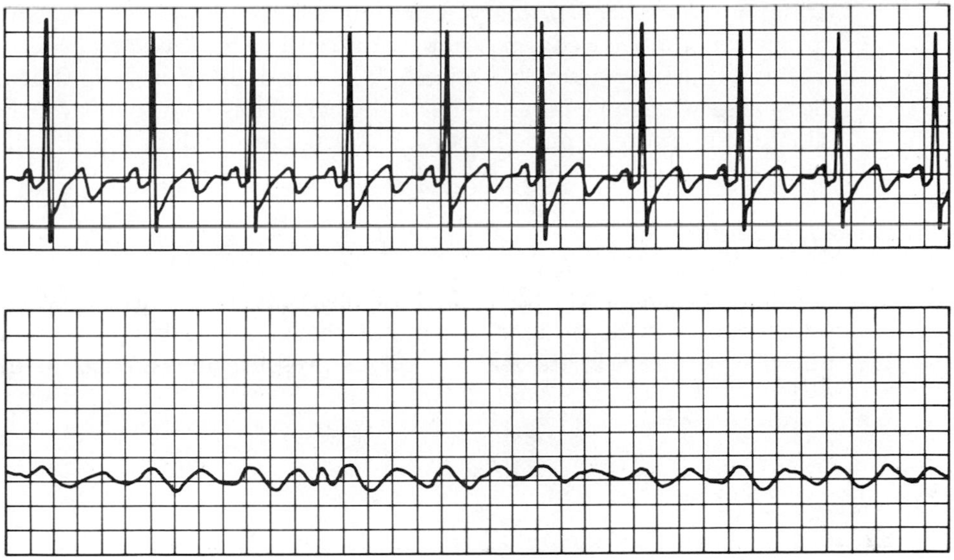

FIGURE 8–8. Right atrial waveform compared with a surface electrocardiogram tracing. Right atrial pressures are monitored on a 0 to 20 mm Hg scale.

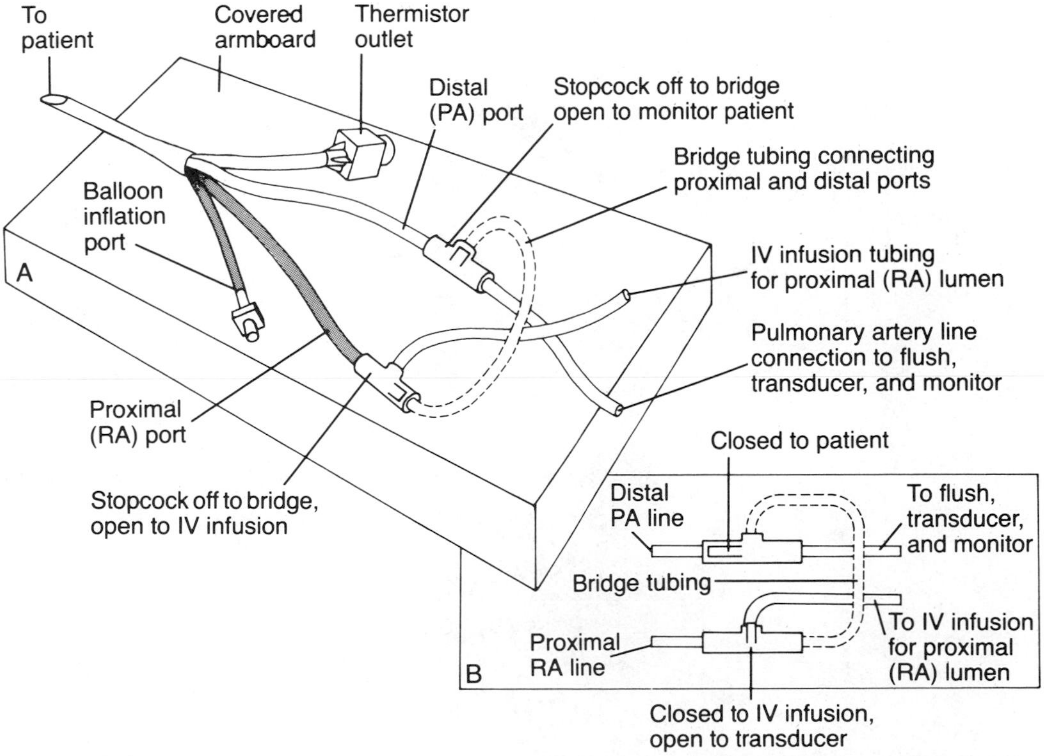

FIGURE 8–9. *A*, Position of stopcocks and set-up for continuous pulmonary artery pressure monitoring with frequent central venous pressure readings. *B*, Position of stopcocks for central venous pressure reading.

atrial pressure. The primary reason is to observe for spontaneous catheter migration into the wedge position, which will be indicated by gradual damping of the pulmonary artery waveform. The secondary reason is that the pulmonary artery diastolic pressure normally correlates well to left ventricular end-diastolic pressure, a more important parameter in the critically ill.

Alternative Techniques

In addition to the above techniques, central venous pressure measurements can be made using a device that acts as a variable pressure volumetric pump in addition to its central venous pressure measuring capability (Fig. 8–10).

COMPLICATIONS

Complications associated with central venous pressure monitoring are essentially the same as those associated with accessing a central vein for any purpose, ie, hyperalimentation, pulmonary artery catheterization, etc. They

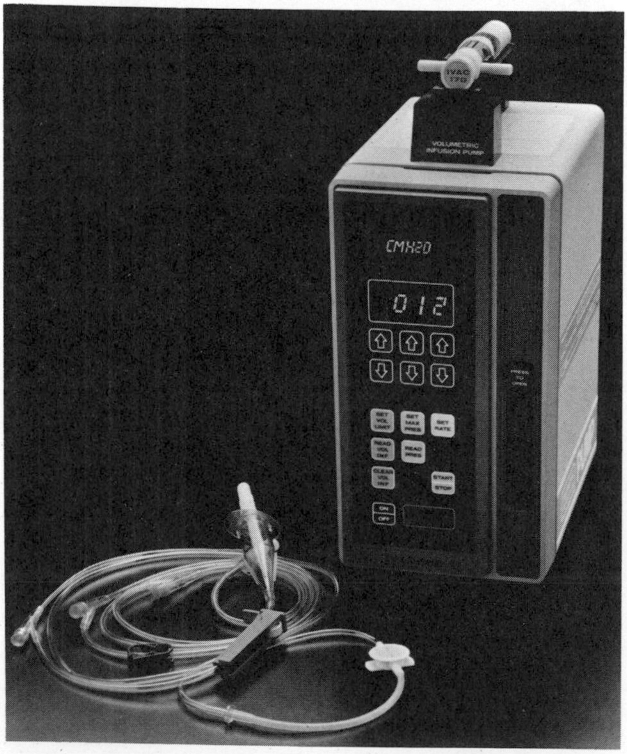

FIGURE 8–10. IVAC Variable Pressure Volumetric Pump, Model 560. A built-in pressure transducer and a sensing disc in the intravenous set measure intermittent central venous pressure. It will be displayed in either cm H_2O or mm Hg, depending on the scale chosen. (Reproduced with permission, IVAC Corporation, San Diego, CA 92138.)

include, but are not limited to, hemorrhage, arrhythmias, local and systemic infection, fluid overload due to improper stopcock positioning, thromboembolic problems, electrical microshocks, air emboli, perforation of the cardiac chambers, and pneumothorax.

Hemorrhagic Complications. Hemorrhage may occur overtly, as in the case of frank bleeding from the insertion site, or covertly, such as hematoma formation deep in body tissue or direct oozing into a body cavity due to distal damage of the involved vessel. The risk of hemorrhage is increased in patients receiving anticoagulant therapy, deficient in clotting factors, having coagulopathies, or having undergone multiple insertion attempts. The likelihood of hemorrhage is reduced when insertion is accomplished via cutdown versus percutaneous technique. It is the responsibility of the caregiver to check for both visible bleeding as well as signs of occult bleeding, such as bruising or swelling. Slow or inconspicuous bleeding into a body cavity may be manifest only as signs of restlessness, apprehension, pallor, tachycardia, or thirst. If hemorrhage continues undetected, uncompensated shock (hypotension) may result. Hemorrhage that is not responsive to applied pressure may necessitate removal of the catheter as well as surgical cutdown at the site of the bleeding for exploration and possible surgical repair of the damaged vessel. Bleeding from the jugular or subclavian veins may be reduced by elevating the patient's head and thorax since this decreases pressure in the veins.

Arrhythmias. Irritation of the right atrial or right ventricular endocardium may precipitate a variety of arrhythmias. Ventricular arrhythmias (ventricular premature beats, ventricular tachycardia) are most common and are associated with spontaneous catheter migration into the right ventricle. The arrhythmia may be precipitated suddenly by turning the patient because this movement may cause the catheter tip to fall against and irritate the ventricular endocardium. Should this occur, the patient should be immediately repositioned; this simple maneuver may terminate the arrhythmia until the catheter is pulled back to the superior vena cava by a physician. A beat-by-beat fluctuation of the water column in the water manometer also indicates ventricular migration. When in doubt, a chest film documents catheter location. To insure safe distance from the right ventricle, the catheter tip should be located in the superior vena cava.

Infectious Complications. All patients with invasive lines must be carefully monitored for any signs or symptoms associated with infection such as fever, chills, redness and tenderness at the site, purulent discharge or pain at or above the insertion site, or the development of an unexplained, elevated white cell count. It is imperative that signs of an inflammatory response be observed and investigated early to prevent septicemia.

Staphylococcus aureus, *S. epidermidis*, gram-negative bacilli, and enterococci are the most common infectious agents associated with contaminated invasive lines.[2] Peripheral insertion sites are at increased risk of sepsis. Pinella, et al[3] reported an increased infection rate (20%) when the antecubital route was used for insertion versus 7% when the subclavian route was chosen.

In addition to poor sterile technique during insertion, with frequent changes of dressings, IV bags, and tubing, the risk of infection increases from improperly capped stopcocks, frequent catheter repositioning, contaminated infusates caused by poor admixture technique when administering medications, and overflow of fluid from the manometer. Immunosuppressed and burn patients are especially susceptible to the development of infections.

Sterile technique is mandatory during insertion, during subsequent dressing changes, and whenever interruption of the system is necessary. The dressing should be changed every 48 hours and PRN. As with all invasive lines, the catheter should be left in place no longer than is absolutely necessary to minimize the potential for sepsis. Hard plastic or pliable manometer sets should be discarded and replaced whenever sterility of the fluid or connecting pieces is in question. If sterility is maintained without question, the manometer sets are changed every 48 hours in conjunction with the routine IV tubing and dressing change.

Should infection occur, the catheter must be removed and the catheter tip sent to the laboratory for culture and sensitivity studies. When removing the catheter for this reason, extra care must be taken to prevent accidental contamination of the tip as it is prepared for the laboratory.

Fluid Overload. Fluid overload is most often caused by failure to reposition the stopcock properly after performing a measurement. When the central venous pressure is measured in conjunction with pulmonary artery pressures using a pulmonary artery catheter, the increased number of stopcocks requiring positioning can increase the incidence of this complication. Increased intravascular volume, even in relatively small amounts, is particularly hazardous in patients sensitive to alterations in fluid balance, such as those with congestive heart failure and renal failure. The symptoms of acute fluid overload will most often present shortly after the volume infusion. The patient may become dyspneic and hypertensive and develop rales as indications of pulmonary edema. Treatment with diuretics is aimed at decreasing the excess volume. Occasionally, institution of rotating tourniquets may be used temporarily. Although not commonly used, phlebotomy may be performed. Careful procedural technique is the key element in prevention of this complication. An infusion control device provides an added safety feature to prevention.

Thromboembolic Complications. Catheter kinking or poor flow of fluid through the catheter can predispose the patient to clot or thrombus formation. Patients at higher risk for the development of thrombosis include those with hypercoaguable states, such as polycythemia, fever, myocardial infarction, cancer, and so on. Any trauma sustained by the vessel wall during or after insertion will also increase the incidence of local thrombosis. A thrombus may present itself as unilateral local edema or neck pain, depending on the catheter insertion site.

The most serious complication associated with catheter thrombosis is the potential detachment of the clot from the vessel wall. The entire clot, or portions of it, can break off and enter the circulating bloodstream. Depending on the size of the embolus and site of potential occlusion, it can cause a variety of complications such as pulmonary emboli, pulmonary infarction, or venous insufficiency.

Forceful flushing of the line should be avoided to prevent the possibility of dislodging any clot that may have formed on the catheter tip. If blood cannot be easily aspirated or free flow of intravenous solution does not occur, suspect the presence of a clot on the catheter tip. When the line is not used for continuous intravenous infusion, eg, the multilumen catheter, intermittent heparin flushes can help prevent thrombus formation. Ideally, an infusion control device is recommended to insure an adequate and consistent flow rate for continuous infusions.

Electrical Microshocks. A pathway directly to the heart exists whenever a patient has a central venous catheter in place. Heart muscle is particularly sensitive to electrical stimulation. Microshocks or electrical currents of less than 1 ampere can travel via this artificial pathway to the myocardium and produce life-threatening dysrhythmias such as ventricular fibrillation. Normally microshocks are imperceptible and do not affect the external body because of the natural defense afforded by the intact skin. The skin also serves as a barrier against leakage current, which is a low level of electrical current found on all electrical equipment. The presence of intravenous lines, severe electrolyte imbalances, moist skin, gel used in attaching electrocardiogram electrodes, and any break in the skin surface decrease the natural resistance afforded by the skin.

General electrical safety guidelines should be observed to decrease the potential for the occurrence of electrical complications such as microshocks. These guidelines include:

1. Protect the catheter from moisture.
2. Use only properly grounded electrical equipment in the patient's environment; this includes using only three-pronged plugs and avoiding the use of cheaters that are used to convert three-pronged plug systems into two-pronged plugs.
3. Provide for routine, qualified inspection of electrical equipment in the room such as the bedside monitoring console as well as portable devices such as infusion pumps, automated blood pressure units, etc. All equipment should be identified as having been inspected by the appropriate department, eg, biomedical engineering, including the date of the inspection.
4. Inspect all cords and plugs for signs of wear such as fraying, cracking or cuts.
5. Use extreme care when handling any liquids, eg, intravenous fluids, near electrical equipment. This includes not storing any liquids on top of any electrical device.
6. Use only dry hands to plug in or disconnect electrical equipment.
7. Remove a plug from a socket by firmly grasping the plug itself, not the cord.
8. Turn the power off before removing any electrical device.
9. Keep all patients as dry as possible, especially high risk patients such as those with diaphoresis or incontinence.
10. Remove all unnecessary electrical equipment from the patient's environment.
11. Plug multiple pieces of electrical equipment into the same outlet

when possible to decrease the chance of a difference in voltage which may cause leakage current to flow through the patient.

12. Do not permit the use of extension cords.

13. Limit the use of a patient's personal electrical equipment, including radios, portable televisions, hair dryers, etc. If used, these pieces of equipment should pass a safety inspection by the biomedical engineer.

Air Embolism. The potential for the occurrence of air emboli exists whenever air bubbles are introduced into the systemic circulation. A venous air embolus can travel through the venae cavae through the right side of the heart and enter the pulmonary circulation. Pulmonary infarction is a possible consequence. An air embolus should be suspected if the patient suddenly develops cyanosis, tachypnea, dyspnea, coughing, or hypotension.

To prevent this possible complication, the patient should hold the breath at end-exhalation whenever the catheter hub and tubing are disconnected. In this way, air cannot enter the circulation because of the protective effect of the increased intrathoracic pressure. Insuring that all connections are secured and clamping the central venous line during necessary interruptions of the system are additional safety precautions to prevent the occurrence of an air embolus.

Perforation of the Cardiac Chambers. Perforation of the right atrium or right ventricle can occur from catheter migration or improper placement during insertion. Documentation of the catheter tip in the superior vena cava following insertion and inspection of subsequent chest films for catheter placement insure proper position. Perforation with hemorrhage into the pericardium (cardiac tamponade) is more likely in patients with elevated right atrial or right ventricular pressures. Any patient with a central venous catheter who suddenly develops distended neck veins, venous hypertension, narrowed pulse pressure, hypotension, distant heart sounds, and pulsus paradoxus should be suspected for cardiac tamponade. The ECG may show decreased voltage and electrical alternans. Treatment is directed at relieving the tamponade through pericardiocentesis or surgical evacuation of the accumulated pericardial blood and repair of the perforation in the atrium or ventricle.

Pneumothorax. The occurrence of pneumothorax as a complication to central venous pressure catheter insertion is increased when the percutaneous versus the cutdown technique is employed. It is also more commonly seen when the internal jugular or subclavian veins are used. A portion of a lung or an entire lung itself may collapse, depending upon the amount of air entering the pleural cavity. Additionally, the potential for blood as well as air entering the pleural cavity exists, creating a hemopneumothorax.

Signs and symptoms of a pneumothorax are abrupt in onset and may include dyspnea, cough, and sharp chest pain. Respiratory chest wall movements will be abnormal or absent on the affected side. If the pneumothorax proceeds uncorrected to a tension pneumothorax, ventilatory status is quickly impaired and cardiac output decreased, and shock may ensue.

Treatment is aimed at removal of air from the pleural cavity, which will be followed by reinflation of the lung or lung segment. This is most often accomplished by closed chest drainage. Supplemental oxygen should be provided. Should the patient experience any pain or discomfort, analgesics should be offered.

REFERENCES

1. Woods SL, Mansfield LW: Effect of body position upon pulmonary artery and pulmonary capillary wedge pressure in non-critically ill patients. *Heart Lung* 1976; 5:83.
2. Bozzetti F: Central venous catheter sepsis. *Surg Gynecol Obstet* 1985; 161:293–299.
3. Pinella JC, Ross DF, Martin T, et al: Study of the incidence of intravascular catheter infections and associated septicemia in critically ill patients. *Crit Care Med* 1983; 11:21–25.

Selected Readings

Andreoli KG, Fowkes VK, Zipes DP, et al: *Comprehensive Cardiac Care*, ed. 4. St. Louis, CV Mosby, 1979.

Beal JM: *Critical Care for Surgical Patients*. New York, Macmillan, 1982.

Berk JL, Sampliner JE: *Handbook of Critical Care*. Boston, Little, Brown, 1982.

Best and Taylor's Physiological Basis of Medical Practice, ed. 11. Baltimore, Williams and Wilkins, 1985.

Braunwald E (ed): *Heart Disease—A Textbook of Cardiovascular Medicine*. Philadelphia, WB Saunders, 1980.

Bullas J: Hemodynamic assessment. *Crit Care Nurse* 1985; 5:73–76.

Cain HD: *Flint's Emergency Treatment and Management*, ed. 7. Philadelphia, WB Saunders, 1985.

Daily EK, Schroeder JS: *Techniques in Bedside Hemodynamic Monitoring*, ed. 3. St. Louis, CV Mosby, 1985.

Fowler NO: *Cardiac Diagnosis and Treatment*, ed. 3. Hagerstown, MD, Harper and Row, 1980.

Guyton AC: *Textbook of Medical Physiology*, ed. 6. Philadelphia, WB Saunders, 1981.

Hurst JW: *The Heart—Arteries and Veins*, ed. 5. New York, McGraw-Hill, 1982.

Kenner CV: *Critical Care Nursing; Body, Mind, Spirit*. Boston, Little, Brown, 1981.

Luckman J, Sorenson KC: *Medical-Surgical Nursing—A Psychophysiological Approach*, ed. 2. Philadelphia, WB Saunders, 1980.

Meltzer LE, Pinneo R, Kitchell R: *Intensive Coronary Care—A Manual for Nurses*, ed. 4. Bowie, MD, Robert J Brady Company, 1983.

Millar S, Sampson LK, Soukup M, et al: *Methods in Critical Care—The AACN Manual*, ed. 2. Philadelphia, WB Saunders, 1985.

O'Boyle CM, Davis DK, Russo BA, et al: *Emergency Care—The First 24 Hours*. E. Norwalk, CT, Appleton-Century-Crofts, 1985.

Palmer PN: Advanced hemodynamic assessment. *Dimensions Crit Care Nurs* 1982; 1:139–144.

Quaal S: *Comprehensive Intra-aortic Balloon Pumping*. St. Louis, CV Mosby, 1984.

Saxton DF: *Addison-Wesley Manual of Nursing Practice*. Menlo Park, CA, Addison-Wesley, 1983.

Scordo K: Hemodynamic monitoring. *Nursing 85* 1985; 15:40–42.

Shoemaker WC, Thompson WL, Holbrook PR: *Textbook of Critical Care*. Philadelphia, WB Saunders, 1984.

Thomas CL (ed): *Taber's Cyclopedic Medical Dictionary*, ed. 15. Philadelphia, FA Davis, 1985.

Trunkey DT, Lewis FR: *Current Therapy of Trauma*. St. Louis, CV Mosby, 1985.

9

Pulmonary Artery Pressure Monitoring

Prior to the availability of invasive bedside hemodynamic monitoring devices, the clinician had only physical signs and symptoms to assess cardiopulmonary function and guide therapy. Unfortunately, clinical findings are typically physical expressions of changes that occur secondary to the initial defect and, as such, are not early or sensitive indications of rapid deterioration or improvement in function. For example, dyspnea, tachypnea, cough, adventitious lung sounds and distended jugular veins are late indicators of left ventricular failure which reflect secondary pulmonary edema and right ventricular failure. In addition, a lag time of several hours may occur between correction of the original disturbance and resolution of clinical findings. Therefore, the clinical picture may be misleading in the critically ill patient, who commonly has rapid changes in cardiopulmonary function. It would obviously be a distinct advantage to have a means of continuous, accurate and immediately monitoring cardiopulmonary pressures and flows for the purpose of diagnosis as well as guiding therapy.

The introduction of central venous pressure (CVP) monitoring in 1962 was the first step in direct cardiac monitoring at the bedside. In the absence of tricuspid valve disease, the CVP is a direct indicator of right ventricular filling pressure (preload). Through knowledge of this value, intravascular volume status and right ventricular function can be evaluated. However, in the presence of flow or pressure abnormalities at any point distal to the CVP catheter tip and proximal to the left ventricle, accurate evaluation of left ventricular filling pressure is impossible. Even given a normal channel from right atrium to left ventricle, correlation between right and left ventricular filling pressure is poor because CVP pressure changes are late to reflect left ventricular dysfunction. (See Chapter 8, Figure 8–1.)

Because the left ventricle is the prime mover of blood, an immediate and accurate means of tracking left ventricular function is essential in managing the critically ill.

The development of the balloon-tipped, flow-directed pulmonary artery catheter by Swan and Ganz in 1970 provided the opportunity for bedside assessment of left ventricular function (pulmonary artery wedge pressure), in addition to pulmonary artery systolic and diastolic pressures. Thus diseases affecting the pulmonary circulation did not prohibit diagnosis of left ventricular dysfunction. Indeed, it now became possible to distinguish cardiogenic from noncardiogenic pulmonary edema.

Several refinements and modifications of the original double-lumen catheter have since been developed. With the more sophisticated catheters, it is now possible to determine cardiac output simply and accurately, record right atrial pressure and, with the parameters obtained, calculate pulmonary and systemic vascular resistance, and monitor mixed venous oxygen saturation as well as pace the atrium and/or ventricles.

However, the utility of this sophisticated monitoring device is only as good as the ability of the clinician to interpret the values and utilize the information to form an active therapeutic plan.

INDICATIONS

The anticipated benefits of any diagnostic, therapeutic, or monitoring modality must clearly outweigh anticipated risks and expense. There is no absolute rule defining the need for the pulmonary artery catheter. Each individual patient circumstance must be carefully considered. Overall, pulmonary artery catheters tend to be more liberally used in teaching-research facilities and more conservatively used in smaller community hospitals.

Generally, the pulmonary artery catheter is indicated in patients in whom cardiopulmonary pressures, flows, and circulating volume require precise, intensive management. Therapeutic goals guided by information obtained from these devices are to 1) maximize cardiac output and tissue oxygenation; and 2) relieve or prevent pulmonary abnormalities such as pulmonary edema.

The general indications for pulmonary artery pressure monitoring are presented in Table 9–1.

CATHETER DESIGN

Catheters are available in a number of sizes suitable for adult and pediatric patients. They range from 60 to 110 cm in length and 4.0 to 7.5 French in caliber. Balloon inflation volumes range from 0.5 to 1.5 ml; the balloon diameters range from 8 to 13 mm. The catheter material is polyvinylchloride, which is pliable at room temperature and will soften further at body temperature. The shaft of the catheter is marked at 10 cm increments by black bands; these aid in determining the location of the catheter tip during

TABLE 9–1. General Indications for Pulmonary Artery Pressure Monitoring

Assessment of Cardiovascular Status and Response to Therapeutic Interventions in:
Complicated myocardial infarction
Cardiogenic shock
Congestive heart failure
Structural defects, such as acute ventricular septal defect
Right ventricular infarction
Valvular dysfunction or disease
Cardiac tamponade/effusion
Pericardial constriction
Perioperative monitoring of the cardiac surgical patient
Shock: All Types if Severe or Prolonged
Assessment of Pulmonary Status and Response to Therapeutic Interventions in:
Cardiogenic or noncardiogenic pulmonary edema (ARDS)
Acute respiratory failure (COPD in crisis, pulmonary embolism, etc.)
Assessment of Fluid Requirements in:
Severe, multiple trauma
Acute renal failure
Large area, deep partial, or full thickness burns
Sepsis
Perioperative Monitoring of Surgical Patients with Major Systems Malfunction

insertion. For example, when the catheter is inserted via the internal jugular vein, advancement to the level of the right ventricle is usually achieved at the 15 to 20 cm mark.

Numerous models offer a wide range of clinical application. In its simplest form, the catheter contains two lumens; one is for transmission of pressures from the catheter tip in the pulmonary artery, the other for balloon inflation. Other more sophisticated models have additional lumina for the purpose of IV infusions, monitoring right atrial pressures, atrial/ventricular pacing, thermodilution cardiac output studies, and/or continuous *in vivo* monitoring of mixed venous oxygen saturation. Catheters are also available with heparin coating, which may reduce catheter related thrombus formation.

The most commonly used catheter for adults is the quadruple-lumen, thermodilution catheter (Fig. 9–1). The distal (PA) port (*A*) opens to a lumen that runs the length of the catheter to terminate at the tip and is used to measure pulmonary artery pressures and pulmonary artery wedge pressures (PWP). Mixed venous blood samples may also be drawn from the distal lumen when the catheter is in the pulmonary artery. Drugs and caustic or hyperosmotic solutions should not be administered through the PA port because a selective and concentrated infusion into a small pulmonary artery segment may result in an untoward local vascular or tissue reaction. The balloon inflation port (*B*) opens to a lumen that terminates within the balloon. The proximal (RA) port (*C*) opens to a lumen that terminates 30 cm from the tip of the catheter. This opening is in the right atrium when the tip of the catheter is in the pulmonary artery. The RA port may be used to monitor RA pressure, administer IV fluids or medications, sample right atrial blood, and receive the injectate solution used for cardiac output studies. The RA port

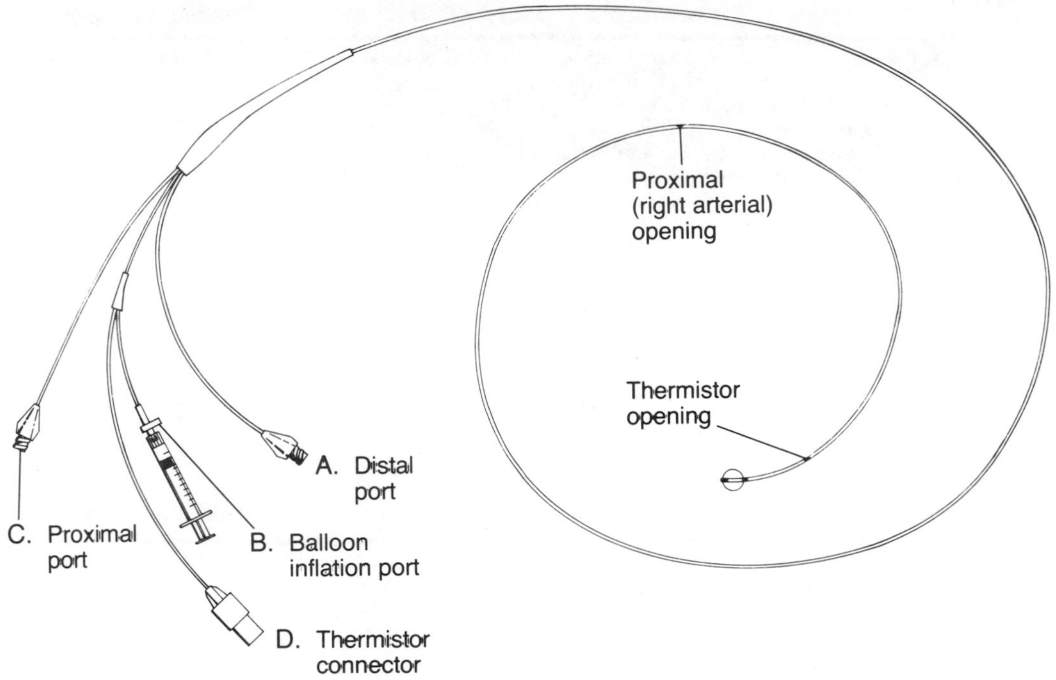

FIGURE 9–1. The #7 French quadruple lumen, thermodilution pulmonary artery catheter.

should not be used for infusion of vasoactive drugs if cardiac output studies are being considered. The thermister port *(D)* incorporates a temperature-sensitive wire that terminates approximately 4 to 6 cm proximal to the tip of the catheter.

METHODS OF INSERTION AND ACCESS SITES

There is no *ideal* method or site for pulmonary artery catheter insertion. Although the method and site are frequently determined by the operator's preference and personal expertise, patient-related factors such as age, body build, areas of regional trauma or burns, the anticipated duration of catheterization, and specific clinical circumstances, such as coagulation or perfusion abnormalities, anticoagulation, and severe pulmonary hypertension, should weigh heavily in the decision making.

There are two approaches for gaining vascular access: (1) the *percutaneous approach:* Following creation of a puncture wound, a sheath introducer is inserted over a guide wire, providing a conduit for the catheter to pass into the lumen of the vein. This approach is commonly used for catheter insertion into the central veins such as the internal jugular or subclavian veins. (2)

The *cutdown approach*. A catheter is directly placed into a surgically isolated, exposed vein. This approach is commonly employed when accessing the basilic or cephalic veins.

When possible, a percutaneous approach is preferable to cutdown because of the increased risk of infection from the latter. When the catheter cannot easily be placed at any given site, rather than risking complications another site should be considered.

The sites used for pulmonary artery catheterization are the same as those used for central venous catheterization (see Table 8–3 and Figure 8–2).

PREPARATION AND SETUP

A very important, often overlooked part of the procedure is patient and family teaching, as well as obtaining informed consent. In the rush and pressure of the critical care environment, one may tend to focus on the technology and equipment so that the patient as a person, as well as the family, is forgotten. The patient is generally acutely ill; thus, the fear of disability and death is present. An invasive procedure that directly involves the heart reinforces the extraordinary nature of the illness. Any discussion with the patient and family should focus on the improved diagnostic, assessment, and treatment/response potentials. Fears and misconceptions should be identified and discussed. A confused or comatose state does not obviate the need to talk to the patient and explain what is being done. The caregiver's touch and voice may be the patient's only contact with reality. On the other hand, a very restless patient may require sedation to limit movement during catheter insertion.

Required Equipment

The specific equipment and setup may vary among institutions. Generally, as experience is gained with pulmonary arterial catheterization, physicians and hospital staff adopt a setup that they find most efficient and with which they are most comfortable.

Chapter 8 (Table 8–4) lists the equipment required for accessing a central vein. In addition the following equipment is required for pulmonary artery catheter insertion and maintenance:

- An IV pole and mainfold
- Sterile three-way stopcocks (5 for monitoring only PA pressure and 7 if PA and RA pressures are monitored)
- A bag of irrigating solution containing 1 to 2 units of heparin per ml of solution (the amount varies with institutions). Normal saline is preferable to dextrose solution because growth of microorganisms of the Enterobacteriaceae group is enhanced by sugar. If a continuous flush device is used for irrigation, macrodrip IV tubing should be utilized instead of microdrip

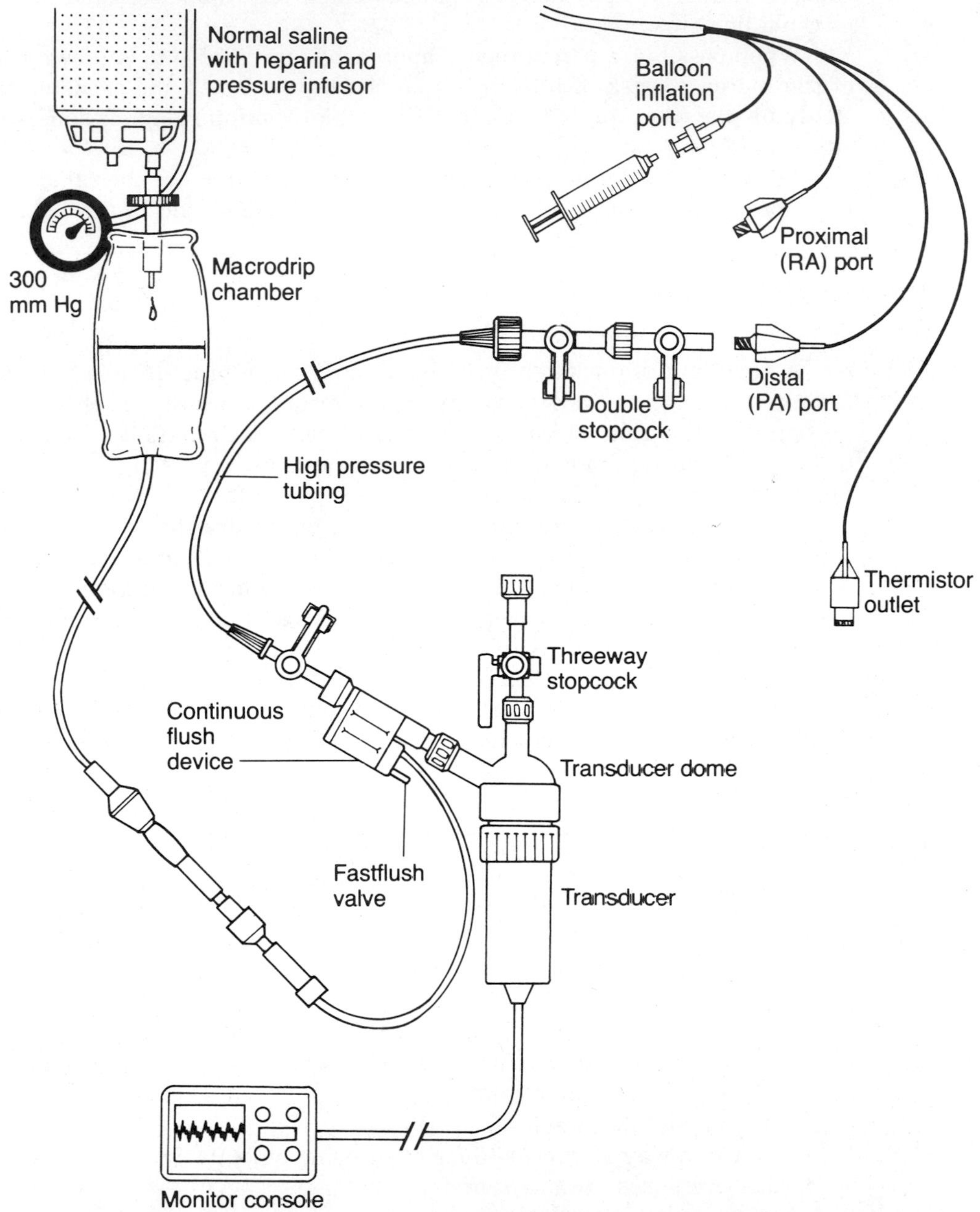

FIGURE 9–2. The components of the pulmonary artery catheter monitoring system. (Adapted from Smith RN: Invasive pressure monitoring. Am J Nurs 1978; 9:1514–1521.)

tubing because of the decreased likelihood of system contamination with air bubbles.

- One transducer with the monitor switch turned *on*. Allow 15 minutes for the transducer to warm up.
- Pressurized connecting tubing
- A small sterile cup or basin of sterile saline to test balloon integrity

Figure 9–2 illustrates the components of the pressure monitoring system.

INSERTION AND FLOTATION

Insertion

Typically, the catheter is advanced at the bedside. However, pulmonary artery catheterization may be performed in any area of the hospital where monitoring and cardiopulmonary resuscitation equipment is available. Whereas each institution or physician has a preferred uniform protocol for insertion, the following principles are generally applicable.

Familiarity with the catheter manufacturer's directions and specifications is mandatory prior to the beginning of the procedure.

Physical assessment and vital signs are obtained immediately before the procedure begins and reevaluated any time during insertion if a change is suspected in the patient's condition.

If the clinical situation allows, an extubated patient should wear a mask to minimize site contamination from oral and nasal flora. All personnel participating in bedside catheter insertion should be dressed in full surgical scrub. Those circulating in the room should wear caps and masks. There is clearly no risk associated with this dress and the added expense is minimal. The benefit of reducing the risk of sepsis in these acutely ill, and often immune-compromised patients, needs no elaboration.

Catheter testing and preparations are done while the patient is being positioned, prepped, and draped. This helps to minimize the time the patient must lie motionless, covered with drapes. The patient is positioned so that accessibility to the insertion site and patient comfort are maximized. Care must also be taken to clear the proposed work area of IV or other tubing, ECG leads, etc. These pieces of equipment are additionally secured so they will not shift into the sterile field during the catheter insertion procedure.

Testing and Preparation of the Pulmonary Artery Catheter. The sterile catheter is removed from its wrappings and the balloon inflated with air to the manufacturer's recommended inflation volume (0.5 to 1.5 ml), which is indicated on the catheter shaft. The balloon is then inspected for symmetrical inflation and protection of the catheter tip, which should be recessed in the center of the inflated balloon with the sensing tip exposed (Fig. 9–3).

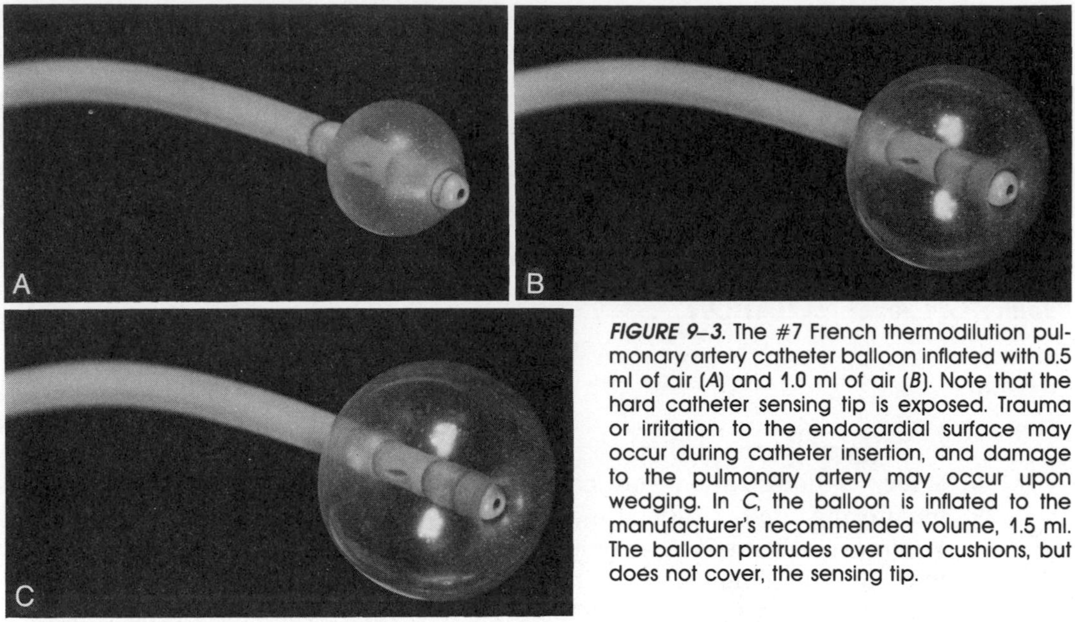

FIGURE 9–3. The #7 French thermodilution pulmonary artery catheter balloon inflated with 0.5 ml of air (*A*) and 1.0 ml of air (*B*). Note that the hard catheter sensing tip is exposed. Trauma or irritation to the endocardial surface may occur during catheter insertion, and damage to the pulmonary artery may occur upon wedging. In *C*, the balloon is inflated to the manufacturer's recommended volume, 1.5 ml. The balloon protrudes over and cushions, but does not cover, the sensing tip.

Fluids should *never* be used as a balloon inflation medium as they may be difficult to retrieve. In addition, the fluid-filled balloon is incompressible, which may stress the walls of the pulmonary vessels. In the presence of communications between right and left sides of the circulation, the patient is at risk for systemic or cerebral air embolization, should balloon rupture occur while in the cardiovascular system. If right to left shunts are suspected, carbon dioxide should be used for balloon inflation rather than air. Carbon dioxide is rapidly absorbed in blood, thus minimizing the risk of cerebral or systemic air embolization. Carbon dioxide also diffuses more easily than air through the Latex balloon. This reduces balloon volume at a rate of approximately 0.5 ml per minute. Therefore, if balloon flotation is significantly prolonged, balloon volume may be lost. When restoration of balloon volume is required, the balloon should be completely deflated before inflating it to its recommended volume to prevent overinflation and possible balloon rupture.

Balloon integrity is further tested by submerging it in a small amount of sterile water or saline and checking for air leaks. The balloon is then passively deflated by removing the syringe from the balloon inflation port. Removal of balloon gas with a syringe may pull the latex balloon into the catheter balloon inflation lumen and risks rupture of the balloon.

Stopcocks are attached to the proximal (RA) and distal (PA) ports. The proximal and distal lumens are flushed with heparinized solution with a syringe attached to one of the stopcock ports. The stopcocks are then closed to keep the flush solution within the catheter lumens.

The outside of the catheter is then wiped with a gauze pad soaked in sterile water or saline. Wetting the catheter prior to advancement helps to reduce vein irritation.

The stopcock at the distal (PA) port is attached to connecting tubing and the heparinized flush solution. These are then attached to the transducer which, in turn, is attached to the pressure monitoring unit. During insertion, the entire length of the catheter is continuously observed to guard against accidental contamination.

When constant observation of the oscilloscope is not possible, the ECG audiosignal is turned on to detect arrhythmias that may occur during balloon flotation. A defibrillator and xylocaine (Lidocaine) are present at the bedside.

Vascular Insertion. A discussion of vascular insertion techniques is not presented in this text. The reader is referred to other texts which give excellent step-by-step instructions for gaining vascular access.[1–4] To avoid complications, insertion must be performed or supervised by an experienced physician. Upon establishing vascular access, the operator introduces the catheter with the balloon deflated into the vein lumen. The distal (PA) lumen is then gently aspirated with the attached syringe to insure free flow of blood and then gently flushed with heparinized solution. The stopcock is then turned to open the PA lumen to the pressure monitoring system.

The catheter is gently advanced into the right atrium. This will usually require 40 to 50 cm (left) and 30 to 40 cm (right) from the antecubital fossa, 10 to 15 cm from the right internal jugular vein, 10 cm from the subclavian vein, and 35 to 45 cm from the femoral vein. Differences in patient size will produce proportional individual variations in these values.

The balloon is inflated upon catheter entry into the right atrium; however, some physicians prefer to inflate the balloon when the catheter tip enters a central thoracic vein. The stream of venous blood aids in directing the balloon, which acts as a sail, into the vena cava and right atrium.

Peripheral Insertion. The catheter is advanced with the balloon deflated until the catheter tip reaches a central thoracic vein. This is documented by respiratory induced fluctuations in the baseline. Should position of the catheter be in question (intrathoracic vs. extrathoracic), the patient is instructed to cough. A marked deflection in the baseline confirms position of the catheter in the thorax (Fig. 9–4).

Central Venous Insertion. The balloon may be inflated as soon as the catheter tip and balloon are introduced into the lumen of the internal jugular, subclavian, or femoral veins. Inflation of the balloon to its *recommended inflation volume* (1.5 ml for the #7 French thermodilution, 0.8 ml for the #5 French double lumen catheter) insures that the balloon extends over, but does not cover, the hard sensing tip, thus protecting the endocardial structures and pulmonary vessels from trauma during insertion (see Figure 9–3*C*). Inflation beyond recommended levels may cause balloon rupture. The bursting volume of the balloon is approximately 3.0 ml.

As the catheter passes from the central venous circulation through the heart, waveforms, characteristic for the chamber being transversed, are

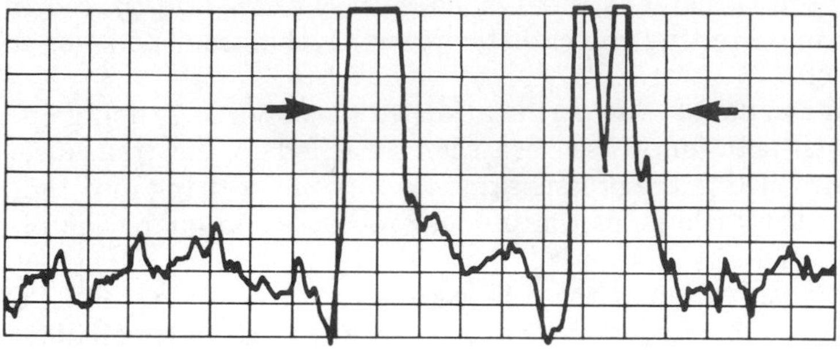

FIGURE 9–4. The catheter sensing tip, now located in the thorax, reflects the marked pressure changes occurring in the chest with coughing (arrows).

encountered. Correlated with the clinical picture and laboratory values, specific clinical judgments and actions can be based on the obtained pressure measurements and shape of the waveforms.

Flotation Through the Cardiac and Pulmonary Vascular Structures

Normally, the passage of the PA catheter from the right atrium to the pulmonary artery wedged position occurs within 10 to 20 seconds. In circumstances of abnormal flow patterns within the heart (tricuspid stenosis/insufficiency and pulmonic stenosis/insufficiency) or elevated right ventricular pressures due to pulmonary disease or low flow states (ischemic heart disease or shock), passage may take longer or flow-direction of the catheter may be difficult. In these special cases, fluoroscopy may be required for successful advancement of the catheter to the pulmonary artery.

The shape of the waveform and pressure values are noted upon entry into each chamber. However, if at any time the obtained values are in doubt, the monitoring equipment must be recalibrated and zeroed, and the lines flushed, lest important therapeutic decisions be based on incorrect information. It must be emphasized that patients in whom pulmonary artery catheterization is indicated frequently have cardiopulmonary dysfunction. Therefore, obtained values may be significantly different than normal values. Table 9–2 summarizes normal and altered pressure values.

Upon entry into the *right atrium,* the following waveform and pressures are observed (Fig. 9–5). The waveform is characterized by continuous oscillations in the baseline relating to *a* and *v* waves. Right atrial pressure is recorded with the monitor in the *mean* mode.

In the absence of tricuspid valve disease, mean right atrial pressure is equal to right ventricular end-diastolic pressure because when the tricuspid valve is open in ventricular diastole, the right atrium and right ventricle openly communicate; therefore, the right atrial *a* wave directly reflects right ventricular end-diastolic pressure. When the tricuspid valve is closed during

TABLE 9–2. Normal and Abnormal Hemodynamic Values

	RIGHT HEART PRESSURE PROFILE
	Right Atrium
NORMAL VALUES	0 to 8 mm Hg
INCREASED	RV failure secondary to left heart dysfunction: Mitral stenosis/insufficiency, left ventricular failure RV failure secondary to factors that increase pulmonary vascular resistance: Pulmonary embolism, hypoxemia, COPD, ARDS, sepsis, shock RV failure due to intrinsic disease: RV infarction, cardiomyopathies Cardiac tamponade/effusion Intravascular volume overload
DECREASED	Hypovolemia
ALTERATIONS IN RA WAVEFORM	Large *a* waves: RV failure, tricuspid stenosis, sporadic appearance in atrioventricular dissociation Large *v* waves: Tricuspid insufficiency
	Right Ventricle
NORMAL VALUES	15 to 25 mm Hg systolic 0 to 8 mm Hg diastolic
INCREASED SYSTOLIC PRESSURE	Factors that increase outflow resistance: COPD, pulmonary embolism, hypoxemia, ARDS, sepsis, pulmonary vascular volume overload due to left heart dysfunction or left-to-right shunts as VSD, or ASD
DECREASED SYSTOLIC PRESSURE	RV failure due to ischemic disease or myopathies
INCREASED DIASTOLIC PRESSURE	All factors that increase RA pressure
DECREASED DIASTOLIC PRESSURE	Hypovolemia
ALTERATIONS IN WAVEFORM	Pulse pressure narrow in severe RV failure, hypovolemia Damped-appearing tracing Pulse pressure wide in ASD or VSD
	PULMONARY CIRCULATION PRESSURE WAVEFORMS
	Pulmonary Artery Wedge Pressure
NORMAL VALUES	4 to 12 mm Hg
INCREASED	Left heart dysfunction: Mitral stenosis/insufficiency, left ventricular failure, decreased left ventricular compliance Intravascular volume overload Tamponade/effusion
DECREASED	Hypovolemia
ALTERATIONS IN WAVEFORM	Large *a* waves: Mitral stenosis, left ventricular failure. Sporadic appearance in atrioventricular dissociation Large *v* waves: Mitral insufficiency
	Pulmonary Artery
NORMAL VALUES	15 to 25 mm Hg systolic 6 to 12 mm Hg diastolic
INCREASED SYSTOLIC PRESSURE	Factors that increase pulmonary vascular resistance: Pulmonary embolism, hypoxemia, COPD, ARDS, sepsis, shock
INCREASED DIASTOLIC PRESSURE	All factors that increase PA systolic pressure: Intravascular volume overload, left heart dysfunction of any cause; LV failure, mitral stenosis/insufficiency, decreased LV compliance (altered volume-pressure relationship) Cardiac tamponade/effusion
PULMONARY ARTERY SYSTOLIC AND DIASTOLIC PRESSURE DECREASED	Hypovolemia
ALTERATIONS IN WAVEFORM	Retrograde *v* waves may distort the PA pressure waveform in acute or severe mitral regurgitation Pulse pressure narrow in tamponade or shock states Pulse pressure wide in VSD or ASD

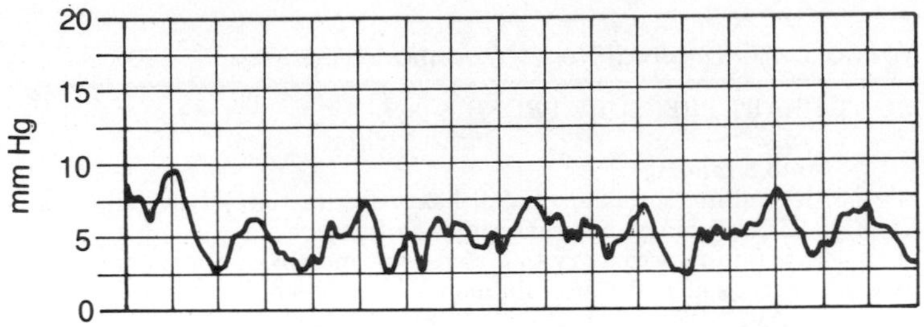

FIGURE 9–5. The right atrial waveform.

ventricular systole, the right atrial pressure associated with atrial filling, the *v* wave, normally rises to a level nearly equal to the *a* wave.

Once the catheter tip is in position in the pulmonary artery, right atrial pressure may be continuously monitored using the proximal lumen attached to a pressure transducer.

Directed by the flow of blood, the balloon enters the *right ventricle* at which time there is a dramatic change in the waveform and peak pressure (Fig. 9–6). The right ventricular waveform is characterized by a steep upstroke ascending to a peak pressure that is normally two to three times higher than the right atrial pressure. The sharp downstroke, without a dicrotic notch, dips and then reaches a baseline that directly records right ventricular end-diastolic pressure. As stated earlier, this is normally equal to mean right atrial pressure.

As the catheter traverses the pulmonic valve and enters the *pulmonary arterial circulation,* another change in waveform and pressure is noted (Fig. 9–7). The shape of the waveform is altered by the presence of a dicrotic notch, relating to pulmonic valve closure, and the recorded pulmonary artery diastolic pressure is higher than right ventricular diastolic pressure. Pulmonary artery systolic pressure is normally equal to right ventricular systolic pressure because the two anatomic areas are in open communication when the pulmonic valve is open. In ventricular diastole, however, the closed pulmonic valve seals off the pulmonary artery from the right ventricle. The increase in pulmonary artery diastolic pressure, compared to right ventricular diastolic pressure, relates to the correlated left atrial pressure added to the normal slight resistance to run-off of blood through the pulmonary vessels.

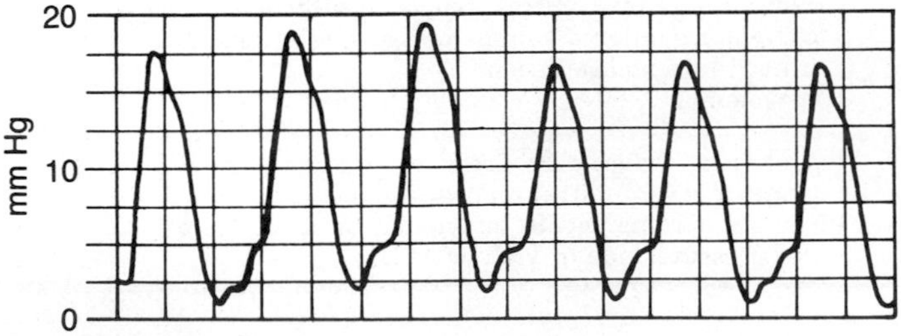

FIGURE 9–6. The right ventricular waveform.

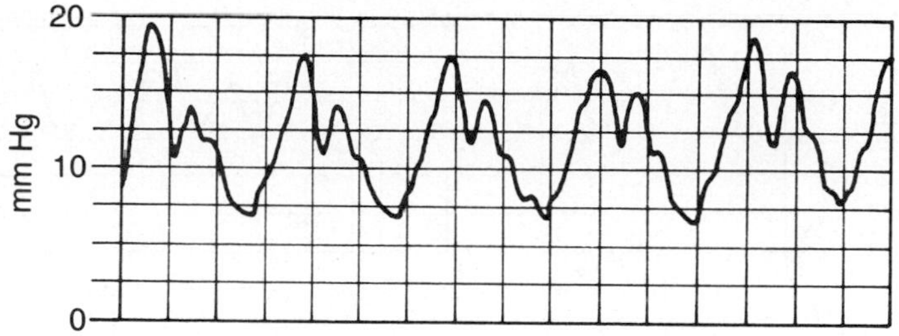

FIGURE 9–7. The pulmonary artery waveform.

The difference is slight, however, because the pulmonary circulation is normally elastic and of low resistance, and left atrial pressure is normally low.

In the pulmonary vascular stream, the inflated balloon continues to act as a sail and is directed into the more peripheral pulmonary circulation (Fig. 9–8). When the inflated balloon lodges (*a*) into a segment of the pulmonary artery that is slightly smaller than the inflated balloon, no blood flows distally to the balloon-occluded segment of the pulmonary circulation. This creates a non-moving column of blood (*b*) which is an extension of the non-moving fluid column within the pulmonary artery catheter and monitoring system. Blood in the non-occluded portion of the pulmonary circulation (*c*) continues to flow into the pulmonary veins and left heart. The catheter sensing tip will record the pressure at the first junction (*d*) where vessels from the occluded and non-

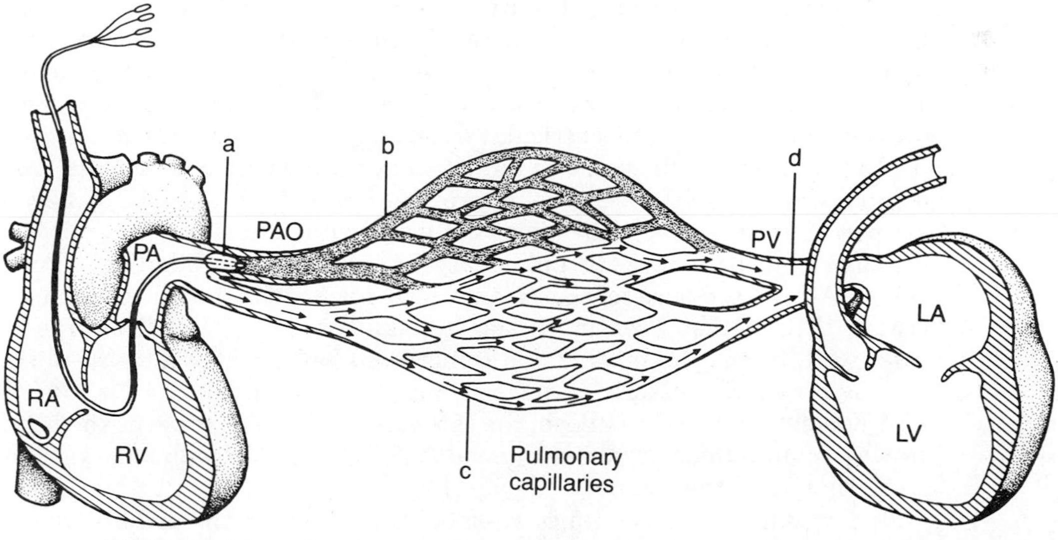

FIGURE 9–8. Schematic representation of the pulmonary artery catheter in the wedged position. From its position in a small occluded segment of the pulmonary circulation, the pulmonary artery catheter in the wedged position allows the electronic monitoring equipment to "look through" a nonactive segment of the pulmonary circulation to the hemodynamically active pulmonary veins and left atrium.

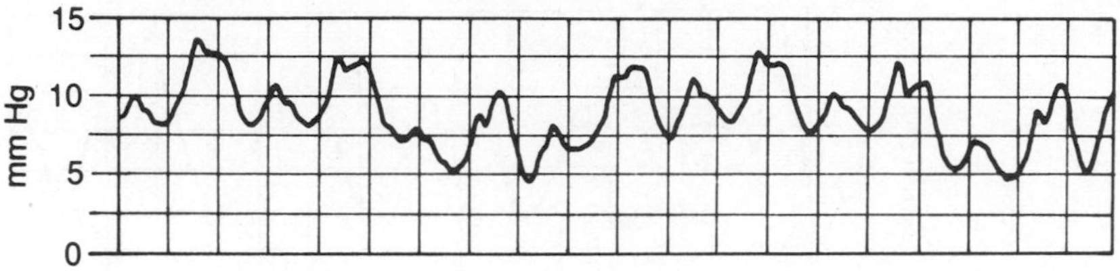

FIGURE 9–9. The pulmonary artery wedge (PWP) waveform.

occluded portion of the pulmonary circulation merge, the pulmonary veins. The catheter sensing tip, therefore, will record the pressure (transmitted backward) from the pulmonary veins which are the next active portion of the pulmonary circulation sensed by the catheter. Hemodynamic events in the pulmonary veins reflect left atrial activity; therefore, as long as there is an open column of blood without flow from the catheter tip to the pulmonary veins, the clinician has a means of assessing left atrial activity at the bedside. Wedging of the catheter, therefore, is associated with a dramatic change from the pulmonary artery waveform to a low amplitude, phasic (*a* and *v* waves) tracing that relates to left atrial pulsations (Fig. 9–9).

When the mitral valve is open in ventricular diastole, there is no obstruction from the catheter tip to the filling left ventricle. Therefore, left ventricular diastolic pressure is also measurable. When the mitral valve closes in ventricular systole, the catheter sensing tip records only the left atrial *v* wave, which relates to left atrial filling against the closed mitral valve, and normally produces no significant pressure change. Consequently, the mean pulmonary artery wedged pressure reflects mean left atrial pressure which in turn reflects left ventricular diastolic pressure (Fig. 9–10).

The balloon should not be allowed to remain inflated in the occluded position beyond 15 seconds or two to three respiratory cycles. Inflation beyond that period of time risks ischemia of the lung segment distal to the catheter, particularly in patients with pulmonary hypertension. In addition, artifactually elevated pressure measurements may result with prolonged wedging because 1) the catheter sensing tip may protrude beyond the balloon into the vessel wall; and 2) the inflated and compressed balloon may alter its shape, thus covering and pressurizing the sensing tip of the catheter.

Upon deflation of the balloon, the catheter recoils back towards the hilum into the main pulmonary artery (usually right), and the pulmonary artery waveform should immediately reappear.

If a wedge tracing continues after balloon deflation, the catheter should be carefully withdrawn by the physician until the recommended balloon inflation volume produces a wedge tracing. If 1.5 ml fails to produce a wedge tracing and the balloon is felt to be intact, the catheter may have slipped back and should be advanced slowly with the balloon inflated.

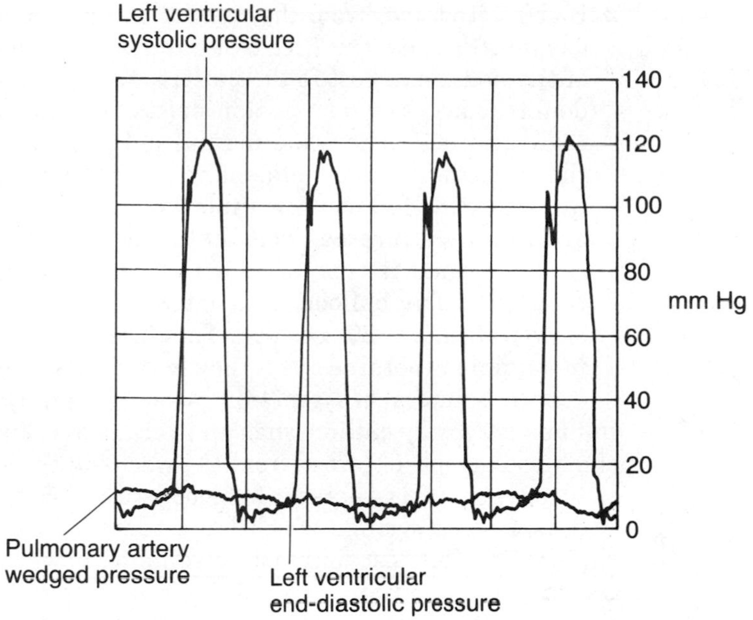

FIGURE 9–10. Simultaneously obtained left ventricular pressure waveform superimposed on the pulmonary artery wedged pressure waveform. Note that the left ventricular end-diastolic pressure, in this middle-aged woman with a normal heart, is equal to mean PWP.

Techniques to Document a True Wedged Position

Following attainment of the wedged reading during insertion, or at any time a wedged reading is in question, the following criteria may be used to verify a true wedge position.

- The pulmonary artery pressure trace flattens to a characteristic left atrial pressure trace immediately upon balloon reinflation (Fig. 9–11). Distinct *a* and *v* waves may not be present; however, an oscillating baseline should be visible. With balloon deflation, the pulmonary artery pressure waveform should immediately return. A significantly less than recommended balloon inflation volume that produces a wedge trace (less than 1.0 to 1.25 ml for a thermodilution catheter) implies that the catheter tip is placed too far peripherally.
- The mean pulmonary artery wedge pressure is lower than the mean pulmonary artery pressure or pulmonary artery diastolic pressure. The pulmonary artery wedge pressure is *never* higher than pulmonary artery diastolic pressure and it represents an artifact if it should occur.

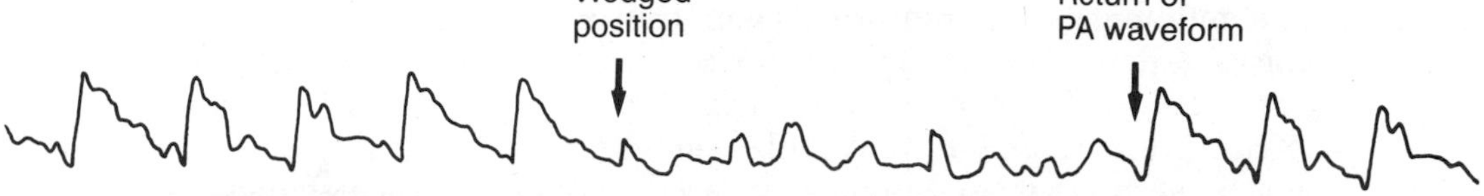

FIGURE 9–11. Balloon inflation stops when the PA tracing flattens to a characteristic left atrial pressure trace (arrow). Upon deflation of the balloon, the PA waveform reappears.

- Blood withdrawn from the wedged catheter should be fully saturated with oxygen. Because the first two criteria are generally reliable, and because of the additional cost to the patient, this procedure is performed only when doubt about catheter position exists such as when giant *v* waves (mitral regurgitation) distort the normal pulmonary artery wedge trace, creating the appearance of a pulmonary artery waveform. Blood samples are obtained in the following manner: With the balloon inflated, 2 ml of blood are rapidly aspirated from the distal (PA) lumen and then discarded. A second syringe is then filled with 2 ml of blood, labelled *PWP aspirate* and then iced. The balloon is deflated and 2 ml of blood are aspirated very slowly (1 ml per 20 seconds). This first sample is discarded and a second 2 ml-sample is obtained very slowly and labelled *PA aspirate* and then iced.

Both samples are sent for blood gas analysis. Blood drawn from the pulmonary artery catheter has an average oxygen saturation of 75%, whereas the blood sample obtained from the wedged position should be fully saturated with oxygen. This represents blood drawn back into the pulmonary artery and aspirating syringe which has undergone oxygenation in the pulmonary capillaries. This test may not be reliable, however, if, in the wedge position, blood is drawn from areas of lung with significant shunting (atelectasis, consolidation from pneumonia) or when positive end-expiratory pressure is applied. In these circumstances, an artifactually low oxygen saturation will be reported. Conversely, rapid aspiration of blood may draw arterialized blood into the syringe when the balloon is deflated and the mixed venous blood sample is obtained. This will produce a false high oxygen saturation for the pulmonary artery blood.

The Pulmonary Artery Diastolic to Pulmonary Artery Wedge Pressure (PAd-PWP) Gradient

The pulmonary artery diastolic pressure (PAd) may be used to assess mean left atrial and left ventricular end-diastolic pressure in patients with a *normal* pulmonary circulation and mitral valve.

In diastole, unaffected by the right ventricular systolic thrust of blood into the pulmonary circulation, the catheter sensing tip in a main pulmonary artery is able to "see through" the pulmonary circulation, which has no valves, to the left atrium. In addition, when the normal mitral valve is open in diastole, the left atrium and left ventricle openly communicate. Pulmonary artery diastolic pressure is 1 to 3 mm Hg higher than pulmonary artery wedge pressure due to the slight resistance to forward blood flow imposed by the pulmonary vasculature. When the catheter is "wedged," there is no forward flow distal to the catheter tip, and the effects of pulmonary vascular resistance will not affect the wedged reading. However, estimation of left atrial pressure or left ventricular end-diastolic pressure from the PAd will not be accurate when pulmonary vascular resistance is elevated (hypoxemia, acidemia, pulmonary embolism, chronic pulmonary hypertension). Indeed, the difference between PAd and PWP may be used as an index in assessing pulmonary vascular resistance. Generally, a PAd-PWP gradient greater than 4 to 5 mm Hg is indicative of increased pulmonary vascular resistance.

Rewedging Protocol

The frequency with which PWP measurements are done will depend on the clinical situation and degree of hemodynamic instability in the given patient. If there is a known good correlation between the PAd and PWP, the PAd may be used to track left atrial pressure and/or left ventricular function. This will reduce the number of balloon inflations that may prolong balloon life and also reduce the risk of pulmonary vascular damage or pulmonary infarction. However, if factors known to alter pulmonary vascular resistance are present, the correlation of pulmonary artery diastolic pressure to pulmonary artery wedge pressure no longer exists, and PWP should be used in assessing left atrial pressure and left ventricular function.

For rewedging, the balloon is slowly inflated while the pulmonary artery waveform is being observed. Inflation is stopped immediately when the PA waveform changes to a PWP waveform. (See Figure 9–11.) Inflation beyond this point risks damage to the pulmonary artery segment. In addition, the distended, compressed balloon may cover and pressurize the sensing tip, resulting in inaccurate readings. Attainment of a wedged trace with less than recommended inflation volume (less than 1.00 to 1.25 ml for a thermodilution catheter) suggests peripheral catheter migration.

Postinsertion Protocol and Importance of Proper Catheter Insertion

Following completion of the insertion procedure, any unusual events (arrhythmia or difficulty in passing the catheter) are recorded along with the type of catheter used for insertion as well as the balloon volume used for flotation and wedging. A postinsertion chest radiograph is then inspected to document catheter placement and also to rule out pneumothorax. When in proper position, the tip of the catheter should not be evident beyond the silhouette of the mediastinal structures. Location beyond that point, together with wedging at decreased balloon inflation volume, indicates placement of the catheter too far into the peripheral pulmonary circulation and may have the following untoward monitoring and clinical implications:

1. Cardiac output measurements may be in error. The thermister should be located in a large, main pulmonary artery or a major subdivision to adequately sample the injected fluid bolus and estimate total cardiac output. If the catheter has migrated peripherally to a smaller pulmonary artery branch, the thermister sensing head may be against the smaller vessel wall or may receive a less than indicative sample of total pulmonary blood flow.

2. Damage to the pulmonary vasculature may occur. The tip of the pulmonary artery catheter normally lies in the right main pulmonary artery. Upon inflation of the balloon, the catheter rapidly moves forward until it wedges. If wedging is accomplished with less than the recommended inflation volume, the hard, unprotected catheter tip may impale on the vessel wall.

3. The catheter may spontaneously migrate into a wedged position.

4. Blood drawn from the pulmonary artery catheter for a "mixed venous specimen" may be contaminated with arterialized blood. Because of the decreased flow rates in the more peripheral vessels, even careful aspiration of blood might draw oxygenated blood from the pulmonary capillaries.

CLINICAL APPLICATIONS OF THE PULMONARY ARTERY CATHETER IN MONITORING THE CRITICALLY ILL

The pulmonary artery catheter is most commonly used in the prevention, diagnosis, and treatment assessment of circulatory failure (due to volume deficits, maldistribution of flow, intrinsic cardiac dysfunction) and pulmonary disorders such as pulmonary edema. Knowledge of the physiologic variables that determine cardiac output and fluid movement into the lung is prerequisite to effective patient management.

Assessment of Variables in Circulatory Function

The determinants of cardiac output are heart rate and stroke volume (see Chapter 2).

HEART RATE

Heart rate and rhythm are monitored routinely in all patients in critical care units. Disturbances in heart rate can be manipulated with drugs or cardiac pacing and adjusted to a level most advantageous for the individual patient.

STROKE VOLUME

Stroke volume, the volume of blood ejected by the heart with each beat, averages 60 to 130 ml. The relationship of stroke volume and heart rate to cardiac output is illustrated in the following equation:

$$\begin{array}{ccccc}\text{Stroke volume} & \times & \text{Heart rate} & = & \text{Cardiac output} \\ 70\text{ ml} & \times & 70 & = & 4900\text{ ml/min}\end{array}$$

In contractile failure, such as occurs in ischemic or fibrotic heart disease, a reduction in stroke volume is the fundamental defect in the equation:

$$\begin{array}{ccccc} \text{Stroke volume} & \times & \text{Heart rate} & = & \text{Cardiac output} \\ 50 \text{ ml} & \times & 70 & = & 3500 \text{ ml/min} \end{array}$$

In mild heart failure, a compensatory increase in heart rate may maintain cardiac output within acceptable levels while the patient is in a resting state.

$$\begin{array}{ccccc} \text{Stroke volume} & \times & \text{Heart rate} & = & \text{Cardiac output} \\ 50 \text{ ml} & \times & 98 & = & 4900 \text{ ml/min} \end{array}$$

It is obvious that a very important indicator of ventricular performance available at the bedside is stroke volume. This can be calculated by dividing cardiac output measured in ml by heart rate:

$$\frac{5000 \text{ ml Cardiac output}}{100 \text{ BPM heart rate}} = 50 \text{ ml Stroke volume}$$

Stroke volume is directly related to the degree of myocardial fiber shortening and reduction in circumferential ventricular size. This is, in turn, affected by preload, afterload, muscular synergy and myocardial contractility.

Preload. Preload refers to the volume or pressure of blood in the ventricle at the end of diastole. A more forceful ventricular contraction occurs in response to a greater degree of stretch (imposed by intraventricular volume) of the myocardial muscle fibers at the end of diastole, up to a physiologic limit. (See ventricular function curve, Chapter 4, Figure 4–12).

A means of measuring ventricular end-diastolic (filling) volume is not available for bedside use. In the *normal* heart, however, exists a good correlation between ventricular filling volume and ventricular filling pressure, which can be measured at the bedside. In the absence of tricuspid valve disease, mean right atrial pressure or central venous pressure (CVP) correlates with right ventricular filling pressure. In the absence of mitral valve disease, mean left atrial pressure and pulmonary artery wedge pressure (PWP) correlates with left ventricular filling pressure. In the absence of pulmonary vascular abnormalities, the pulmonary artery diastolic pressure also correlates with left ventricular filling pressure. For the diseased heart, the upper physiologic limit for improving left ventricular function usually occurs when a left ventricular filling volume produces a pressure of 15 to 18 mm Hg. Beyond that critical limit, the potential exists for decreasing ventricular performance as well as producing pulmonary congestion and edema.

PRELOAD MEASUREMENT AS A MEANS OF EVALUATING INTRAVASCULAR VOLUME STATUS. In patients with normal ventricular compliance and cardiac function, a simultaneous increase in pulmonary artery wedge pressure, right atrial pressure, pulmonary artery diastolic pressure, and cardiac output indicates an increase in intravascular volume. Conversely, a decrease in the above values indicates a decreased circulating blood volume. Thus intravascular volume changes are generally met with the same direction changes in intracardiac and pulmonary vascular pressure measurements.

INFLUENCE OF PRELOAD ON MYOCARDIAL OXYGEN CONSUMPTION. Myocardial oxygen consumption (MVO_2) increases in direct proportion to the diameter of the heart. For example, if heart size doubles due to ventricular failure, MVO_2 can be expected to double. This clearly has potential adverse effects on the ischemic-prone heart. If, however, intraventricular volume and heart size are reduced through the use of diuretics or venodilator agents, myocardial oxygen consumption can be expected to decrease.

From the above discussion, it can be seen that assessment of ventricular performance is possible by evaluation of ventricular filling pressure and its relationship to cardiac output. In addition, manipulation of ventricular performance and myocardial oxygen consumption is possible by pharmacologic and/or fluid therapy adjustments in preload. Overall, the *optimal* preload level for the left ventricle is that which produces an adequate cardiac output without causing pulmonary edema or worsening an ischemic process.

INFLUENCE OF ALTERED VENTRICULAR COMPLIANCE ON PRELOAD. In the diseased heart, ventricular filling volume and pressure may not correlate because ventricular compliance is altered and must be taken into account. As ventricular compliance increases (dilated cardiomyopathy), a large increase in ventricular filling volume may be accompanied by a small change in filling pressure. On the other hand, in the stiff, noncompliant ventricle of ischemic or fibrotic heart disease, the ventricular filling pressure will be increased disproportionately to the ventricular filling volume. Hence, a left ventricular filling pressure less than 12 mm Hg may be associated with a significant decrease in cardiac output in the diseased (acute myocardial infarction) heart, while values of 4 to 12 mm Hg are compatible with an adequate cardiac output in the normal heart.

INFLUENCE OF VENTRICULAR FAILURE ON THE VENTRICULAR FUNCTION CURVE. With ventricular failure, the output of the ventricle (stroke volume) usually decreases. Because the ventricle empties inadequately with each beat, the filling volume and pressure of the ventricle increase and are usually proportionate to the severity of failure. Patients with myocardial dysfunction, however, have only a small increase in stroke volume with increases in ventricular filling pressure, which are manifested by flatter, depressed function curves (see Chapter 4, Figure 4–12). Evaluation of ventricular filling pressure and its relationship to cardiac output, therefore, allows the detection of ventricular failure before clinical manifestations of heart failure are present. In addition, the efficacy of therapeutic interventions for impending or overt failure may be immediateliy assessed.

Afterload. Afterload relates to the resistance or pressure against which the ventricle must eject its contents. Afterload for the right and left ventricles is affected by pulmonary artery and aortic diastolic pressure, and the resistance to blood flow through the pulmonary and systemic circulations as determined by vascular tone. As afterload increases, stroke volume falls and myocardial oxygen consumption increases proportional to the increased pressure work of the heart. As afterload decreases, stroke volume increases and myocardial oxygen consumption decreases. Afterload is difficult to measure. However, measurements of systemic vascular resistance (SVR) and pulmonary vascular resistance (PVR), which are derived calculations and not direct measurements, provide a guide to the level of right and/or left ventricular afterload.

DETERMINANTS OF VASCULAR RESISTANCE. As described in Chapter 4, blood flow in the vascular system is primarily determined by two factors:

- The pressure gradient between the two ends of the system. The rate of flow is directly proportional to the inflow minus the outflow pressure gradient. A decrease in arterial pressure and/or an increase in venous pressure may reduce flow rates and have the potential to produce circulatory failure.
- The degree of resistance to blood flow through the vascular system. The resistance to flow is the result of friction between flowing blood and vessel walls. The diameter of the vessel is the principal factor determining resistance to blood flow; the rate of flow through a vessel is proportional to the fourth power of the radius of the vessel. For example, if vasoconstriction decreases the radius of an arterial bed by half, resistance to flow increases 16 times. As a result of this vasoconstriction, the arterial diastolic pressure proximal to the constricted vasculature bed will increase; however, flow distal to that segment of the circulation may fall predisposing to capillary underperfusion and tissue ischemia.

Systemic vascular resistance (SVR) is the average or total resistance to blood flow in the entire systemic circulation. Not measurable by direct means, SVR is calculated from pressure differences at either end of the circulation and measurements of blood flow. Clinically, this is done by dividing mean arterial pressure minus central venous (RA) pressure (the pressure gradient across the systemic vascular bed) by cardiac output (the rate of flow through the vascular bed). The result is multiplied by 80, a conversion factor for adjusting the value to the basic physical unit used to express resistance; dynes second/cm^{-5}. For this conversion, pressure in mm Hg is changed to dynes/cm^{-2} and flow in liters/minute changed to cm^{-3}/second. The formula for calculating SVR is:

$$\underset{\text{dyne sec/cm}^{-5}}{\text{SVR}} = \frac{\text{Mean arterial pressure} - \text{Central venous pressure}}{\text{Cardiac output}} \times 80$$

Given a patient with a mean arterial pressure of 90 mm Hg and a right atrial pressure of 5 mm Hg and a cardiac output of 5 liters per minute:

$$\underset{\text{dyne sec/cm}^{-5}}{1360} = \frac{90 \text{ mm Hg} - 5 \text{ mm Hg}}{5 \text{ liters/min}} \times 80$$

Normal values range from 770 to 1500 dyne sec/cm^{-5}. Decreased values suggest a generalized vasodilator reaction. Increased values relate to generalized vasoconstriction. This calculated value has diagnostic importance and may be used as a guide to therapy: vasodilator vs vasopressor therapy.

Factors that decrease SVR (decrease left ventricular afterload) include vasodilator therapy, hyperdynamic septic shock, cirrhosis, aortic regurgitation, anemia, and anaphylactic and neurogenic shock. Factors that increase SVR (increase left ventricular afterload) include hypovolemia, hypothermia, low cardiac output syndromes, and excessive catecholamine secretion.

When calculating SVR, it is important to remember that this value represents an average of the resistance of all vascular beds. It does not reflect regional differences in vascular resistance and blood flow. For example, significant increases in renal vascular resistance may occur without significant increases in SVR as cardiac output begins to fall.

Pulmonary vascular resistance (PVR) is the total resistance to blood flow in the pulmonary circulation. It is calculated by dividing mean pulmonary arterial pressure minus pulmonary artery wedge pressure (the pressure gradient across the pulmonary vascular bed) by cardiac output (the rate of blood flow through the pulmonary circulation) and multiplying by 80.

$$\underset{\text{dyne sec/cm}^{-5}}{\text{PVR}} = \frac{\text{Mean pulmonary artery pressure} - \text{PWP}}{\text{Cardiac output}} \times 80$$

For example, given a mean pulmonary artery pressure of 15 mm Hg, a PWP of 8 mm Hg, and a cardiac output of 5 liters per minute:

$$\underset{\text{dyne sec/cm}^{-5}}{112} = \frac{15\text{ mm Hg} - 8\text{ mm Hg}}{5\text{ liters/min}} \times 80$$

Because the pulmonary circulation is normally a highly compliant, low resistance circulation, values will be considerably less than SVR. Normal values range from 20 to 120 dyne sec/cm^{-5}. However, this variable may not always reflect changes relating only to changes in pulmonary vascular tone. For example, changes in left atrial pressure, which commonly occur in the critical care setting, will influence this calculation.

Factors that may increase pulmonary vascular resistance (increase right ventricular afterload) include pulmonary emboli, cardiogenic and noncardiogenic pulmonary edema, sepsis, acidemia, hypoxemia, idiopathic primary pulmonary hypertension, and congenital or valvular heart disease. Factors that may decrease pulmonary vascular resistance (decrease right ventricular afterload) include vasodilator therapy, as well as correction of oxygenation deficits or acidemic states.

Muscular Synergy. Muscular synergy cannot be evaluated at the bedside. However, it is known that the organized contraction pattern of the ventricle may be impaired by regional ischemia, conduction disturbances, ventricular aneurysm arrhythmias or ventricular dilatation; correction is directed at the cause and may vary from simple termination of a ventricular arrhythmia to surgical resection of a ventricular aneurysm.

Contractility. This describes the inotropic state of the myocardium which relates to the velocity and extent of muscle contraction regardless of preload and afterload. The slope of the ventricular function curve can be altered by changes in contractility. Positive inotropic agents (digitalis, dopamine, dobutamine) produce a steeper function curve and shift it upward while negative inotropic agents (calcium channel or beta blocking agents) produce a flattened, depressed function curve (see Chapter 4, Figure 4–12). Pharmacologic agents affecting contractility also have effects on preload, afterload, or both (see Chapter 13). Contractility cannot be measured at the bedside although the effects on the ventricular function curve and perfusion status of the patient can be appreciated.

Indexed Parameters in Assessing Circulatory Function

Body Surface Area. A person's size may affect hemodynamic parameters. For example, the heart's output suitable to meet the metabolic needs of a large body needs to be greater than that for a small body. It is known that cardiac output increases nearly in proportion to the body surface area. Therefore, as a more accurate means of assessing tissue perfusion, hemodynamic parameters may be *indexed* by body surface area. That is, flow rates measured in liters or milliliters are related to square meter of body surface area rather than the entire body. The average adult male weighing 70 kg has a body surface area of approximately 1.7 square meters. The body surface area for each individual may be obtained by the use of a nomogram such as the DuBois Body Surface Chart which utilizes height and weight to calculate body surface area (see Chapter 10, Figure 10–1).

Cardiac Index (CI). This calculated value provides the means by which cardiac output of different persons can be compared with each other, eliminating the variable of differences in body weight. Clearly, a cardiac output of 4 liters per min. may be quite adequate for a resting, elderly female weighing 95 pounds, but would be inadequate for a young, resting male who weighs 250 pounds. Cardiac index is the cardiac output per square meter of body surface area; the average is 3.4 liters/minute/m^2, while the range is 2.5 to 4.2 liters/minute/m^2. Typically higher in youth and diminishing with age, at ten years of age it averages approximately 4.0 liters/minute/m^2, but at eighty years of age it averages about 2.5 liters/minute/m^2.[5] This value is calculated by dividing cardiac output by body surface area.

$$\frac{CO}{BSA} = CI$$

Assessment of Variables in Pulmonary Edema

In the absence of cardiopulmonary disease, pulmonary artery diastolic pressure, pulmonary capillary hydrostatic pressure, pulmonary venous pressure, left atrial pressure and left ventricular end-diastolic pressure are nearly equal. Knowledge of one, therefore, assumes knowledge of all.

Since pulmonary capillary hydrostatic pressure, as estimated by pulmonary artery wedge pressure, is the principal determinant of fluid shift from the pulmonary capillaries into the lung tissue and alveoli, knowledge of this value is of major significance in the assessment and management of pulmonary congestion and edema. In people with normal plasma oncotic pressure and pulmonary capillary permeability, values below 18 mm Hg are almost always associated with dry lungs.[6] At values of 20 to 30 mm Hg, fluid enters the lung tissue and may be associated clinically with tachypnea, dyspnea, wheezing, crackles, and cough. With levels in excess of 30 to 35 mm Hg, florid pulmonary edema ensues and is incompatible with survival beyond a few hours.[6]

Several clinical exceptions to the tolerance of the listed pressure values are commonly encountered. Patients with chronic pulmonary hypertension, such as that due to mitral stenosis or insufficiency, may tolerate elevated pressure levels with considerably less fluid shift and, therefore, have fewer clinical signs and symptoms. On the other hand, patients with the adult respiratory distress syndrome (ARDS) due to increased pulmonary capillary permeability develop severe pulmonary edema with pulmonary artery wedge pressures in the normal range.

POTENTIAL PROBLEMS AND PITFALLS IN OBTAINING ACCURATE PRESSURE MEASUREMENTS

A number of clinical circumstances are known to produce errors or inconsistencies in obtained hemodynamic parameters.

Body Position

The patient is often placed in the supine position to measure hemodynamic parameters based on the assumption that this position is necessary to obtain accurate values. However, certain clinical circumstances, such as pulmonary edema or increased intracranial pressure, necessitate continued elevation of the head and thorax. In these situations, flat positioning of the patient may precipitate a crisis. Repeated position changes may also be disturbing to the patient and interrupt rest.

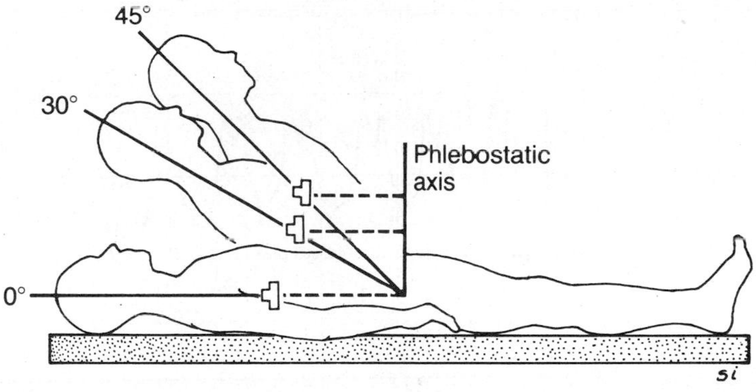

FIGURE 9–12. The air-fluid interface of the transducer dome must be leveled to the phlebostatic axis each time the level of the head and thorax is changed.

It has been shown that the backrest position may vary within a range of 0 to 20 degrees without markedly affecting pulmonary artery and pulmonary artery wedge pressure measurements.[7] If the patient's condition requires upper body elevation beyond this range, some inaccuracy in obtained values may result. However, directional changes in parameters are more important than absolute values. The important principle to remember is that the transducer air-fluid interface must be leveled to the phlebostatic axis each time the level of head elevation is changed (Fig. 9–12). Overall, technique should be as consistent as possible each time hemodynamic measurements are done.

Cardiac Dysfunction

Accurate interpretation of values may be difficult; the close relationship between pulmonary artery wedge pressure, left atrial pressure, and left ventricular end-diastolic pressure may not exist in the following circumstances.

Mitral Regurgitation. In acute or severe mitral regurgitation, the *v* wave associated with systolic regurgitant flow may make interpretation of the pulmonary artery wedge tracing difficult. In fact, the pulmonary artery wedge tracing may imitate the pulmonary artery tracing. To differentiate between pulmonary artery or pulmonary artery wedge, the ECG strip may be superimposed on the balloon-deflated and balloon-inflated tracings. The *v* wave of the wedge waveform will be located later in the cardiac cycle than in the pulmonary artery systolic wave (Fig. 9–13).

Left Ventricular Dysfunction. To insure optimum performance (which may still be inadequate), an impaired ventricle is very dependent on the atrial kick to maximize ventricular filling at end diastole. This may be associated with a heightened *a* wave on the PWP trace; however, the mean PWP and left atrial pressure may not increase proportionately with the

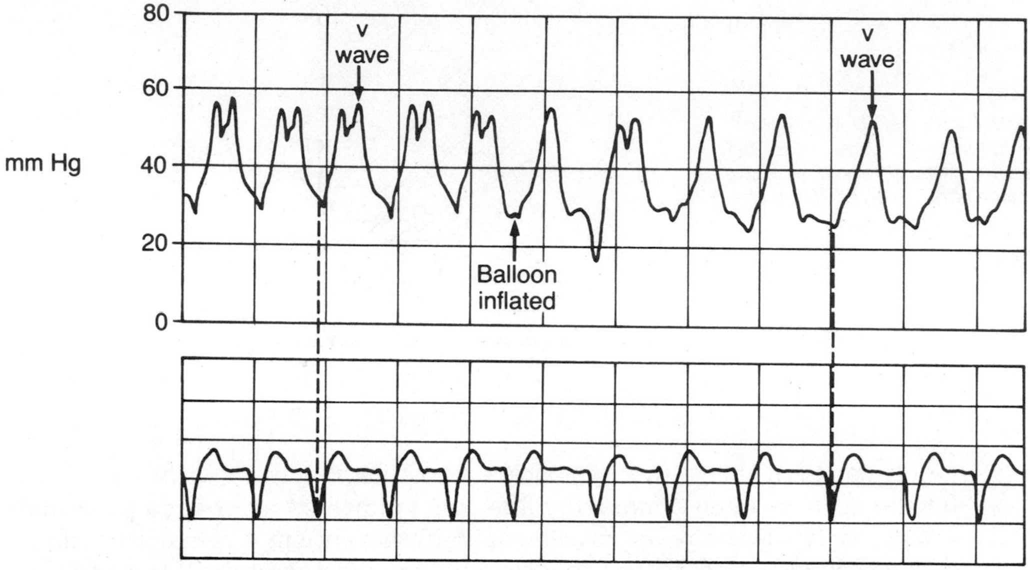

FIGURE 9–13. Simultaneous ECG and PAP and PWP pressure tracing in a patient with mitral regurgitation. Note the giant *v* wave distorting the PA waveform, thus giving it a notched appearance. Upon inflation of the PA catheter balloon, only the giant *v* wave is seen in the wedge position. The *v* wave is located later in the cardiac cycle than the PA systolic peak. (Courtesy of Cedars-Sinai Medical Center, Department of Hemodynamics.)

increased left ventricular end-diastolic pressure (LVEDP). The relationship of left ventricular end-diastolic pressure to PWP seems to become less reliable at LVEDP greater than 15 to 20 mm Hg. For example, at a very high LVEDP of 30 to 35 mm Hg, the PWP may be 5 to 10 mm Hg less. Whereas the mean PWP no longer accurately reflects the true LVEDP for monitoring purposes, this effect is physiologically desirable because left atrial contraction can increase LVEDP without a proportionate increase in pulmonary capillary hydrostatic pressure, thus limiting the risk of pulmonary edema.

In both of the above circumstances (mitral regurgitation, LV dysfunction), the pulmonary artery wedge *a* wave pressure closely approximates the true left ventricular end-diastolic pressure.

Mitral Stenosis, Left Atrial Myxoma. Obstruction within the left atrial chamber by tumor mass or a stenotic mitral valve precludes interpretation of left ventricular filling pressure. The measured mean PWP, however, is reflective of pulmonary capillary hydrostatic pressure, the primary determinant of fluid movement into the lung.

Catheter Whip (Fling, Noise)

Catheter whip represents an artifact, seen as spikes superimposed on the pulmonary artery pressure waveform, which may make accurate pressure measurements impossible. The following are possible causes of and remedies for this artifact.

Hyperdynamic Heart. In hyperdynamic cardiovascular states (early sepsis, catecholamine administration or excess), the force of right ventricular contraction may be sufficiently powerful to cause the catheter to pulsate within the pulmonary artery with each beat of the heart. This causes the fluid within the catheter lumen to vibrate, which records as a noisy tracing. Devices can be incorporated into the system that filter out the high frequency artifact.

Excessive Catheter Length. A loop of catheter in the right ventricle may cause pulsating catheter movement and related disturbances of the waveform. A reduction in the length of catheter within the ventricle may substantially reduce or eliminate the noise.

Location of the Catheter Tip near the Pulmonic Valve. The high velocity, turbulent flow in this anatomic area may produce a whip artifact. Forward flotation of the catheter by the physician to the right or left main pulmonary artery may eliminate this disturbance.

External Sources of Noise. If a length of catheter or connecting tubing lies across the patient's chest, precordial movements or movement of the thorax related to breathing, shivering, etc. may accelerate fluid within the monitoring system and create noise. The catheter and connecting tubing should be placed away from the area of movement.

If the whip artifact cannot be eliminated, the recorded pulmonary artery systolic and diastolic pressures are not reliable. The mean pressure is the least unreliable, and directional changes in mean pressure may be utilized as a guide to assessment.

Ventilatory Effects on Pulmonary Artery Measurements

Effects of Normal, Quiet, Spontaneous Breathing. Intravascular pressures within the thorax and intracardiac pressures are affected by the pressure on the outer wall of these structures, which can be assumed to be the same as pleural pressure. During normal, quiet breathing, inspiration and expansion of the lung requires a slight subatmospheric pleural (intrathoracic) pressure, while exhalation and deflation of the lung slightly increases pleural pressure. These cyclic changes in intrathoracic pressure are transmitted to the intravascular pressure tracing, creating a minimally wandering baseline whose inspiratory troughs and expiratory peaks relate to the respiratory cycle. The recorded mean PWP is minimally affected by these slight pressure changes. The pressure at end-expiration is referred to that of the atmosphere. At this time, there is minimal air flow and variation in pleural pressure to reflect on the catheter tip in the pulmonary vessel. Therefore, pressures obtained at end-expiration would not be contaminated by extravascular pressures.

Effects of Labored Breathing. If lung compliance is decreased (ARDS, cardiogenic pulmonary edema) or if airflow resistance is increased (bronchitis, asthma), much greater swings in pleural pressure are required to move air in and out of the lungs. As a result, the PAP and PWP baseline will fluctuate widely with ventilatory movements. If the PA systolic and diastolic pressures are obtained from a digital readout, the monitor will read the inspiratory troughs and expiratory peaks as the PA waveform follows the respiratory induced *roller coaster* excursions. This results in inconsistent and inaccurate recordings, which will make accurate interpretation of PAP and PWP difficult if not impossible.

To provide a stable baseline, it might seem reasonable to ask the patient to momentarily stop breathing at the end of a normal exhalation. If readings were taken at this point, intravascular pressures would not be contaminated by pressure changes surrounding the vessels and heart. Unfortunately, this may be impossible for the critically ill or dyspneic patient. In addition, most people hold their breath against a closed glottis (Valsalva maneuver), which increases intrathoracic pressure and produces a falsely high pulmonary vascular pressure measurement.

Reading PAP and PWP on the portion of the waveform that corresponds with end-expiration provides an accurate means of obtaining PAP and PWP measurements[8, 9] (Fig. 9–14).

The preferred method of identification of this point for measurement of PAP and/or PWP utilizes a calibrated pressure tracing taken from a strip-chart recorder. If a calibrated paper tracing is not available, end-expiratory pressure measurements can be obtained from a calibrated oscilloscope screen.

Other Pulmonary Variables That May Influence Pressure Measurements. Gravity influences the distribution and flow of blood in the lungs. Pulmonary artery pressures increase progressively down the lung whereas alveolar pressures are about equal throughout the lung. West's[10] zone model illustrates the relationship of alveolar pressures and gravitational forces to pulmonary vascular pressure and blood flow (Fig 9–15).

The uppermost portion of the lung is in Zone 1 in an upright human being. This is the apex, an area with potentially no pulmonary arterial blood flow because alveolar pressure exceeds pulmonary artery and venous pressures. In this circumstance, a wedged catheter that has, per chance, moved to the upper segment of the lung will not reflect left heart pressures since the catheter tip must have a patent vascular lumen to "look through" to the left atrium. Instead, the catheter tip will reflect only alveolar pressures. In reality, flotation upward would be an unusual event as gravity directs blood flow, and the inflated pulmonary artery catheter, downward. Zone 1 conditions may prevail over a greater segment of the lung, however, if pulmonary vascular pressures are decreased due to hypovolemia or if alveolar pressure is increased due to alveolar air trapping or mechanical ventilation, particularly if positive end-expiratory pressure (PEEP) is applied (see *Effect of Mechanical Ventilation*).

The center portion of the lung is in Zone 2. Here alveolar pressure is less than pulmonary artery pressure but greater than pulmonary venous pressure.

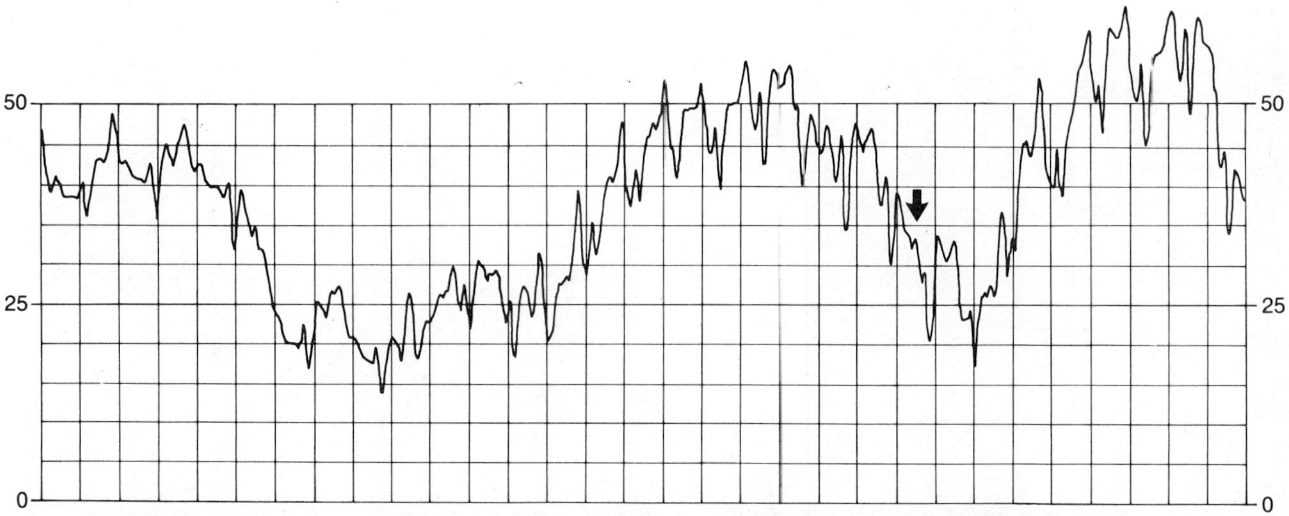

FIGURE 9–14. Marked respiratory variation in the baseline of a PWP trace in a 64-year-old woman with mitral stenosis. Note the marked negative deflection associated with inspiration and positive deflection associated with exhalation. The recorded PWP value is at end-exhalation (arrow).

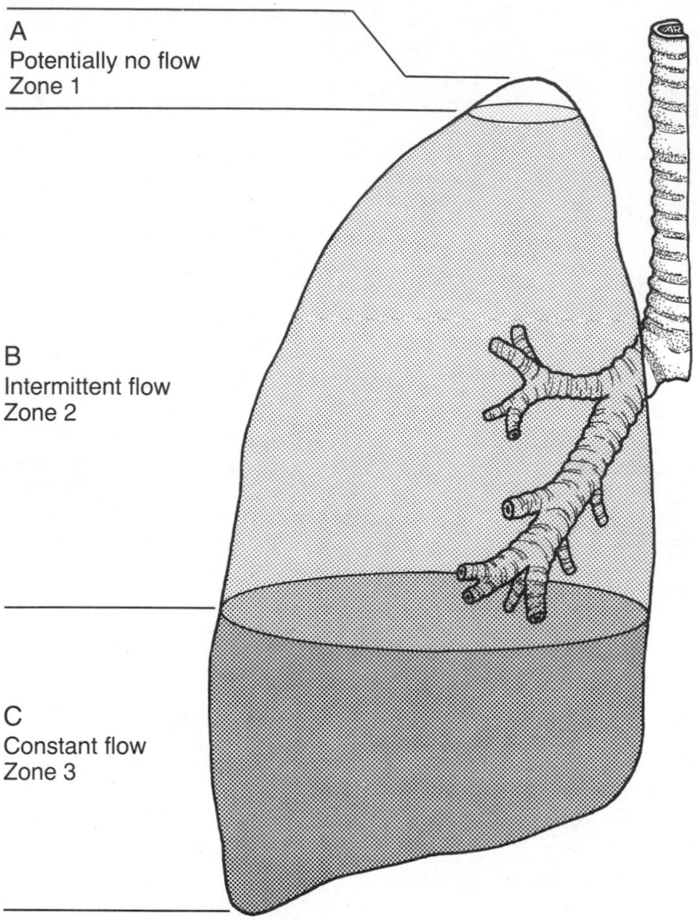

FIGURE 9–15. West's Zone Model: The Relationship of Alveolar Pressure and Gravitational Forces to Pulmonary Vascular Pressures and Blood Flow. *A*, Zone 1, The least gravity-dependent area of the lung where, theoretically, there is no blood flow because pulmonary artery and venous pressure is less than alveolar pressure. *B*, Zone 2, Pulmonary artery systolic pressure is greater than alveolar pressure, but alveolar pressure is greater than pulmonary venous pressure. Since pulmonary artery pressures (systolic and diastolic) and alveolar pressures (inspiration and expiration) are phasic, the changing perfusion/ventilation pressures allow only intermittent flow. *C*, Zone 3, The gravity dependent area of lung where, under normal circumstances, pulmonary artery and venous pressure always exceed alveolar pressures and blood flow is constant.

Note: These are not anatomically fixed zones but rather *functional* zones. Any anatomic part of the lung may take on the characteristics of Zone 1, 2, or 3 depending on alterations in hemodynamic (increased or decreased pulmonary blood volume and pressures) and ventilatory status (PEEP, CPAP, alveolar air trapping).

Since alveolar pressures are phasic, the changing intra-alveolar pressures could allow the Zone 2 wedged catheter to "see through" the pulmonary circulation during end-expiration and inspiration (when alveolar pressure is at its lowest point) and accurately reflect left atrial pressure. During expiration, however, the elevated alveolar pressure may pinch the pulmonary capillaries and veins, and the wedged catheter may register only alveolar pressure. This would produce an erroneously high mean PWP.

At the bottom of the lung, Zone 3, pulmonary artery and venous pressures are greater than alveolar pressure. A constantly open vascular channel from the PA catheter tip to the left atrium allows the PWP to reflect accurately left atrial pressure. In supine patients, most of the lung fulfills Zone 3 conditions.

Erroneous or inconsistent measurements may be due, therefore, to rewedging of the catheter tip in different parts of the lung, circulatory volume changes such as hypovolemia, and/or factors that increase alveolar pressures.

To insure Zone 3 conditions for accurate reflection of left atrial pressure by the wedged catheter, identification of consistent left atrial *a* and *v* waves should be possible. A damped wedge tracing suggests Zone 1 or 2 conditions if the fluid-filled monitoring equipment is known to be patent. A cross-table lateral chest film can determine a catheter position that is in question (high in the lung above left atrial level).

Effects of Mechanical Ventilation on Pulmonary Artery Pressure Measurements. The airway and pleural pressures for the machine-induced breaths are positive pressure breaths and are markedly different from those of spontaneous, normal breaths, which essentially represent negative pressure breathing. These positive changes in airway pressure reflect on the heart and vascular structures of the thorax. The more compliant the lungs, the more the positive airway pressures will be reflected on the cardiovascular structures. This has the potential to confound accurate measurement and interpretation of hemodynamic parameters for three reasons.

- The excursions of the baseline reflect the pressure fluctuations that relate to the ventilator mode used on the patient (Fig. 9–16). When the ventilator delivers the machine breath, the monitored PAP and PWP will increase. However, the pressure at end-expiration should be the same as with spontaneous breathing. Therefore, PAP and/or PWP should be measured at end-expiration.
- Mechanical ventilation has the potential to decrease cardiac output inversely proportional to mean airway pressure given that the effective circulating blood volume remains constant. Secondary to the increased average intrathoracic pressure and loss of the thoracic pump, there is a decrease in venous return to the heart and consequent reduction in ventricular filling volume. In addition, the positive pressure surrounding the heart may produce a tamponade effect on the ventricles, thereby further interfering with diastolic filling. Because of perivascular and pericardial compression, however, the CVP, mean PAP, and PWP may physically rise. Since intravascular volume, not pressure, is important in determining stroke volume, cardiac output may fall despite normal or elevated RA pressures or PWP. In other words, pressures that appear to be normal may be insufficient to insure adequate ventricular filling and cardiac output because the volume/pressure relationship has been distorted by positive pressure breathing.
- Positive alveolar pressure may increase Zone 1 and 2 conditions, especially if pulmonary artery pressures are low. If a Zone 1 or 2 condition develops, the PWP measured no longer accurately reflects LA pressure but is contaminated, entirely or partially, by alveolar pressure.

Patients with severe airways obstruction (COPD, asthma) tend to develop alveolar air trapping with hyperinflation and are particularly likely to increase Zone 1 and 2 conditions. The effects on pressure measurement are especially pronounced in the highly compliant lungs of the COPD patient because the elevated alveolar pressures are readily transmitted to the pleural space and cardiovascular structures. PAP and PWP may thus be deceptively high in the presence of a decreased ventricular filling volume.

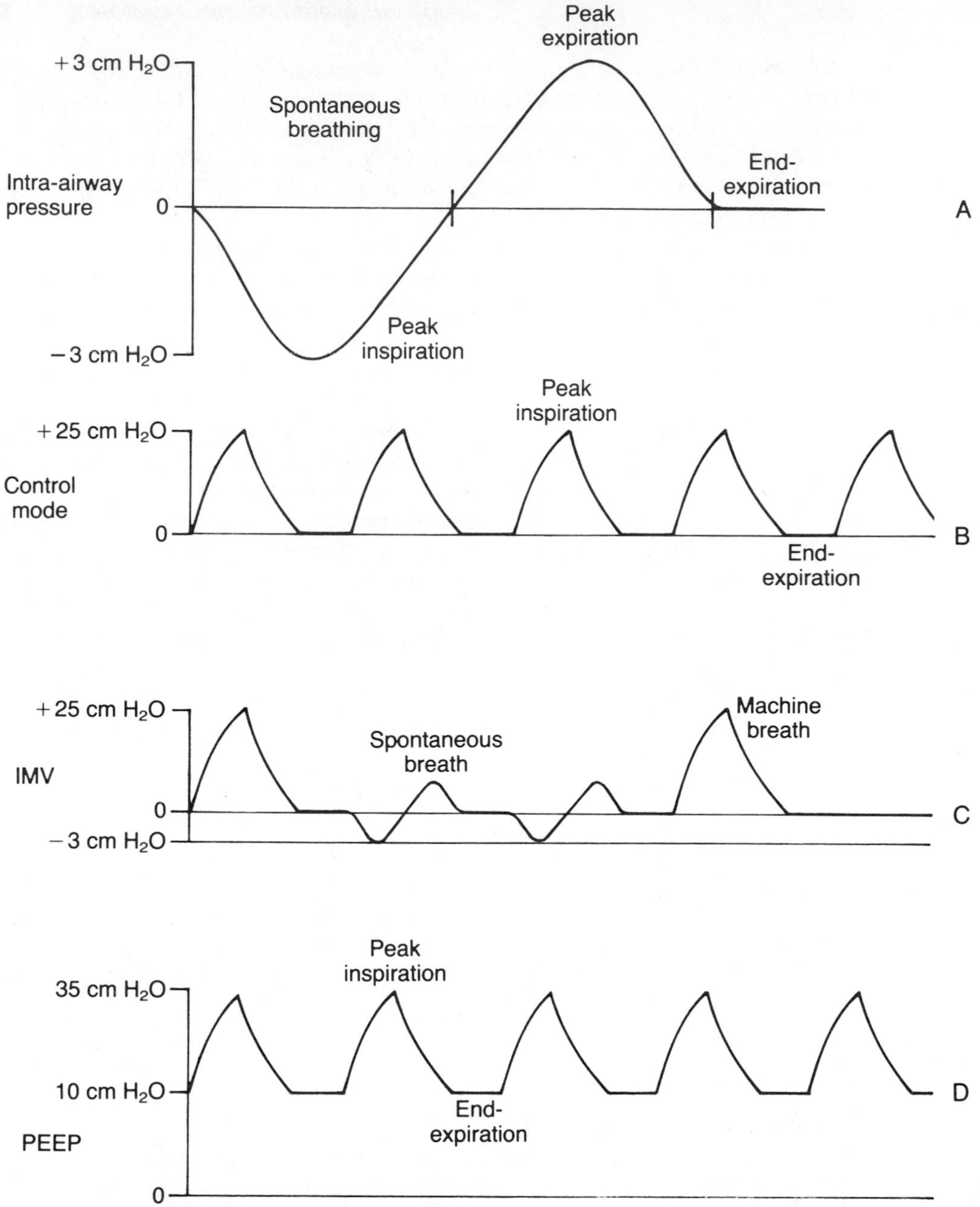

FIGURE 9–16. Airway pressure curves for spontaneous and ventilator (machine) breathing. *A, Spontaneous breathing.* A negative airway pressure draws fresh air into the lungs whereas a positive airway pressure forces expired air out of the lungs to the atmosphere. *B, Control mode.* Used for apneic patients, the ventilator completely determines ventilatory rate and tidal volume. A positive pressure pushes the prescribed tidal volume into the patient's lungs. *C, Intermittent mandatory ventilation* (IMV). The patient's spontaneous breaths are interspersed with a prescribed number of ventilator breaths. *D, Positive end-expiratory pressure* (PEEP). While being machine-ventilated, the patient's pressure at end-expiration is maintained at a positive value, most commonly in a range of 8 to 15 cm H_2O.

Effects of Positive End-Expiratory Pressure (PEEP) or Continuous Positive Airway Pressure (CPAP) on PA Pressure Measurements. If the patient has positive end-expiratory pressure applied from PEEP or CPAP, all of the effects on hemodynamic and pressure measurements described above will be exaggerated. One would expect that the intracardiac and intravascular pressures would be increased approximately porportional to the increases in pleural pressure. There are discrepancies, however, in the results of studies investigating the PWP/LAP/LVEDP relationship with the use of PEEP. The variability in findings may relate to differences in the ventilatory mode being used, intravascular volume, catheter location, individual lung compliance and the level of positive alveolar pressure. Generally, at PEEP levels of 10 cm H_2O or less, the PWP accurately reflects LAP and LVEDP. However, at levels of PEEP greater than 10 to 15 cm H_2O, there tends to be an increasing but uncertain disparity between PWP/LAP/LVEDP, as well as an increasing risk of cardiovascular compromise.

The following techniques have been suggested to insure more accurate measurements of LAP or LVEDP by wedged readings when the patient is being maintained on ventilatory support, particularly with PEEP or CPAP.

- Pressure surrounding the heart and vessels can be estimated to be one third to one half of alveolar pressure (1 mm Hg = 1.36 cm H_2O). This calculated pressure is then subtracted from the PWP measurement.

For example:

PEEP applied = 15 cm H_2O (11 mm Hg)
Measured PWP = 18 mm Hg
1/2 of 11 mm Hg PEEP = 5.5 mm Hg pressure surrounding the heart and blood vessels

Therefore,

18 mm Hg measured PWP
− 5.5 mm Hg PEEP applied perivascular and pericardial pressure
12.5 mm Hg true PWP reading

Because lung compliance and the effects of PEEP differ from patient to patient, reliability of this technique cannot be assured.

- In some institutions, mechanical ventilation or the use of PEEP is discontinued for the measurement of PAP or PWP. This technique has significant weak points. Because mechanical ventilation, especially with PEEP, produces pressure changes in the thorax which affect blood flow, removing the patient from the ventilator produces a sudden change in hemodynamics. Venous return is suddenly increased (autotransfusion effect), ventricular diastolic dynamics are changed, and PEEP-applied compression of the pulmonary capillaries is relieved. Thus, more blood empties into the left ventricle. The measured pressures then reflect a hemodynamic state that exists only when the patient is removed from the ventilatory support. One is interested only in the hemodynamic events while the patient is being properly supported. In addition, there is risk of suddenly overloading the left ventricle and pulmonary circulation. When CPAP or PEEP are removed, loss of alveolar stability and small airway collapse may immediately result in a precipitous decrease in P_aO_2, which may seriously threaten tissue oxygenation.

- The effects of PEEP or CPAP may be judged by measuring the changes in PWP or PAP with each increase in PEEP during the PEEP trial. Unfortunately, this only addresses the effect of applied extravascular pressure on the intravascular pressure measurements and does not take into account the additional factors of hemodynamic changes, possible pulmonary capillary compression by PEEP-distended alveoli, and the altered ventricular volume/pressure relationship.
- Measurement of intrathoracic pressure, using an esophageal balloon or a fluid filled pleural catheter with subtraction of this value from measured PWP, has been proposed. Unfortunately, differing areas of compliance in the lung may exert nonuniform pressures on the heart and vessels. In addition, this technique involves further invasive instrumentation with its associated risks to the patient.

In summary, mechanical ventilation, especially with high alveolar pressures, may interfere with accurate measurement and interpretation of hemodynamic data through two mechanisms: transmission of extravascular pressures to the intravascular structures and catheter tip and/or intermittent or complete obstruction from the pulmonary arterioles to the pulmonary venules by PEEP-compressed capillaries. The difficulties and uncertainties in measurement of true LA or LVEDP in this circumstance underscores the importance of evaluation of changes in pressure measurements and the relationship of these changes to alterations in clinical and laboratory data rather than reliance on a single absolute measurement.

MONITORING PROBLEM IDENTIFICATION AND SOLUTION

The absolute accuracy of the recorded pressure measurements is difficult to determine. Therefore, if consistency is used in obtaining values, and if waveform morphology and measurements are as anticipated for the clinical setting and do not change without apparent clinical reason, the measurements are accepted. Distortion of the monitored waveforms, inaccurate pressure measurements, or the inability to obtain pressure measurements may occur as a result of numerous factors.

Marked Changes in Pressure Measurements or Inappropriate Pressures

Numerical values that have suddenly changed and/or do not fit the clinical picture should be suspect for inaccuracy and investigated. Causes include:

Positional Changes. If the upper part of the patient's body has been raised or lowered, but the transducer has not been re-referenced to the phlebo*static* level (the standard anatomic reference level at which the catheter tip is assumed to be) significant errors in pressure measurements may occur. For example, for each inch the transducer is located *below* this level, an error of 1.86 mm Hg *above* the true reading will be introduced; conversely, a falsely *low* 1.86 mm Hg reading will be obtained for each inch the transducer is *above* the phlebo*static* level. This is particularly important when measuring pressures in the central circulation where an error of as little as 5 mm Hg may result in significant errors in diagnosis and therapy.

Inaccurate Static Reference Points (ie, zero and calibration). The zero reference point is established by turning the stopcock off to the patient and open to air (the transducer dome is open to atmospheric pressure). When checking the accuracy of the zero point, the protective caps should be removed from the venting ports. Otherwise, the protective caps may obstruct the port and prevent equilibration of the transducer to atmosphere.

The calibration point is tested by comparing the digital and oscilloscope display with a known pressure from a mercury column (see Chapter 6). Typically, a pressure scale and amplifier setting of 40 mm Hg is used for pulmonary artery pressure monitoring. To insure accurate hemodynamic measurements, an important principle to remember when setting up, zeroing, and calibrating the monitoring system is "garbage in = garbage out."

Inability to Obtain a Wedged Reading

If a wedge waveform does not follow balloon inflation with the proper amount of air, balloon rupture or retrograde slippage of the catheter into the pulmonary trunk or right ventricle should be suspected. A chest x-ray may be required to document backward slippage. Once documented, catheter advancement and redirection of the inflated balloon more peripherally by the physician allows rewedging.

Damped Pressure Tracing

If the amplitude of the waveform decreases (lower systolic pressure and/or elevated diastolic pressure), the patient should immediately be assessed for physiologic alterations such as shock. If it is determined that the patient's condition is stable, technical causes of a damped waveform should be investigated, including:

1. Air in the tubing.
2. Clotted blood at the catheter tip or within the catheter lumen. Inadequate line irrigation due to a leaky irrigation solution pressure bag (less than 300 mm Hg pressure) may predispose to clot formation.
3. Kinking or knotting of the catheter or tubing.
4. A loose connection with a small leak in the system. This may be associated with the appearance of blood backing up from the pulmonary artery catheter.

5. Incorrect calibration.
6. Spontaneous catheter migration into a near-wedged position.
7. Catheter tip positioned against the vessel wall.
8. Amplifier setting in the wrong pressure range, eg, a pulmonary artery pressure monitored at an arterial pressure scale (200 mm Hg) may appear severely damped.
9. A loose or cracked transducer dome or air in the dome.

No Waveform

The complete absence of a waveform may be due to:

1. Pulmonary artery transducer improperly engaged in the monitor outlet or engaged in the wrong outlet.
2. Defective transducer.
3. Large leak in the system—blood will very likely be backing up from the pulmonary artery catheter.
4. Loose or cracked transducer dome or air in the dome.
5. Stopcock turned to the wrong position.
6. Amplifier is on zero or off.
7. Catheter lumen or catheter tip is fully clotted.

After it has been determined that the altered waveform and/or pressure are not the result of physiologic changes, incorrect transducer reference point, incorrect amplifier setting, or faulty connection of cables to monitor, a systematic approach should be used to identify and solve the problem. This begins as simply and non-invasively as possible and with the most common sites of disturbance. If necessary, investigation may then proceed to more complex and manipulative approaches to trouble-shooting.

Problems are most frequently located within the fluid-filled portion of the system; therefore, the transducer dome and tubing are first inspected for the presence of blood, kinks (this may require removal of dressings), and air bubbles as well as tight fit at connection sites, appropriate position of stopcocks or defects such as cracks in the transducer dome. The pressure bag should also be checked for adequate inflation pressure—300 mm Hg.

If air bubbles or blood is seen in the tubing, the system is gently aspirated with a syringe until blood from the pulmonary artery appears. This insures that clotted blood or air has been cleared from the line. The line is then gently flushed with irrigating solution. Aspiration or irrigation should not be undertaken if there is a possibility that the catheter has spontaneously wedged because of the risk of damage or rupture to the distal pulmonary artery segment. If the transducer dome is the source of the problem, it is flushed of air or blood or changed if defective.

If the problem cannot be visibly identified proximal to the catheter, it may be within the length of the catheter, at the catheter tip, or may relate to catheter position. If gentle aspiration followed by flushing does not improve the waveform, the catheter tip may be resting against the vessel wall. Turning

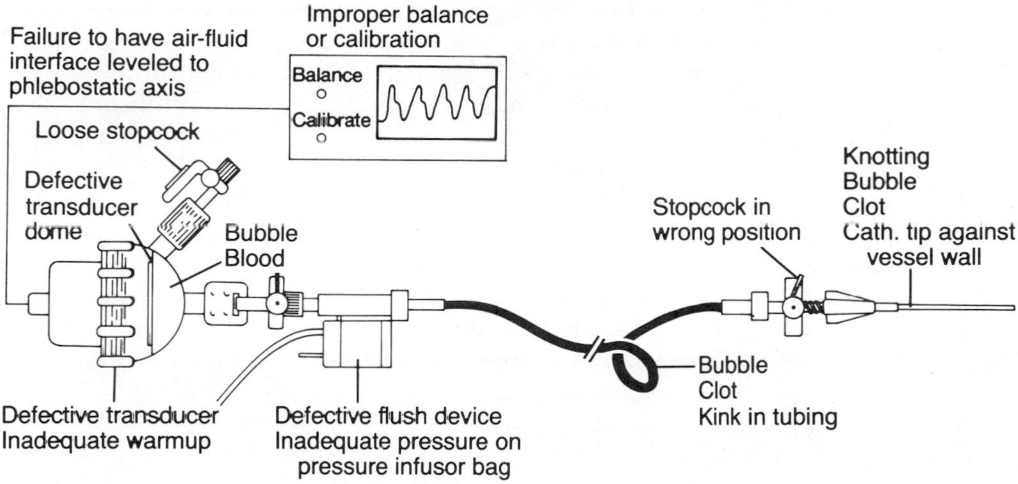

FIGURE 9–17. A step-by-step approach to problem source identification begins noninvasively with the most common sites of disturbance.

the patient to the left or right side, or patient coughing, may move the catheter tip away from the vessel wall. A fully clotted catheter (difficulty in withdrawing blood and inability to flush the line) frequently requires replacement. The catheter should not be force-irrigated because the obstructing thrombus may be propelled forward and become a pulmonary embolism. Spontaneous wedging, or kinks or knots within the heart or great vessels, may require chest x-ray for diagnosis. If spontaneous wedging is verified, the catheter is withdrawn carefully until a wedged waveform reappears upon balloon reinflation to the recommended volume. Intracardiac knots may be eliminated utilizing fluoroscopic manipulation of the catheter or may require removal of the catheter via transvenous or surgical routes.

If the fluid-filled components of the monitoring system are found to be free of problems, the monitoring instruments are checked. The present transducer is replaced by a transducer known to be in good working condition. The pressure transducer is a delicate and expensive instrument and deliberate care during cleansing and assembly can do much to maintain accuracy and prolong transducer life. If the original problem persists, the monitoring consoles are tested and exchanged. Figure 9–17 illustrates possible problem sites encountered with pulmonary artery pressure monitoring.

REMOVAL OF THE PULMONARY ARTERY CATHETER

To minimize the incidence of complications during removal, the catheter is withdrawn with the balloon deflated; withdrawal is never forced when resistance is encountered. Following catheter removal, the patient is watched for any changes in cardiopulmonary function.

Although the reported incidence of complications encountered with catheter removal is low, some may be associated with significant functional impairment or death. In one reported case, a thrombus was apparently stripped off the PA catheter during removal and embolized across a ventricular septal defect into the cerebral and coronary circulations.[11]

Owing to the small but very real potential for major complications associated with catheter removal, therefore, the author recommends that removal be performed only by a physician. While the insertion of a catheter may be an urgently needed procedure, its removal is not, and waiting the few hours until a physician is available has little clinical significance.

COMPLICATIONS

Any procedure that introduces a foreign body into the circulation introduces risks to the patient. The role of the caregiver in preventing complications relates not only to the purely moral issue of doing no harm, but also to reducing time and cost of the hospital stay. The following guidelines may contribute significantly to reducing the incidence of complications encountered with pulmonary artery catheterization.

1. Insertion and flotation should be performed or supervised by an experienced physician.

2. Scrupulous attention should be paid to manufacturer's recommendations for catheter placement and maintenance.

3. The pulmonary artery catheter should be used only as long as the patient's condition requires pulmonary artery pressure monitoring. The PA catheter should *not* be left in place as a venous access site or for central venous pressure monitoring.

All complications related to accessing central veins and line placement may occur with pulmonary artery catheterization. (See Chapter 8, Complications of Central Venous Catheterization.) The following are additional complications specific to pulmonary artery pressure monitoring.

Arrhythmias

Atrial and ventricular arrhythmias, due to irritation of the endocardium by the catheter, may occur any time during catheter flotation and maintenance. The incidence of arrhythmias, particularly ventricular ectopy, however, is greatest during catheter insertion. This underscores the importance of careful ECG monitoring during flotation and the immediate availability of equipment for cardiopulmonary resuscitation.

The incidence of arrhythmias is significantly higher in patients with predisposing conditions (acute ischemic disease, shock, hypoxemia, ventricular failure, acidosis, hypocalcemia, hypokalemia, hypomagnesemia, or digitalis toxicity). For this reason, whenever possible, arrhythmia risk factors should be corrected prior to catheter insertion. The risk of arrhythmias may be additionally minimized by minimizing flotation time. In addition, inflating the balloon to its recommended volume insures that the hard catheter tip will be cushioned by the inflated balloon, thus reducing endocardial stimulating effects. No circumstance, other than tricuspid or pulmonic stenosis, justifies flotation of the balloon with less than the manufacturer's recommended inflation volume.

Ventricular ectopy may also occur if the catheter tip slips back into the right ventricle after being placed in the pulmonary artery. Backward slippage will be associated with the appearance of a right ventricular waveform (absence of the dicrotic notch and a lower end-diastolic pressure) on the pulmonary artery trace. Temporarily inflating the balloon to its recommended volume may redirect the catheter to the pulmonary artery position. If redirection cannot be accomplished by the physician and the arrhythmia continues, the pulmonary artery catheter should be promptly removed.

Balloon Rupture

Inflation of the balloon is typically associated with a feeling of resistance. Absence of this resistance, coupled with a failure to wedge, suggests balloon rupture. The one time introduction of 0.8 to 1.5 ml of air into the pulmonary circulation is not harmful; however, additional injections of air may have deleterious effects. Therefore, a piece of tape labeled *balloon rupture* should be applied to the balloon inflation port so that other hospital personnel will not repeat the attempt to wedge.

The latex material of the balloon gradually loses elasticity and weakens as it absorbs lipoproteins from the blood. Balloon life may additionally be shortened by multiple inflations (the average balloon can withstand approximately 72 inflations), manual removal of air from the inflated balloon, and exceeding the balloon inflation volume.

A monitoring problem occurs with balloon rupture because the pulmonary artery wedge pressure measurement is no longer available. However, if there is a good correlation between the pulmonary artery diastolic and pulmonary artery wedge pressure, the pulmonary artery diastolic pressure may be used to track left atrial pressure.

Potential patient risks associated with balloon rupture include embolization of balloon fragments into the distal pulmonary circulation and, in the presence of right to left shunts, cerebral or systemic air embolization. If a right to left shunt is suspected, carbon dioxide should be used for balloon inflation instead of air.

Bundle Branch Block

A right bundle branch block may suddenly occur during insertion or maintenance of the pulmonary artery catheter. Ordinarily, this has no clinical significance. However, patients with preexisting left bundle branch block may develop complete heart block. Therefore, a pacemaker insertion tray or external cardiac pacemaker should be immediately available. Mechanical irritation of the conduction tissue or damage to the bundle of His during catheter passage is believed to be the cause.

Knotting

Knotting of the pulmonary artery catheter may occur within the vascular space, cardiac chambers, around intracardiac structures, and other intravascular catheters. Knotting is more likely to occur with the use of a small caliber pulmonary artery catheter when the catheter is repeatedly withdrawn and readvanced, when the patient has dilated cardiac chambers, and/or when an excessive length of catheter has been inserted. During flotation, no more than 10 to 15 cm of catheter should be required to obtain a pulmonary artery trace after the right ventricular pressure tracing has appeared. The insertion of excessive length predisposes to the formation of loops or kinks which may then form knots.

Knotting should be suspected when resistance is encountered during withdrawal of the catheter. When gentle traction is applied to the catheter, the presence of a pulse-by-pulse tug suggests involvement of the tricuspid valve apparatus. The pulmonary artery waveform may also appear damped and is not improved by flushing. Chest x-ray confirms the diagnosis.

The knotted catheter may be removed transvenously, or unknotted by a physician by fluoroscopic manipulation of the catheter. However, guidewire placement, venotomy or thoracotomy and cardiotomy may be required for catheter removal.

Damage to Cardiac Structures

Structural damage to the pulmonic and/or tricupsid valve apparatus has been reported with pulmonary artery catheterization. Clinically significant valve dysfunction is less common than autopsy evidence of valvular damage.

Preventive measures include: 1) avoiding prolonged catheterization; 2) withdrawing the catheter with the balloon deflated; and 3) never forcing movement of the catheter when resistance is encountered.

Infectious Complications

Several physical characteristics of the pulmonary artery catheter and factors associated with its use increase the potential for local and systemic

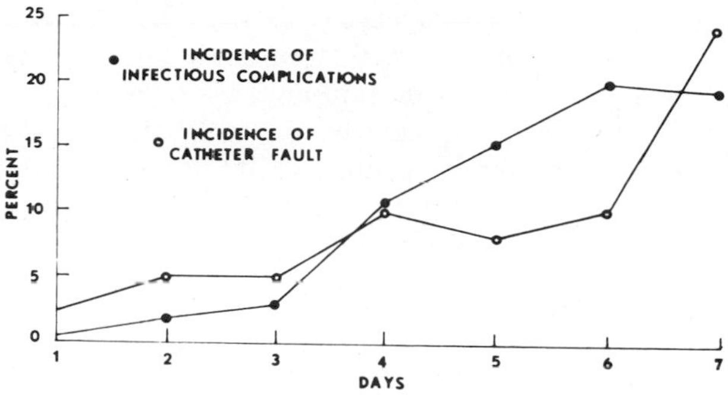

FIGURE 9–18. Incidence of infectious complications and catheter fault as related to PA catheter indwelling time. Catheters maintained longer than 72 hours had a significantly higher incidence of both infectious complications and catheter fault. (From Sise MJ, et al: Complications of the flow-directed pulmonary artery catheter: A prospective analysis in 219 patients. *Crit Care Med* 1981; 9:317.)

infections (see Chapter 12). These factors include: 1) the intracardiac location of the catheter; 2) the frequent breaks in the closed system for withdrawal of blood samples and/or injection of fluid boluses for thermodilution studies; 3) the repeated manipulations of the catheter (ie, repositioning); 4) the possibility of spontaneous migration of the catheter with entry of a nonsterile portion of the catheter into the vascular system; 5) the thrombogenic and adherence characteristics of the polyvinylchloride catheter for microorganisms; and 6) the critically ill, often immune-compromised state of the patient who is a candidate for pulmonary artery catheterization.

The ubiquitous threat of infectious disease is insidious because the causative agents (microorganisms) are invisible to the naked eye. There is a tendency to believe (consciously or unconsciously) that that which cannot be seen is either not there or is inconsequential. Further, the effects of line or wound contamination are typically not physically expressed as site infection or septicemia until 24 to 48 hours after the incident that allowed contamination of tissue or blood; therefore, the cause and effect relationship of infectious disease is not always well established. The patient is said to have become "septic" as though by some unfortunate twist of fate.

Sepsis is a major and often avoidable cause of morbidity and mortality in the critically ill patient population. It is incumbent on the caregiver, therefore, to use meticulous sterile technique during insertion and maintenance, to keep cardiac output studies, blood withdrawals, and catheter repositioning maneuvers to a minimum, to be keenly alert to any signs of infection, and to remove the catheter as soon as possible. It has been shown that the incidence of infectious complications as well as catheter fault (balloon rupture, thermistor malfunctions, luminal obstruction) progressively increase with increases in catheter indwelling time (Fig. 9–18).

Thromboembolic Complications

Any catheter in the vascular system can promote thrombus formation, particularly in patients who have prolonged circulatory impairment. The polyvinylchloride pulmonary artery catheter is additionally known to initiate a thrombogenic response. The clot can form anywhere along the length of the pulmonary artery catheter and may also cover the catheter tip. The incidence of clot formation appears to be far greater than what would be indicated by clinical evidence. For example, one study found postmortem and venographic evidence of internal jugular vein thrombosis at the catheter insertion site in 22 of 33 patients, none of whom were symptomatic.[12]

The clinical and monitoring implications of catheter-related thrombosis include the following:

- Extensive clot material in the area of the catheter tip may occlude the pulmonary vessels distal to the catheter tip, resulting in ischemic injury to the lung.
- A thrombus anywhere in the systemic veins, right heart, or pulmonary arterial system can dislodge or fragment and produce pulmonary emboli.
- Subclavian venous thrombosis may interfere with venous drainage from the head and/or same side upper extremity. This will be clinically evidenced as unilateral jugular venous distension and/or upper extremity edema.
- The accuracy of pulmonary artery pressure or thermodilution cardiac output measurements may be adversely affected by the presence of a thrombus over the pulmonary artery pressure sensing tip or thermistor bead.

The presence of a clot may be detected by: 1) consistently damped pressure tracing without evidence of peripheral migration; 2) poor infusion of IV fluids or flush solution via the proximal (RA) or distal (PA) port; or 3) an increase in pulmonary artery systolic and diastolic pressure, with a widening of the PAd-PWP gradient without apparent cause. The latter should raise suspicion of pulmonary embolism.

Prevention of thrombus formation entails consideration of anticoagulation in patients at risk for a hypercoagulable state if pulmonary artery pressure monitoring is prolonged or if catheter insertion is known to have been traumatic. Heparin-bonded catheters may reduce catheter thrombogenicity. Continuous infusion of a heparinized saline solution (2 to 3 ml per hour) helps prevent clot formation in the lumen or around the catheter tip. Additional manual flushes may be required in patients known to be hypercoagulable. If clotting of the proximal or distal sensing port is suspected, gentle aspiration of clotted blood followed by gentle irrigation may clear the line.

Pulmonary injury or infarction, if small, may be asymptomatic and may go unrecognized. Clinical signs, if present, include hemoptysis, shooting or stabbing chest pain, cough, and x-ray findings of an unexplained density distal to the catheter tip.

Pulmonary Complications

Pulmonary complications include pneumothorax, pulmonary infarction, and damage and/or rupture of the pulmonary artery.

Pneumothorax. Although discussed in complications of central venous pressure monitoring, pneumothorax is mentioned in relation to pulmonary artery pressure monitoring because of its frequency. For example, in one study of 320 pulmonary artery placements done in 219 patients, 10 major complications occurred.[13] Of these, six were pneumothoraces; five occurred at catheterization of new sites; and one at a pre-existing CVP access site. The postcatheter insertion chest radiograph should be carefully inspected not only for line placement but also for the presence of pneumothorax.

Pulmonary Ischemic Injury or Infarction. After mechanical occlusion of the pulmonary artery, the likelihood of pulmonary infarction is increased in patients with pulmonary venous hypertension or inadequacy of the bronchial collateral circulation (fibrotic lung disease, COPD).

Predisposing factors to pulmonary artery catheter-related lung injury include:

- Persistent wedging of the pulmonary artery due to spontaneous forward migration into a small peripheral branch of the pulmonary artery. Following insertion, the pulmonary artery catheter warms to body temperature and softens. The pulsatile action of blood flow may move the softened catheter more peripherally until any excessive catheter loop tightens or the uninflated balloon spontaneously wedges in a vessel slightly smaller than the catheter tip. A significant decrease in balloon inflation volume (less than 1.00 to 1.25 ml for the thermodilution catheter) suggests peripheral migration.
- Persistent or prolonged inflation of the balloon in the wedged position. This may produce a larger area of pulmonary ischemic injury because a more central branch of the pulmonary arterial circulation remains obstructed. In this circumstance, the obtained value is of uncertain accuracy anyway as the balloon may herniate over the sensing tip, or the catheter tip may be pushed against the vessel wall.

Ischemic injury to the lung due to persistent wedging may be prevented by: 1) never leaving the catheter in the wedge position longer than 15 seconds—2 to 3 respiratory cycles; 2) continuously monitoring the pulmonary artery waveform, carefully observing for changes in waveform and pressure; 3) insuring that a clearly defined (not damped) pulmonary artery waveform returns when the wedged balloon is deflated; and 4) inspecting the postcatheter insertion chest x-ray, and subsequent x-rays to verify correct position of the catheter tip. With balloon deflation, the catheter recoils into a main pulmonary artery. In the correct position, the catheter tip should not be visible beyond the mediastinal silhouette.

If peripheral migration is suspected, the catheter should be withdrawn slowly and carefully until a full (or near full) inflation volume produces a PWP trace.

Damage or Rupture of a Pulmonary Artery Segment. The spectrum of pulmonary artery injuries may vary from clinically undetectable injury to life-threatening hemorrhage. Possible causes of pulmonary vascular injury include:

- Spontaneous distal migration of the catheter with damage to the pulmonary vessel by the uncushioned, unprotected catheter tip. As the catheter advances into the narrower lumen of a more peripherally located vessel, the pulsatile action of blood flow may cause the catheter tip to rhythmically strike against the vessel wall, ultimately resulting in erosion or perforation.

- Flotation utilizing less than the manufacturer's recommended inflation volume or rewedging that requires less than full inflation volume. Normally, when in the pulmonary artery position, the catheter lies in a main, usually right, pulmonary artery. With the onset of balloon inflation, the balloon moves rapidly forward. If the catheter has migrated to a smaller distal vessel, wedging occurs with a smaller balloon inflation volume and the hard, unprotected catheter tip may spear the distal vessel wall. In addition, asymmetrical balloon inflation, which typically occurs in a peripherally located catheter during prolonged balloon inflation, may cause the catheter tip to push into the vessel wall.
- Overinflation of the balloon in a vessel too small to accommodate the excessive volume. This typically occurs when the catheter has migrated to a smaller peripheral vessel and the previously used volume of gas for balloon inflation is injected for rewedging. Lateral pressure may damage or rupture the pulmonary arterial wall.
- Forced irrigation of the distal (PA) lumen of the pulmonary artery catheter. Vascular damage or rupture is particularly likely to occur if the catheter is wedged or located in a peripheral vessel.

Any condition that produces chronic pulmonary hypertension (mitral valve disease, COPD) increases the risk of vascular damage or rupture because the distended pulmonary vessels allow the catheter to lodge more peripherally. In addition, inflation of the balloon in these fragile, noncompliant vessels may alter balloon shape and cause the catheter tip to protrude into the vessel wall. Additional risk factors include advanced patient age and stiffening of the catheter with hypothermia. Systemic anticoagulation or blood dyscrasias increase the risk of severe hemorrhage.

Clinically, the patient may be asymptomatic if only mild damage to the pulmonary artery occurs. Vascular rupture may present with minimal blood-tinged sputum. At the other end of the clinical spectrum, massive hemoptysis may quickly lead to shock and death. If hemoptysis is scanty, it may be difficult to differentiate pulmonary artery rupture from infarction. However, aspiration of air through the distal (PA) lumen is indicative of pulmonary artery rupture.

Conservative management with close observation of clinical status and vital signs may suffice if minor damage is incurred and the patient's condition is stable. With significant, active bleeding, the patient is placed with the affected side (usually right) down to prevent spillage of blood into the uninvolved lung. Endotracheal intubation and ventilation and/or emergency thoracotomy with resection of the involved lung lobe may be required.

The following guidelines should prevent damage or rupture of the pulmonary artery:

1. Do not advance the catheter with the balloon uninflated.

2. Carefully obtain PWP measurements by *slowly* inflating the balloon while continuously observing the pulmonary artery waveform. Inflation is stopped immediately when the pulmonary artery trace changes to a wedged

pressure trace (see Fig. 9–11). If less than recommended volume is required to wedge, the catheter should be pulled back by the physician.

3. Do not inflate the balloon with fluid because the incompressible balloon increases stress on the vessel wall.

4. Keep wedging time and the number of balloon inflation/deflation cycles to a minimum. If a close pulmonary artery diastolic/wedge pressure relationship exists, pulmonary artery diastolic pressure may be used to assess left atrial pressure.

5. Position the catheter tip in a central pulmonary vessel so that the full or nearly full recommended inflation volume produces the wedge waveform.

6. Avoid excessive catheter manipulation.

7. Avoid irrigating the pulmonary artery lumen under high pressure. This is sometimes attempted when it is assumed that the damped trace is the result of a clot at the catheter tip. If a clot is indeed present, it may be distally propelled, producing a pulmonary embolism. On the other hand, the damped tracing may be due to spontaneous wedging, and forced irrigation may produce rupture of the pulmonary artery.

8. Remove or reposition the catheter if hemoptysis occurs to prevent the catheter from further injuring the lung.

Although studies have been conducted to determine the incidence of complications associated with pulmonary artery catheterization, the true incidence is unknown and may be underestimated for several reasons. A single center study indicates the number of complications only at the institution participating in the study. Moreover, the number of complications is influenced by institutional protocol for catheter insertion and maintenance. Since knowledge that a study examining the incidence of complications is being conducted may influence caregivers to be more fastidious with technique of insertion and maintenance, this may bias the outcome. Therefore, the results of a single study cannot be applied to medical practice as a whole since insertion and management techniques may vary widely among institutions and, for that matter, within an institution among practitioners. Another reason that complications may be underestimated is that a minor complication, such as a small pulmonary embolism or infarction, may go unrecognized.

Although pulmonary artery catheterization offers distinct assessment and management advantages, it is not a completely benign procedure. When its use is being considered, clearly the anticipated benefits to the patient should outweigh anticipated risks. Unfortunately, the likelihood of complications tends to increase as the patient becomes more seriously ill. Consequently pulmonary artery catheterization should be used with extreme caution in patients with bleeding tendencies, hypercoagulable states, immunosuppression (especially granulocytopenia), or recurrent sepsis, or in patients who are anticoagulated or have hemorrhagic blood disorders.

REFERENCES

1. Civetta JM: Pulmonary artery catheter insertion. In Spring CL (ed): *The Pulmonary Artery Catheter; Methodology and Clinical Application.* Baltimore, University Park Press, 1983, pp 21–55.

2. Daily EK, Schroeder JS: Venous and pulmonary arterial pressure monitoring. In *Techniques in Bedside Hemodynamic Monitoring*, ed 3. St. Louis, CV Mosby Company, 1985, pp 57–61.
3. Keefer JR, Barish PG: Pulmonary artery catheterization. In Blitt CD (ed): *Monitoring in Anesthesia and Critical Care Medicine*. New York, Churchill-Livingstone, 1985, pp 188–193.
4. Urbach DR, Rippe JM: Pulmonary artery catheter, placement and care. In Rippe JM, Irwin RS, Alpert JS, et al: *Intensive Medicine*. Boston, Little, Brown, 1985, pp 47–50.
5. Guyton AC: Cardiac output, venous return and their regulation. In *Textbook of Medical Physiology*, ed 7. Philadelphia, WB Saunders Company, 1986, p 272.
6. Swan HJC, Ganz W: Balloon flotation catheters, their use in hemodynamic monitoring in clinical practice. *JAMA* 1975; 233:865–867.
7. Woods SL, Laurend DJ, Grose BC, et al: Effect of backrest position on pulmonary artery pressures in acutely ill patients. *Circulation* 1980; 62:111–184.
8. Riedinger MS, Shellock FG, Swan HJC: Reading pulmonary artery and pulmonary wedge pressure waveforms with respiratory variations. *Heart and Lung* 1981; 10:675–678.
9. Civetta JM: Pulmonary artery catheter insertion. In Sprung CL (ed): *The Pulmonary Artery Catheter; Methodology and Clinical Application*. Baltimore, University Park Press, 1983, pp 67–68.
10. West JB, Dollery CT, Naimark A: Distribution of blood flow in isolated lung; Relation to vascular and alveolar pressures. *J Appl Physiol* 1964; 19:713–724.
11. Devitt JH, Noble WH, Byrick RJ: A Swan-Ganz catheter–related complication in a patient with Eisenmenger's syndrome. *Anesthesiology* 1982; 57:335.
12. Chastre J, Cornud F, Bouchama A, et al: Thrombosis as a complication of pulmonary artery catheterization via the internal jugular vein. *N Engl J Med* 1982; 306:278–281.
13. Sise MJ, Hollingsworth P, Brimm JE, et al: Complications of the flow-directed pulmonary-artery catheter: A prospective analysis in 219 patients. *Crit Care Med* 1981; 9:315–318.

SUGGESTED READINGS

Bone RC: Monitoring respiratory and hemodynamic function in the patient with respiratory failure. In Kirby RR, Smith RA, Desaultels DA (eds): *Mechanical Ventilation*. New York, Churchill-Livingstone, 1985.

Boysen PG: Hemodynamic monitoring in the adult respiratory distress syndrome. *Clin Chest Med* 1982; 3:157–169.

Cerra F, Milch R, Lajos TZ: Pulmonary artery catheterization in critically ill surgical patients. *Ann Surg* 1973; 177:37–39.

Daily EK, Schroeder JS: *Techniques in Bedside Hemodynamic Monitoring*. ed 3. St. Louis, CV Mosby Company, 1985.

Donovan KD: Invasive monitoring and support of the circulation. *Clin Anesthesiol* 1985; 3:909–953.

Gore JM, Alpert JS, Benotti JR, et al: *Handbook of Hemodynamic Monitoring*. Boston, Little, Brown, 1985.

Guyton AC: Physics of blood, blood flow, and pressure: Hemodynamics. In *Textbook of Medical Physiology*, ed 7. Philadelphia, WB Saunders, 1986.

Halpenny CJ: Systemic and pulmonary circulations. In Underhill SL, Woods SL, Sivarajan ES, et al (eds): *Cardiac Nursing*. Philadelphia, JB Lippincott, 1982.

Keefer JR, Banash PG: Pulmonary artery catheterization. In Blitt CD (ed): *Monitoring in Anesthesia and Critical Care Medicine*. New York, Churchill-Livingstone, 1985.

Matthay MA: Invasive hemodynamic monitoring in critically ill patients. *Clin Chest Med* 1983; 4:233–249.

Pierson DJ, Hudson LD: Monitoring hemodynamics in the critically ill. *Med Clin North Am* 1983; 67:1343–1360.

Puri VK, Carlson RW, Bander JJ, et al: Complications of vascular catheterization in the critically ill. *Crit Care Med* 1980; 8:495–499.

Sise MJ, Hollingsworth P, Brimm JE, et al: Complications of the flow-directed pulmonary-artery catheter: A prospective analysis in 219 patients. *Crit Care Med* 1981; 9:315–318.

Sprung CL: *The Pulmonary Artery Catheter: Methodology and Clinical Application.* Baltimore, Universtiy Park Press, 1983.

Sprung CL, Schein RMH: Pulmonary artery catheterization. In Sprung CL, Grenvic A (eds): *Invasive Procedures in Critical Care.* New York, Churchill-Livingstone, 1985.

Swan-Ganz Monitoring Systems. American Edwards Laboratories, Santa Ana, CA.

Swan HJC, Ganz W, Forrester J, et al: Catheterization of the heart in man with use of a flow-directed balloon-tipped catheter. *N Engl J Med* 1970; 283:447–451.

Swan HJC, Ganz W: Complications with flow-directed balloon-tipped catheters. *Ann Intern Med* 1979; 91:494.

Swan HJC, Ganz W: The Swan Ganz catheter: Past and present. In Blitt CD (ed). *Monitoring in Anesthesia and Critical Care Medicine.* New York, Churchill-Livingstone, 1985.

Understanding hemodynamic measurements made with the Swan-Ganz catheter. American Edwards Laboratories, Santa Ana, CA.

Urbach DR, Rippe JM: Pulmonary artery catheter placement and care. In Rippe JM, Irwin RS, Alpert JS, et al (eds): *Intensive Care Medicine.* Boston, Little, Brown, 1985.

10

Monitoring Cardiac Output

LINDA A. YACONE, RN, BS, CCRN

The provision and transport of oxygenated blood to the body at the cellular level is a complex process, prerequisite for sustaining life itself. The cardiopulmonary system fulfills the role as pump and transporter in sustaining this vital supply. The quantity of blood delivered to the systemic circulation is known as the cardiac output. Its value is represented in both time and volume, resulting in a measurement of liters per minute. The normal resting range for the cardiac output is 4 to 8 liters/minute.[1]

Measurement of cardiac output remains an important assessment of left ventricular performance. Various techniques are available but all require skill and expertise on the part of the health practitioner. This procedure should be adequately covered in orientation to the critical care setting both in theory and in clinical practice under the supervision of experienced personnel.

Presently, three methods are utilized to calculate cardiac output. They include the Fick oxygen consumption method, the indicator-dilution method, and the thermodilution method. All three methods are discussed, with major emphasis on the thermodilution method as the primary bedside technique.

FACTORS AFFECTING CARDIAC OUTPUT

Cardiac output is a product of stroke volume times heart rate. Stroke volume is the amount of blood ejected by the left ventricle with each contraction. It is approximately 60 to 130 ml. Variations in heart rate, stroke volume, and/or other physiologic alterations may significantly influence cardiac output. Factors affecting stroke volume include preload, afterload, and the inotropic state of the heart. At the cellular level, changing needs and demand for oxygenation also influence cardiac output.

EFFECTS OF ANATOMIC SHUNTING

In the absence of underlying pathology such as anatomic intracardiac shunts, the cardiac output for both pump chambers of the heart, the right and left ventricles, is essentially the same. If the output of either ventricle increases or decreases for any reason, the output for the other adjusts to match the change and a new dynamic equilibrium is established. In the presence of anatomic shunting, however, disparate right and left ventricular end-diastolic pressures and outputs of these respective chambers can occur. In left to right anatomic shunts (eg, atrial septal defects and ventricular septal defects), pulmonary blood flow is increased and pulmonary artery oxygen saturation is greater than that expected in mixed venous blood. Right to left anatomic shunts (eg, congenital aortic arch obstruction, tetralogy of Fallot, etc.) produce unsaturated arterial blood. For example, the major anatomic abnormalities associated with tetralogy of Fallot are pulmonic stenosis and a ventricular septal defect. When the stenosis results in great resistance to pulmonary artery outflow, a right to left shunt occurs through the ventricular septal defect. This produces unsaturated arterial blood which is manifested in the form of cyanosis.

CLINICAL APPLICATION

Cardiac Output

Cardiac output measurement is extremely useful in the critical care setting. Its clinical usefulness lies in its ability to help assess patient perfusion status and response to therapy. It provides a quick means of evaluating hemodynamic status and provides the necessary information to calculate cardiac index. For example, when the cardiac output is markedly reduced, signs of tissue hypoperfusion will be present. At this point arterial blood pressure may or may not reflect the low cardiac output. Since blood pressure is the product of cardiac output and systemic vascular resistance, systemic vascular resistance can increase and produce a normal or increased blood pressure despite an unchanged or low cardiac output. It is also possible for a patient with a decreased systemic vascular resistance to have hypotension and a normal or increased cardiac output, the blood pressure reflecting a low systemic vascular resistance. When a cardiac output measurement is added to other data such as pulmonary artery pressures, systemic vascular resistance, arterial blood pressure, and so on, it can help develop and guide a truly therapeutic program for the critically ill patient since isolated pieces of data can be misleading.

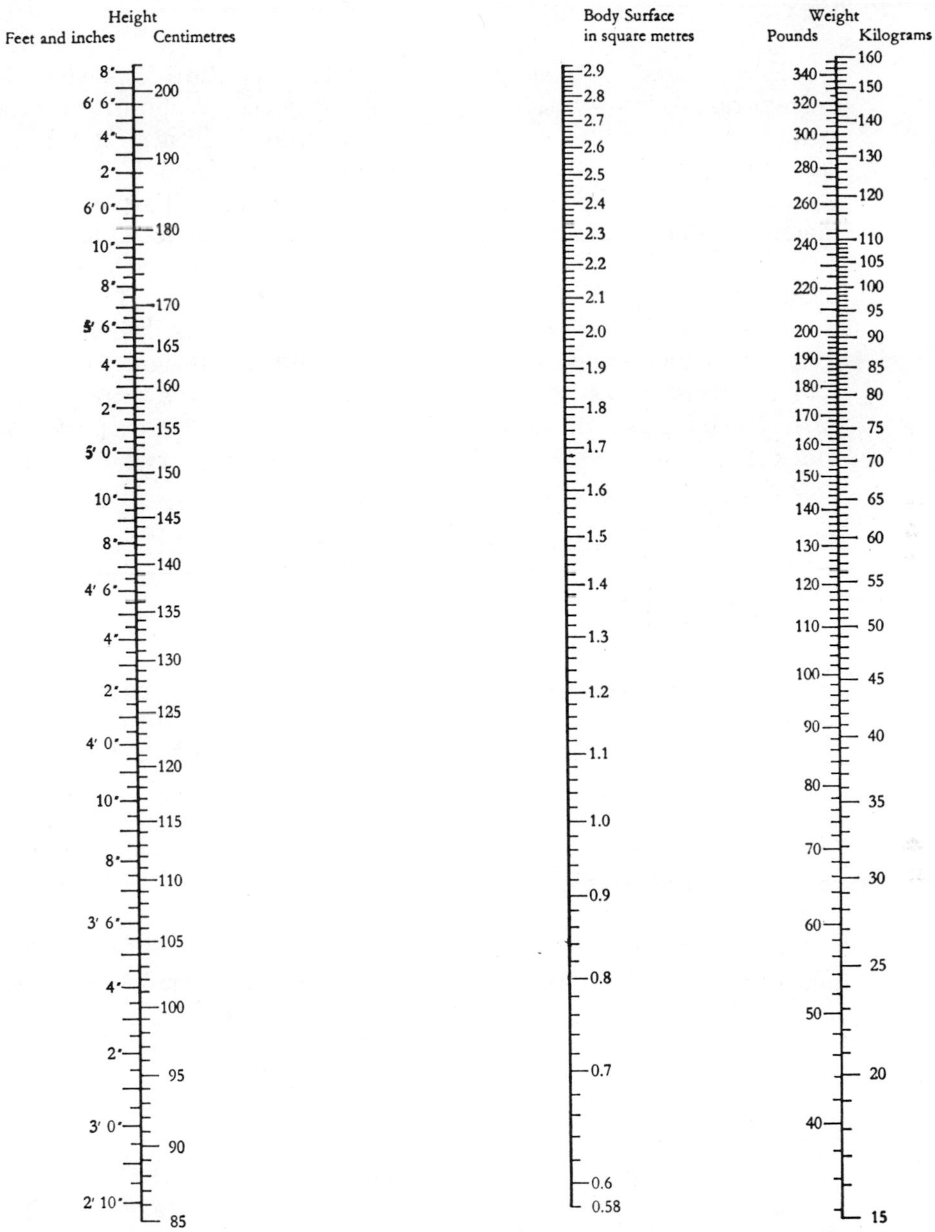

Figure 10–1. A body surface chart. To find the body surface area of a person, locate the height in feet and inches, or centimeters, on Scale I and the weight in pounds, or kilograms, on Scale III and place a ruler between these two points. The ruler will intersect on Scale II at the person's body surface area. (From Meschan I, Ott DJ: *Introduction to Diagnostic Imaging.* Philadelphia, WB Saunders, 1984.)

Cardiac Index

Parameters such as pulmonary artery pressure measurements have normal ranges irrespective of individual body size. When interpreting cardiac output measurements, it is necessary to take body size into account. This "adjustment" is considered when calculating the cardiac index—the cardiac output divided by the body surface area. Its value is reported in liters/minute/meter^2. The body surface area can be obtained by the use of a nomogram such as the Dubois Body Surface Chart, which plots height and weight to calculate body surface area (Fig. 10–1).

The normal range for a cardiac index is 2.5 to 4.2 liters/minute/meter^2.

The cardiac index is an extremely useful calculation since it represents a more precise measurement of blood flow relative to a square meter of body surface area. Since it is a more precise indicator of tissue perfusion, cardiac index is the more useful guide in evaluating circulatory status and response to therapy.

METHODS OF CALCULATING CARDIAC OUTPUT

Three methods are commonly used to calculate cardiac output: Fick oxygen consumption, indicator-dilution, and thermodilution. All three methods bear explanation; however, emphasis will be given to the latter since this is the method most often used clinically.

Fick Oxygen Consumption Method

The "standard" to which other methods are compared is the Fick oxygen consumption method because of its extreme accuracy. This technique is employed more commonly in the cardiac catheterization laboratory and research settings than at the patient's bedside. It does not have practical clinical application because it is time consuming and requires additional personnel. In addition, when not performed correctly, this technique carries a greater chance for error than the other two methods.

The Fick oxygen consumption method is based on the principle described by Adolph Fick in 1870 that the total uptake or release of a substance by an organ is the product of the blood flow through that organ and the arteriovenous difference of that substance.[2] In this method of cardiac output calculation, the organ is the lung and the substance measured is oxygen. This concept is expressed in the following formula:

$$\text{Cardiac output (liters/minute)} = \frac{\text{Oxygen consumption (ml/min)}}{\text{Arteriovenous oxygen content difference (ml/dl blood)}}$$

The oxygen consumption for a normal, resting adult is approximately 220 to 290 ml/minute. Oxygen consumption is calculated by analyzing the oxygen content difference of inspired minus expired air which is collected in a bag over a 3-minute period. One hundred ml of arterial blood contains approximately 19 ml of oxygen (19 vol percent), whereas 100 ml of mixed venous blood contains approximately 15 ml of oxygen. In other words, for every 100 ml of blood perfusing the tissues, normally 4 to 5 ml of oxygen are consumed or removed. Substituting for the formula:

$$\frac{240 \text{ ml/min}}{(19 \text{ ml} - 15 \text{ ml})/\text{dl}} = \frac{240 \text{ ml/min}}{4 \text{ ml/dl}} = 6{,}000 \text{ ml/min or 6 liters/min cardiac output}$$

One disadvantage of the Fick method is that the patient must remain in a steady metabolic state, outside the sphere of sudden intervening variables. Such variables can affect oxygen consumption and arterial and mixed venous oxygen content, thereby, interfering with an accurate reflection of cardiac output. For example, if oxygen consumption—a reflection of the metabolic state—is increased suddenly by shivering, extreme emotional stress, pain, etc., or if arterial content is suddenly altered by a decrease in oxygen saturation, an inaccurate cardiac output will result. Normally the metabolic needs of the tissues require 25 to 40 percent extraction of oxygen from the arterial blood. Venous blood returning to the heart, therefore, usually is approximately 60 to 75 percent oxygen saturated. When the cardiac output is decreased (valve dysfunction; myocardial infarction), less blood flows to the body resulting in less delivered oxygen; the tissues attempt to compensate for this decrease by extracting more oxygen from available blood. Therefore, mixed venous blood will have a lower oxygen content if the cardiac output is low. This produces a wide arterial-venous oxygen content difference, a variable which the Fick method of analysis utilizes in determining cardiac output.

When using the Fick technique, the expired air and blood samples must be obtained at the same time. The room oxygen content must be measured with an oxygen analyzer. The patient then breathes into a collection bag so that an analysis of expired oxygen can be made. Samples of blood from the pulmonary artery are also obtained to measure mixed venous oxygen content. Arterial oxygen content must also be measured, usually accomplished by obtaining a peripheral blood sample from either the brachial or femoral artery. The Fick method requires great skill and precision to maintain the patient's steady metabolic state and to perform the blood sample withdrawals and calculations. Thus, it is not a practical bedside method. It is, however, the most accurate method available to evaluate patients with low cardiac outputs.

Indicator-Dilution Method

The second method used to measure cardiac output is the indicator or dye dilution method. This technique is also used more commonly in cardiac catheterization laboratories and research settings. It is usually accomplished by a single injection of a nontoxic indicator dye such as indocyanine green. The presence and amount of the indicator dye are measurable at a distal point in the circulation from the injection site. For example, 1 ml of the dye solution is injected into the pulmonary artery where it mixes with venous blood. This injection must be followed by an immediate flush of intravenous solution to clear the injection line and stopcock ports of any potential remaining dye solution. Failure to do so could produce erroneous results. The blood/dye solution passes a sampling site such as the brachial artery which is further downstream in the circulation. Peripheral arterial blood samples are withdrawn from this specified site via an arterial line in a continuous fashion at a set rate. This concentration of blood and dye solution can be measured accurately and plotted on a time/concentration curve. The values obtained are then recorded on paper until recirculation has occurred. A computer is usually used to perform the necessary calculations. The results are then immediately available and can be calculated much faster than by the Fick method. Because this technique requires great precision in the calculation of volume and time, the preparation and injection of the indicator dye solution, and the insertion of catheters in the pulmonary and peripheral arteries, it too is not a practical bedside procedure. It is also not the recommended method for any patient with an intracardiac shunt since an intact cardiac chamber is necessary for the blood and indicator dye to mix before the downstream sample is obtained.

Thermodilution Method

The thermodilution method is currently the most widely clinically used technique to calculate cardiac output. It was first described by Fegler in 1954[3] but did not gain widespread acceptance until the development and routine application of the pulmonary artery catheter in hemodynamic assessment of the critically ill. The principle behind the thermodilution method is similar to the indicator-dilution principle. A specific quantity of known indicator solution, in this case a solution with a temperature different from blood temperature, is injected into the proximal (RA) port of the thermodilution pulmonary artery catheter. It is injected rapidly and smoothly as a bolus into the right atrial chamber where it mixes with the blood. The patient's baseline blood temperature is recorded by the cardiac output computer prior to the injection. The temperature of the mixed blood (a combination of indicator solution and blood) is also recorded further downstream in the pulmonary artery by a thermistor bead located at the tip of the pulmonary artery catheter. The cardiac output is plotted as the difference in temperatures on a time/temperature curve. The cardiac output is plotted on a horizontal axis and temperature differential on a vertical axis. A normal curve is shown in Figure 10–2. The top or peak of the curve represents the lowest temperature or greatest temperature differential between the baseline blood temperature

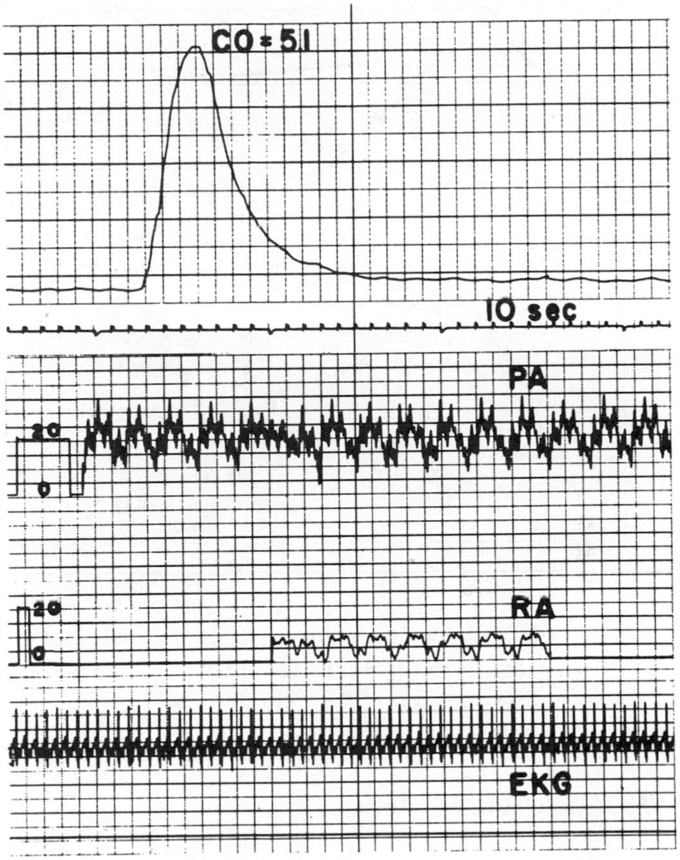

Figure 10–2. A normal thermodilution curve with pulmonary arterial (PA) and right atrial (RA) pressures using a balloon-tipped flow-directed thermodilution catheter. The scales at the left calibrate pressure from 0 to 20 mm Hg. (Reproduced by permission from Grossman W: Cardiac Catheterization and Angiography (ed 2). Philadelphia, Lea & Febiger, 1980, p 82.)

and the injectate and blood as it passes the tip of the catheter and is sensed by the thermistor bead. The curve then drops back to baseline as the indicator solution washes out of the pulmonary artery and the temperature of the blood in the pulmonary artery returns to normal.

The volume of cardiac output is inversely proportional to the area observed under the curve. A high cardiac output will characteristically have a small area under the curve. This is due to a rapid blood flow through the heart (Fig. 10–3*A*). In a low cardiac output, the opposite is true (Fig. 10–3*B*). The area under the curve is large, representing the slower blood flow in the heart. Figure 10–3*C* represents a normal cardiac output curve. Faulty technique may cause an artifactual curve variation (Fig. 10–3*D*). The peak may be notched or the upstroke may not be well defined and slow. When this occurs, the measurement results should be discarded and the procedure repeated.

After the calculations are performed internally, the final cardiac output measurement is displayed on the front panel of the cardiac output computer.

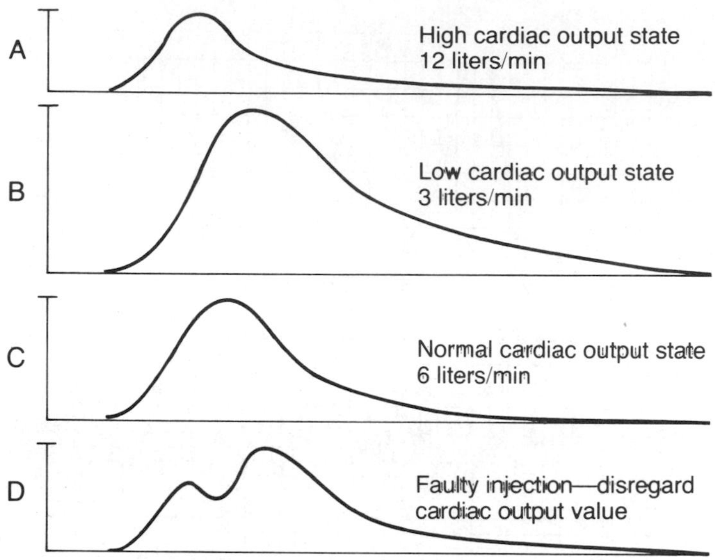

Figure 10–3. Variations in cardiac output thermodilution curves. (Copyright Hewlett-Packard Company. Reproduced with permission.)

It can be performed easily by one person at the patient's bedside. When performed by a skilled operator, the technique can be done quickly and has a high degree of reproducibility.

PROCEDURAL REVIEW

Presently two systems are available for use with the pulmonary artery thermodilution catheter: an open injectate delivery system and a closed injectate delivery system.

Open Injectate Delivery System

The open injectate delivery system is the most popular currently in use today.

Equipment. Assuming the prior insertion of a thermodilution pulmonary artery catheter, special equipment needed to perform a cardiac output measurement includes a cardiac output computer (Fig. 10–4); a number of these are available (American Edwards Laboratories, Gould, Critikon, Hewlett-Packard, etc.). Also needed are a minimum of five 10-ml sterile, plastic syringes; injectate solution—depending on the technique used, one or two 100-ml bags of normal saline or 5% dextrose in water are necessary. These are the two acceptable injectate solutions since other types of fluids have varying specific heats and densities, graduate or basin with ice/slush solution at 0 to 4°C (if the iced injectate method is chosen); mechanical injector gun

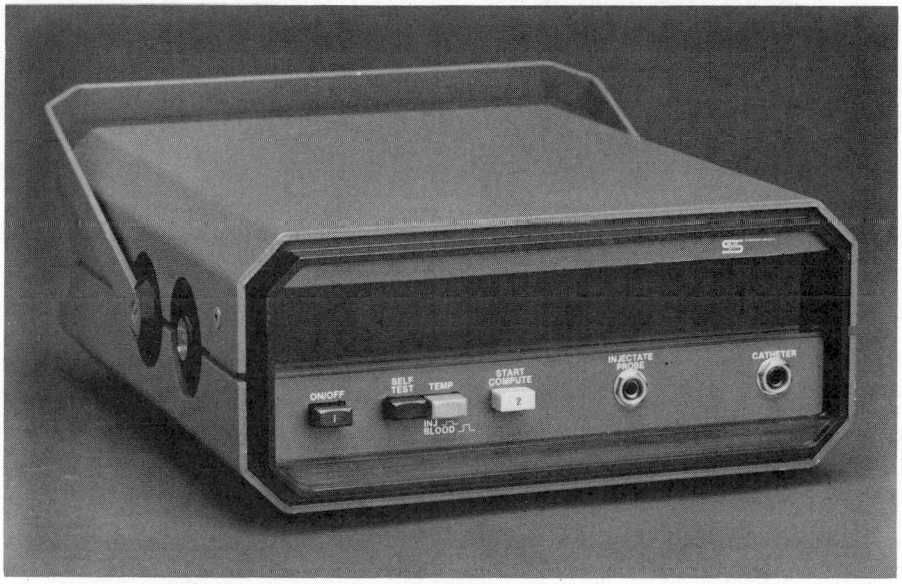

Figure 10–4. The Sorenson Cardiac Output Computer, Number 41212-01. (Reproduced by permission from Sorenson Research, Salt Lake City, UT.)

with CO_2 cartridges (optional); injectate temperature probe; and catheter connecting cable.

Procedure. The procedure should be explained to the patient when feasible. This will help decrease unnecessary anxiety and elicit cooperation. Depending on the individual situation, the family should be included in the explanation.

As with all procedures, hand-washing is an important first step to decrease the chance of contamination and infection. Sterile gloves for an additional precaution against contamination should be considered, especially if the patient is known to be immune-compromised.

The positioning of the patient must be assessed. When using the thermodilution technique, a backrest position of less than or equal to 20 degrees should not alter the cardiac output.[3, 4] However, many of these patients are on pharmacologic therapy such as potent vasodilators, which by causing increased peripheral venous pooling can produce orthostatic hypotension with relatively slight changes in position. If doubt exists as to the reliability of a reading and the patient is able to tolerate positional changes, two cardiac output procedures should be performed, one with the patient supine and one with the patient's head elevated, to ascertain any differences.[4, 5]

The correct position of the thermodilution catheter should be ascertained prior to injection. The catheter tip must be in the main pulmonary artery. After insertion, positioning is confirmed by chest radiograph. It would not be practical to obtain chest films prior to each cardiac output measurement since they are usually performed several times daily. Distal migration is suggested by balloon wedging that requires significantly less than the manufacturer's recommended balloon inflation volume. Changes in the shape of the waveform are also indicative of balloon displacement. Catheter position checking is also done as a safety measure since current leakage from the thermistor bead can induce ventricular arrhythmias if it is in the right ventricle when it is connected to the cardiac output computer. An improper catheter placement will produce inaccurate values.

The balloon on the pulmonary artery catheter must be deflated prior to injecting any solution for a cardiac output reading.

Most cardiac output computers need to be turned on manually. The computer can be used with either wall current or battery power. If using wall current, it may be necessary to set a line voltage selector on the back of the unit. The line voltage regulator must be appropriately set. As always, electrical safety guidelines should be observed. Cardiac output computers should be inspected routinely by a biomedical engineering service. Batteries should be left in the recharging mode when not in use to prolong their life.

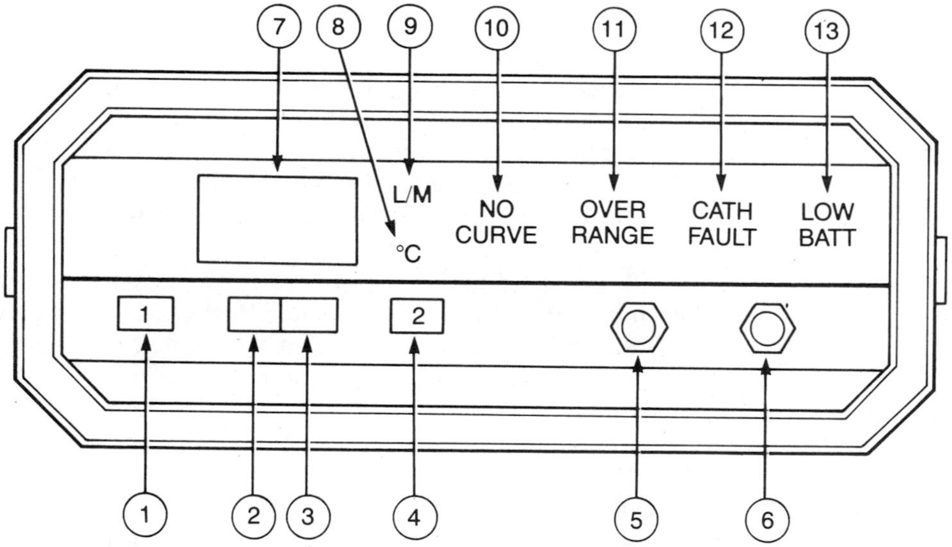

1. On/off power button
2. Self-test button
3. Blood temp or injectate temp button
4. Start computer button
5. Injectate probe input
6. Catheter connecting cable input
7. C.O. in liters/min or blood/inj. temperature in C
8. C light on when blood or injectate temp is displayed
9. L/M indicator
10. No curve indicator
11. Over range indicator
12. Catheter fault indicator
13. Low battery indicator

Figure 10–5. Operational information for the Sorenson Cardiac Output Computer, Number 41212-01. (Reproduced by permission from Sorenson Research, Salt Lake City, UT.)

TABLE 10–1. Iced Injectate Preparation

1. Fill graduate or basin with ice slush solution.
2. Connect the injectate probe to the cardiac output computer so that the computer can sense the injectate temperature.
3. Fill a minimum of five syringes with the desired injectate solution. This must be done as precisely as possible. A protective cap on each syringe will help prevent possible contamination. When aseptically prepared on a sterile field, with use of a sterile cap, mask, gown, and gloves, these syringes will remain sterile for at least 36 hours.[6] Although only three syringes are necessary to perform the cardiac output measurement, prepare a fourth in case of a questionable result with one injection or a possible contamination; use the fifth syringe to check the temperature of the iced syringes.
4. Insert the injectate probe into one of the syringes filled with injectate solution. After the plunger is removed and the probe inserted, stand the syringe upright in the ice slush bath. The computer will test the injectate temperature via the injectate temperature probe. An alternative procedural variation is to place two bags of injectate solution in the ice slush bath. Insert the injectate probe into one bag to check temperature and fill the syringes with solution from the other bag.
5. Attach the catheter connecting cable to the thermistor port of the thermodilution catheter and to the cardiac output computer. This connection site can be identified readily and is protected by a red removable cap on the end of the pulmonary artery catheter thermistor lumen. Remove when connecting the cable from the cardiac output computer and replace it when the cardiac output measurement is completed.
6. Press the appropriate button on the cardiac output computer to determine the injectate temperature. (Some units have separate thermistors for sensing injectate temperature during injection, making this an unnecessary step.) The temperature of the iced injectate solution should read between 0 and 4° C. This may require chilling the solution for 45 minutes to 1 hour before an adequate temperature may be reached.
7. Inspect each syringe for the presence of air bubbles. Failure to remove air bubbles prior to injection could cause air emboli as well as interfere with reliable test data.

A self-test mechanism is available on the cardiac output computer (Fig. 10–5). This causes the cardiac output computer to generate an internal cardiac output curve. Proper functioning can be verified by a designated numerical or digital design display on the unit itself. A calibration knob adjustment may be performed to lock in the correct numerical information.

Either iced or room temperature saline or $D^{5}W$ is acceptable as an injectable solution. Preparation of both solutions is shown in Tables 10–1 and 10–2.

The patient's blood core temperature may be obtained by pressing the appropriate button on the cardiac output computer. This information is held internally by the computer.

The computation constant, a number predetermined by the manufacturer to provide accurate results by taking catheter length, volume of injection, and temperature of injectate into consideration, is "dialed into" the computer.

TABLE 10–2. Room Temperature Injectate Preparation

1. Two 100-ml bags of the desired solution are necessary.
2. Place the injectate temperature probe into one of the bags to serve as the control temperature. The other bag is used for solution withdrawal.
3. Fill syringes with injectate solution using sterile technique. Be sure the volume is accurate.
4. Follow steps 5 through 7 from the iced injectate procedure (Table 10–1).

7F-110 cm

Volume Injected	Iced (0-5°C)	Room Temp. (19-25°C)
10 ml	922	911
7 ml	639	620
5 ml	441	437
3 ml	260	260

8F-110 cm

Volume Injected	Iced (0-5°C)	Room Temp. (19-25°C)
10 ml	880	894
7 ml	586	618
5 ml	404	440
3 ml	228	260

7F-85 cm

Volume Injected	Iced (0-5°C)	Room Temp. (19-25°C)
10 ml	972	911
7 ml	660	620
5 ml	465	437
3 ml	265	260

Figure 10–6. Sample computation constants as seen on the Sorenson Cardiac Output Computer, Number 41212-01. (Reproduced by permission from Sorenson Research, Salt Lake City, UT.)

The computation constants available are displayed on the cardiac output computer for reference (Fig. 10–6).

A prepared syringe is attached to the right atrial or proximal port of the thermodilution catheter. For this purpose, a stopcock is often added to the port so that the line may be kept patent by a continuous intravenous infusion and the procedure for a cardiac output necessitates only a turn of the stopcock.

The START COMPUTER button on the computer is activated. When the computer signals READY, a bolus of prepared solution is injected smoothly, and rapidly. It should be injected within approximately 4 seconds.[7] A mechanical injector gun may be used for this step. Although it does minimize handling of the syringes, which could interfere with test results, it offers no particular advantage over manual injection when the procedure is done by experienced personnel.[5]

The cardiac output computer will display the results on a digital panel. Most computers do not have a built-in memory to recall previous cardiac output results so the data should be written down immediately upon reviewing the digital display. Activation of any of the buttons on the front panel would erase the data.

The continuous intravenous infusion must be resumed by turning the stopcock to the open position This is easily overlooked and could result in line thrombus formation.

The procedure is repeated three times. An average of these three injections is used to determine the cardiac output. The readings should fall within the same range; if not, a technical error may have occurred and the fourth syringe should be used to perform an additional measurement. It is necessary to wait approximately 1½ to 2 minutes between injections in order for the patient's blood temperature to return to normal.

Closed Injectate Delivery System

Closed injectate delivery requires a special delivery system, such as the CO-Set system (American Edwards Laboratories, Santa Ana, CA) (Fig. 10–7). Although this system can be used with either iced or room temperature injectate, a recent study by Barcelona et al[8] found that the iced solution provided more reliable cardiac outputs. This system requires a cooling container with attached injectate delivery tubing. The bulk of the system is its primary disadvantage. The injectate solution is delivered with a syringe attached to the proximal injectate hub. The injectate probe is attached to the cardiac output computer and a special attachment, the flow-through housing, where it senses and records the injectate temperature. This is a completely closed system and that remains its primary advantage because it potentially reduces the risk of infection and contamination.

SPECIAL CONSIDERATIONS

Regardless of the system used to calculate cardiac output, several special considerations must be kept in mind.

Many cardiac output computers accommodate internally to the effects of respiratory variation on blood temperature. If the patient is on ventilatory

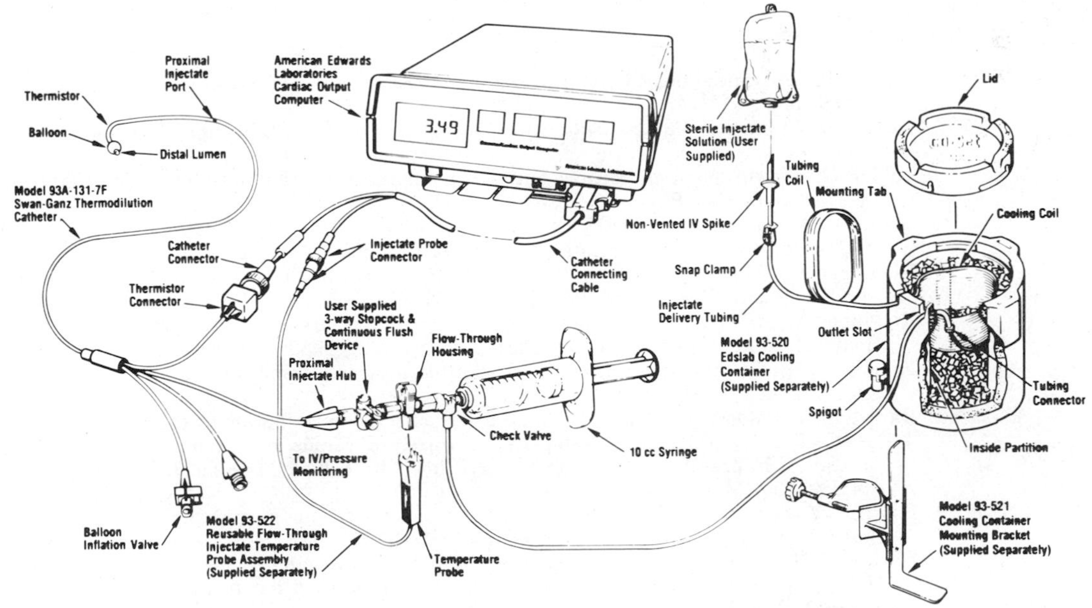

Figure 10–7. CO-Set II, Closed Injectate Delivery System, Cold Injectate. (Reproduced by permission from American Edwards Laboratories, Santa Ana, CA, copyright 1985.)

support, there may be a phasic relationship between cardiac output and airway pressure. If three injections are made at evenly spaced intervals and an average taken, it is possible to record cardiac output accurately.[9] The variation in outputs can be artifactual but probably not to the extent to produce clinically significant inaccurate data.

The volume of injectate solution used should take into consideration the patient's disease process. Lower volumes should be used with renal patients, pediatric patients, or in any situation in which fluid overload is a concern (eg, congestive heart failure).

Iced or room temperature injectate solutions are both acceptable.[10, 11] Room temperature injection does have the advantage of easier preparation with regard to time involved and less chance for accidental spills or electrical hazards from spilled ice. It is also less expensive.

To decrease the chance of damage by accidental spilling into or onto the instrument, neither the fluid nor other items should be stored on the cardiac output computer itself.

Pulmonary artery thermodilution catheters with side port extensions pose potential sources of error when calculating cardiac output. Results can be affected by the volume and temperature of the infusion through the side port or by the sheath covering the proximal port. This is most common with internal jugular or subclavian vein insertions.[4]

After the thermodilution catheter has been in place for 24 to 48 hours, the cardiac output reported value can increase. This is due to loss of sensitivity of the catheter to the cold injectate as it becomes coated with plasma proteins.[12]

REFERENCES

1. Palmer PN: Advanced hemodynamic assessment. *Dimensions of Critical Care Nursing* 1982; 1:139–144.
2. Grossman W: *Cardiac Catheterization and Angiography*. ed. 2. Philadelphia, Lea & Febiger, 1980.
3. Fegler G: Measurement of cardiac output in anaesthetized animals by Thermo-dilution method. *2 J Exper Physiol* 1954; 39:153–164.
4. Grose BL, Woods SL, Laurent DJ: Effect of backrest position on cardiac output measured by the thermodilution method in acutely ill patients. *Heart Lung* 1981; 10:661–665.
5. Riedinger MS, Shellock FG: Technical aspects of the thermodilution method for measuring cardiac output. *Heart Lung* 1984; 13:215–222.
6. Riedinger MS, Shellock FG, Shah PK, et al: Sterility of prefilled cardiac output syringes maintained at room and ice temperature. *Heart Lung* 1985; 14:8–11.
7. Kadota LT: Theory and application of thermodilution cardiac output measurement: A review. *Heart Lung* 1985; 14:605–616.
8. Barcelona M, Patague L, Bunoy M, et al: Cardiac output determination by the thermodilution method: Comparison of ice-temperature injectate versus room-temperature injectate contained in prefilled syringes or a closed injectate delivery system. *Heart Lung* 1985; 14:232–235.
9. Snyder JV, Powner DJ: Effects of mechanical ventilation on the measurement of cardiac output by thermodilution. *Crit Care Med* 1982; 10:677–681.
10. Shellock FG, Riedinger MS: Reproducibility and accuracy using room-temperature vs. ice-temperature injectate for thermodilution cardiac output detemrination. *Heart Lung* 1983; 12:175–176.
11. Vennix CV, Nelson DH, Pierpont GL: Thermodilution cardiac output in critically ill patients: comparison of room-temperature and iced injectate. *Heart Lung* 1984; 13:574–578.
12. Boysen PG: Adult respiratory distress syndrome. *Clin Chest Med* 1982; 3:159.

SELECTED READINGS

Andreoli KG, et al: *Comprehensive Cardiac Care* ed 4. St. Louis, CV Mosby, 1979.

Beal JM: *Critical Care for Surgical Patients.* New York, Macmillan Publishing Co, 1982.

Berk JL, Sampliner JE: *Handbook of Critical Care.* Boston, Little, Brown, 1982.

Best and Taylor's Physiological Basis of Medical Practice. ed 11. Baltimore, Williams and Wilkins, 1984.

Braunwald E, et al: *Heart Disease—A Textbook of Cardiovascular Medicine.* Philadelphia, WB Saunders, 1980.

Bullas J: Hemodynamic assessment. *Crit Care Nurs* 1985; 5:73–76.

Cain HD: *Flint's Emergency Treatment and Management.* ed 7. Philadelphia, WB Saunders, 1985.

Daily EK, Schroeder JS: *Techniques in Bedside Hemodynamic Monitoring.* ed 3. St. Louis, CV Mosby, 1985.

Fowler NO: *Cardiac Diagnosis and Treatment.* ed 3. Philadelphia, WB Saunders, 1981.

Guyton AC: *Textbook of Medical Physiology.* ed. 6. Philadelphia, WB Saunders, 1981.

Hurst JW, et al: *The Heart—Arteries and Veins.* ed 5. New York, McGraw-Hill Book Company, 1982.

Kenner CV: *Critical Care Nursing; Body, Mind, Spirit.* Boston, Little, Brown, 1981.

Luckmann J, Sorenson KC: *Medical-Surgical Nursing—A Psychophysiological Approach.* ed 2. Philadelphia, WB Saunders, 1980.

Meltzer LE, Pinneo R, Kitchell R: *Intensive Coronary Care—A Manual for Nurses.* ed 4. Bowie, MD, Robert J. Brady Company, 1983.

Millar S, et al: *Methods in Critical Care—The AACN Manual.* ed 2. Philadelphia, WB Saunders, 1985.

O'Boyle CM et al: *Emergency Care—The First 24 Hours.* E Norwalk, CT, Appleton-Century-Crofts, 1985.

Palmer PN: Advanced hemodynamic assessment. *Dimensions of Critical Care Nursing 1982;* 1:139–144.

Quaal S: *Comprehensive Intra-Aortic Balloon Pumping.* St. Louis, CV Mosby, 1984.

Saxton D, et al: *Addison-Wesley Manual of Nursing Practice.* Reading, MA, Addison-Wesley, 1983.

Shoemaker WC, Thompson WL, Holbrook PR: *The Society of Critical Care Medicine: Textbook of Critical Care.* Philadelphia, WB Saunders, 1984.

Continuous Monitoring of Mixed Venous Oxygen Saturation

11

KATHLEEN WHITE, RN, MS, CCRN

The purpose of the cardiopulmonary system is to deliver sufficient quantities of oxygen to meet the needs of the tissues. This principle led to the efforts of the past two decades to understand, monitor, and manage cardiac and pulmonary function. So were born artificial airways, mechanical ventilation, and arterial blood gas analysis, followed by pulmonary artery catheters, hemodynamic assessment, and cardiac output manipulations. Arterial blood gas analysis provides information on pulmonary function to permit appropriate adjustments in treatment to improve oxygenation. Hemodynamic data provide information on cardiac output, which can then be manipulated according to its determinants—preload, afterload, contractility, and heart rate. To what extent cardiopulmonary function actually meets the tissue needs for oxygen, however, cannot be known based on cardiopulmonary data alone. A method for evaluating the tissue need for oxygen and the adequacy of the cardiopulmonary system in meeting that need seemed the next logical step in monitoring. This led to the development of the most recent technology in critical care assessment, continuous monitoring of mixed venous oxygen saturation ($S\bar{v}O_2$).

OXYGEN SUPPLY

Chapter 2, Pulmonary Anatomy and Physiology, presented the concept of oxygen transport (sometimes referred to as oxygen supply) as the movement of oxygen content (CaO_2), which consists of oxygen dissolved in plasma (PaO_2) and oxygen attached to hemoglobin (SaO_2), by the flow of blood (cardiac output) to the tissues. An equation is used to express this transport (or supply) of oxygen to the tissues:[1–8]

$$
\begin{aligned}
O_2 \text{ Supply} &= \text{Arterial oxygen content} \times \text{Cardiac output} \times 10 \\
&= ([\text{Hgb} \times SaO_2 \times 1.36] + [PaO_2 \times 0.0031^*]) \times CO \times 10 \\
&= ([15 \times 0.98 \times 1.36] + [100 \times 0.0031]) \times CO \times 10 \\
&= (20 \text{ vol. }\%) \times 5 \times 10 \\
&= 1000 \text{ ml/min}
\end{aligned}
$$

Where a. 1.36 is the number of milliliters of oxygen each gram of hemoglobin can carry, and
b. the constant 10 is used to convert the measure of hemoglobin from gm/dl to gm/1000 ml of blood.

When oxygen arrives at resting tissues, dissolved oxygen diffuses out of the capillaries and into the cells, according to the diffusion gradient between them.[1, 5] At the arteriolar end, PO_2 normally begins at 100 mm Hg. With cell PO_2 normally less than 5 mm Hg, dissolved oxygen diffuses out of the vessels and into the cells according to the diffusion gradient. When blood reaches the venous end of the capillary bed, the PO_2 is reduced to 40 mm Hg. As described by the oxyhemoglobin dissociation curve, the reduction in PO_2 prompts the dissociation of oxygen from hemoglobin, which replenishes capillary PO_2 and prevents reduction in capillary PO_2 to such low levels that they lessen the diffusion gradient, which would in turn slow the movement of oxygen into the cells. Because the oxygen attached to hemoglobin is responsible for replenishing dissolved oxygen (PO_2) which diffuses out of the vessels, it is apparent that the PO_2 of the capillary is as good as the oxygen standing behind it attached to hemoglobin. Once the cells receive what they need (approximately 250 ml/min at rest), the blood enters the venous tree to return to the heart with a PO_2 of 40 and with the hemoglobin, on the average, still 75 percent saturated (Fig. 11–1).[11]

The Venous Oxygen Reserve

The oxygen that returns to the heart is referred to as the venous oxygen reserve and is described by the following equation:

$$
\begin{aligned}
O_2 \text{ Reserve} &= \text{Venous oxygen content} \times \text{Cardiac output} \times 10 \\
&= ([\text{Hgb} \times S\bar{v}O_2 \times 1.36] + [P\bar{v}O_2 \times 0.0031]) \times CO \times 10 \\
&= ([15 \times 0.75 \times 1.36] + [40 \times 0.0031]) \times CO \times 10 \\
&= (15 \text{ vol. }\%) \times 5 \times 10 \\
&= 750 \text{ ml/min}
\end{aligned}
$$

The amount of oxygen represented by the dissolved state, PvO_2, represents a very small percentage ($< 2\%$) of the total amount of oxygen that returns unused to the heart. The major store of venous oxygen is found attached to

*Because PO_2 represents only 2 percent of the total amount of oxygen in the blood, the other 98 percent being attached to hemoglobin, PO_2 is often omitted from the equation to simplify the mathematics.[9, 10]

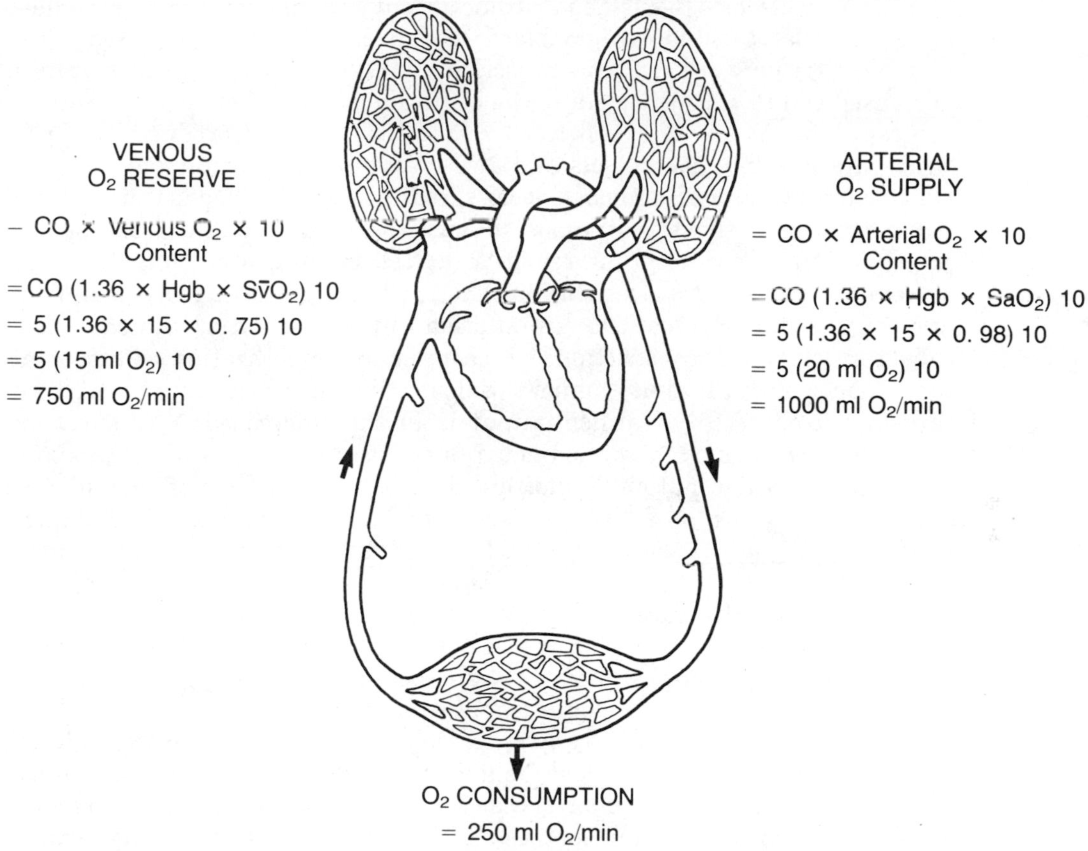

FIGURE 11–1. Oxygen supply, oxygen consumption, and oxygen reserve.

hemoglobin. The venous oxygen content of 15 vol. % multiplied by a resting cardiac output of 5 LPM accounts for a total venous oxygen reserve of 750 ml/min.

The venous reserve of oxygen could serve as the major oxygen source for the tissues when demands for oxygen increase (as in exercise). The venous oxygen reserve, however, is not the first and primary fuel source when routine increases in oxygen demand occur. Furthermore, the venous reserve is not as abundant with oxygen as one would think. When circulation ceases, for example, the total amount of oxygen in the venous reserve is only enough to sustain the body for three to four minutes. Rather than utilize this limited but important store of oxygen, working cells that need more oxygen depend instead on an increase in oxygen supply.

Physiologic Means of Increasing Oxygen Supply

The body initiates numerous physiologic steps to increase the supply of oxygen to meet increased oxygen needs of the tissues.[12–14] These steps involve hemodynamic efforts to augment cardiac output and involve respiratory efforts to insure that the more rapid blood flow is kept fully oxygenated. First, increased tissue work (such as muscle activity, digestion of food) results in decreased cell PO_2, thus widening the diffusion gradient between the cell and the capillary. Meanwhile, cell work results in increased production of CO_2, which diffuses into the vessels and also creates a more acidic environment. Decreasing PO_2 and pH promotes local vasodilation. Afterload is thus reduced, a hemodynamic effect that tends to increase cardiac output. Second, the arrival of increased PCO_2 at sensitive aortic, carotid, and central nervous system receptors stimulates a sympathetic discharge to increase heart rate and contractility. Sympathetic stimulation to the vasculature of nonworking cells results in vasoconstriction, which promotes mobilization of blood into the venous return, to thus augment preload. With increases in preload, heart rate, and contractility, cardiac output is further increased. With maximal exercise, these hemodynamic maneuvers can result in as much as a sixfold increase in cardiac output. Conditioned athletes have been found to have cardiac outputs as high as 30 liters per minute at maximal exercise. Changes in cardiac output, therefore, are clearly not controlled by the heart but rather by the tissues, according to their needs for oxygen.[5]

Sympathetic discharge to the respiratory center stimulates increased rate and depth of breathing, which insures that the blood flowing more quickly through the pulmonary vasculature is exposed to oxygen and that oxygen saturation of arterial hemoglobin is maintained.

When tissue needs for oxygen increase—such as with exercise, work, increased metabolic rates of fever, shivering, and so on—the normal physiologic response is to increase oxygen supply and preserve the venous reserve. The increase in supply to meet the increased demand of exercise can be illustrated by the equation in Table 11–1, wherein cardiac output has increased to 15 liters per minute to provide oxygen to tissues whose consumption has increased to 1000 ml/min.

With the increase in cardiac output, oxygen supply is increased threefold. With the additional supply, the working tissues consume four times that of

TABLE 11–1. Normal O_2 Supply, Consumption, and Reserve

At Rest:				
Arterial O_2 supply	−	O_2 Consumption	=	Venous O_2 reserve
$CaO_2 \times CO \times 10$	−	250 ml/min	=	$CvO_2 \times CO \times 10$
$(Hgb \times 1.36 \times SaO_2) \times CO \times 10$	−	250 ml/min	=	$(Hgb \times 1.36 \times SvO_2) \times CO \times 10$
$(15 \times 1.36 \times 0.98) \times 5 \times 10$	−	250	=	$(15 \times 1.36 \times 0.75) \times 5 \times 10$
1000 ml/min	−	250	=	750 ml/min
During Exercise:				
Arterial O_2 supply	−	O_2 Consumption	=	Venous O_2 reserve
$CaO_2 \times CO \times 10$	−	1000 ml/min	=	$CvO_2 \times CO \times 10$
$(15 \times 1.36 \times 0.98) \times 15 \times 10$	−	1000 ml/min	=	$(15 \times 1.36 \times 0.65) \times 15 \times 10$
3000 ml/min	−	1000 ml/min	=	2000 ml/min

TABLE 11–2. Examples of O_2 Supply/Demand Imbalances with Subsequent Use of the Venous Oxygen Reserve

Hypoxemia				
$CaO_2 \times CO \times 10$	−	250 ml/min	=	$CvO_2 \times CO \times 10$
$(Hgb \times 1.36 \times SaO_2) \times CO \times 10$	−	250 ml/min	=	$(Hgb \times 1.36 \times S\bar{v}O_2) \times CO \times 10$
$(15 \times 1.36 \times 0.80) \times 5 \times 10$	−	250 ml/min	=	$(15 \times 1.36 \times 0.55) \times 5 \times 10$
816 ml/min	−	250 ml/min	=	566 ml/min
Anemia				
$(8 \times 1.36 \times 0.98) \times 5 \times 10$		250 ml/min	−	$(8 \times 1.36 \times 0.52) \times 5 \times 10$
533 ml/min	−	250 ml/min	=	283 ml/min
Heart Failure				
$(15 \times 1.36 \times 0.98) \times 2 \times 10$		250 ml/min	=	$(15 \times 1.36 \times 0.37) \times 2 \times 10$
400 ml/min	−	250 ml/min	=	150 ml/min
Heart Failure and Pulmonary Edema				
$(15 \times 1.36 \times 0.80) \times 2 \times 10$	−	180 ml/min	=	$(15 \times 1.36 \times 0.36) \times 2 \times 10$
326 ml/min	−	180 ml/min	=	146 ml/min
Excessive O_2 Demands				
$(15 \times 1.36 \times 0.98) \times 8 \times 10$	−	1000 ml/min	=	$(15 \times 1.36 \times 0.37) \times 8 \times 10$
1600 ml/min	−	1000 ml/min	=	600 ml/min

the resting state in order to meet the oxygen demands of exercise. Only minimal use of the venous oxygen reserve (the second source of oxygen in time of need) has occurred. Enough oxygen has been delivered to the capillaries that even with the fourfold increase in tissue oxygen consumption, the hemoglobin returns to the heart still 65% saturated (within the limits of normal).[12, 15] Assuming no abnormal shift in the oxyhemoglobin dissociation curve, an $S\bar{v}O_2$ of 65% implies that dissolved oxygen, PO_2, was maintained above 35 mm Hg. The increase in oxygen supply not only maintained the oxygen diffusion gradient at the tissue level but also preserved the venous oxygen reserve.

Clearly, in the critical care unit, some patients are unable to increase oxygen supply to match increased demands (Table 11–2). The most unstable patients are those whose supply system (CO, SaO_2, Hgb) is incapable of meeting even resting demands. When supply fails to meet demand, the tissues "extract" more oxygen, ie, more dissolved oxygen moves out of the capillaries.[13, 15] This prompts the desaturation of hemoglobin, whose rate of delivery to the tissues is already inadequate to replenish capillary PO_2.[15, 16] Falling capillary PO_2 results in a lessened diffusion gradient and thus slowed movement of oxygen into the cells, When cell consumption of oxygen falters due to the inadequate diffusion gradient, cell demand for oxygen cannot be met. At this point anaerobic metabolism and lactic acidosis occur.[3, 7, 13]

Since change in O_2 saturation is prompted by change in PO_2—especially on the venous end of the oxyhemoglobin dissociation curve, where small changes in PO_2 result in significant change in O_2 saturation—and since $S\bar{v}O_2$ is depleted only when O_2 supply fails to meet demand, it becomes apparent that $S\bar{v}O_2$ monitoring might serve as a sensitive barometer to O_2 supply/demand status. If $S\bar{v}O_2$ decreases, reflecting a use of the venous reserve, the clinician could then deduce that O_2 demands were in excess of O_2 supply, the determinants of which are cardiac output, hemoglobin, and SaO_2.

TECHNOLOGY OF $S\bar{v}O_2$ MONITORING

In 1981, Oximetrix (Mountain View, California) introduced a pulmonary artery catheter capable of customary hemodynamic measurements (pulmonary artery pressure, pulmonary artery wedge pressure, central venous pressure, cardiac output) as well as continuous monitoring of mixed venous oxygen saturation. $S\bar{v}O_2$ is measured by reflection spectrophotometry through fiberoptics housed in the catheter. One fiberoptic transmits narrow wavebands of light down the catheter and out the catheter tip, which is positioned in the pulmonary artery. Light that strikes the red blood cells is absorbed and reflected, according to the saturation of the hemoglobin, toward the receiving fiberoptic in the catheter. This information is then transmitted through a cable to a microprocessor, which interprets the signal, averages the computed $S\bar{v}O_2$ over a 5-second interval, and continuously reports the $S\bar{v}O_2$ on a digital display and on a slow (4 inches/hr) trend recorder.

Venous blood is considered "mixed" once it has circulated through the right side of the heart and has reached the pulmonary artery. Mixed venous blood represents an average of venous effluents from all parts of the body. Measurement of hemoglobin saturation in any other venous structure, for example the superior vena cava or right atrium, could result in fluctuations in $S\bar{v}O_2$, as sampling of specific venous effluents could occur. The hemoglobin saturation of venous blood from the heart, for example, is approximately 30% and from the kidneys, 91%.[17] The oxygen saturation of mixed venous blood is normally 60 to 80%.

Mixed venous oxygen saturation may also be monitored intermittently by obtaining serial samples of blood drawn from a pulmonary artery catheter. The technique for obtaining a mixed venous blood sample is outlined in Table 11–3.

Interpreting Change in $S\bar{v}O_2$

Impairment of the cardiopulmonary system jeopardizes the ability of the patient to supply adequate amounts of oxygen to the tissues (see Table 11–2). Continuous monitoring of $S\bar{v}O_2$ permits on-going assessment of oxygen supply/demand balance. A decrease in $S\bar{v}O_2$ signals use of the patient's venous reserve and the need to investigate the extent of the patient's oxygen demands as well as the status of his or her oxygen supply (CO, Hgb, SaO_2).

In the patient with respiratory dysfunction/failure (eg, ARDS, pulmonary edema, pulmonary embolism), $S\bar{v}O_2$ can be used primarily as a reflection of SaO_2. Physiologically, a decline in SaO_2, and thus arterial oxygenation,

TABLE 11–3. Obtaining Mixed Venous Blood Gas Samples

Equipment

Heparinized blood gas syringe (usually 3-ml syringe with 1 ml of heparin)
Syringe cap
10-ml syringe for clearing line before sampling
10-ml syringe for clearing line after sampling
Cup of ice

Procedure

Wash hands
Prepare blood gas syringe
1. Draw up 1 ml of heparin and coat inside of syringe
2. Expel excess heparin, leaving heparin to fill the dead space in the hub of the syringe

Locate the sampling stopcock connected to the distal port of the pulmonary artery catheter
Attach 10-ml syringe
Turn stopcock OFF to the flush solution
Using 10-ml syringe, aspirate 5 ml to clear the line of flush solution. Close stopcock to the halfway position. Remove and discard syringe
Attach blood gas syringe
Open stopcock again to the distal port and aspirate sample slowly. Aspirating too rapidly may "arterialize" the sample, ie, withdrawing blood backward from the alveolar level, where blood is reoxygenated. Also, applying too much suction on the pulmonary artery may collapse the vessel, making it impossible to collect the sample
Close stopcock and remove blood gas syringe. Hold syringe upright and expel any air in the syringe. Cap the syringe and roll it gently to mix the blood with the heparin. Cap and submerge in ice immediately
Attach sterile syringe to stopcock. Open stopcock to the flush solution, and irrigate into the syringe until stopcock is clear. Turn stopcock OFF to the sampling port. Remove and discard the syringe, cap the port with sterile cap or plug
Flush line until traces of blood are removed
Check bedside oscilloscope to confirm presence of pulmonary artery waveform and patency of line
Label the specimen/lab slip with:
1. patient name and ID number
2. type of sample: mixed venous blood gas
3. date and time sample was drawn
4. type and amount of oxygen therapy
5. patient's temperature

Expedite delivery of the sample to the laboratory

prompts compensatory mechanisms to insure supply by increasing cardiac output. If the patient cannot augment the cardiac output in order to compensate for the SaO_2 deficit in the O_2 supply equation, then supply will fail to meet demand and the venous oxygen reserve ($S\bar{v}O_2$) will be used.[18] The best example of decreased $S\bar{v}O_2$ as a reflection of a decreased SaO_2/PaO_2 can be seen during endotracheal suctioning (Fig. 11–2). Suctioning technique that does not include hyperoxygenation or hyperinflation before suctioning can deplete the patient's SaO_2/PaO_2. With this impairment in oxygen supply, the patient will utilize greater amounts of the venous reserve, as seen by a prompt decline in $S\bar{v}O_2$. Restoration of the oxygen source/mechanical ventilator usually replenishes SaO_2/PaO_2, resulting in a prompt restoration of $S\bar{v}O_2$.

$S\bar{v}O_2$ monitoring has been used in combination with continuous arterial PO_2 and SaO_2 monitoring (eg, ear oximetry) to reveal both the status of oxygen supply/demand and the status of SaO_2, as one of the four possible

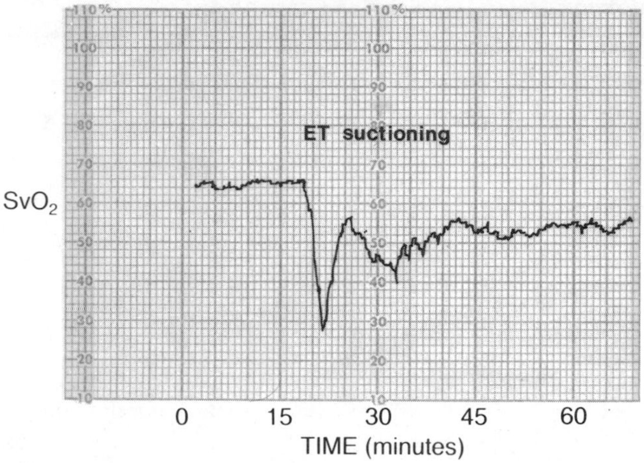

FIGURE 11–2. Effect of endotracheal suctioning $S\bar{v}O_2$.

contributors to an oxygen supply/demand imbalance. Once therapy for respiratory dysfunction is begun (ie, endotracheal intubation, mechanical ventilation, positive end-expiratory pressure adjustments, diuresis), improvements in $S\bar{v}O_2$ can be interpreted as improvement in oxygen supply (ie, improvement in SaO_2/PaO_2)[19] or a reduction in oxygen demand (eg, decreased work of breathing), or both. These $S\bar{v}O_2$ interpretations often reduce the need for arterial blood gas sampling and cardiac output measurements during adjustments in therapy.

Patients with decreased hemoglobin, whether chronic or acute, are also forced to compensate for the deficit in O_2 supply by increasing cardiac output.[7] If cardiac output is unable to make up for the deficit in hemoglobin such that supply fails to meet demand, $S\bar{v}O_2$ will be accessed. For this reason, $S\bar{v}O_2$ can be used to track change in hemoglobin in the patient at risk for bleeding. Decline in hemoglobin tends to create a slow, downward trend in $S\bar{v}O_2$, seen over several hours rather than minutes (Fig. 11–3). Identification of this trend in $S\bar{v}O_2$ prompts an assessment of $S\bar{v}O_2$ and cardiac output as possible causes. Those being ruled out, hemoglobin should then be measured.

As a reflection of cardiac output, $S\bar{v}O_2$ monitoring can be in some cases a sensitive assessment technique. Anything that jeopardizes cardiac output (eg, myocardial infarction, open heart surgery, ischemic heart disease, myocardial depressant medications) may not only compromise oxygen supply at rest but also prohibit the compensatory increases in cardiac output that are necessary to satisfy increased oxygen needs of working tissues.[6,7] A cardiac output that is adequate at rest may be inadequate when activity increases. Again, supply that fails to meet demand results in the use of the venous oxygen reserve. From this standpoint, $S\bar{v}O_2$ can be used as a sensitive indicator of how well the cardiac output is able to keep up with the tissues' demand for oxygen.

In the patient with cardiac compromise, decline in $S\bar{v}O_2$ can be interpreted as a decline in oxygen supply or an increase in oxygen demand that exceeds

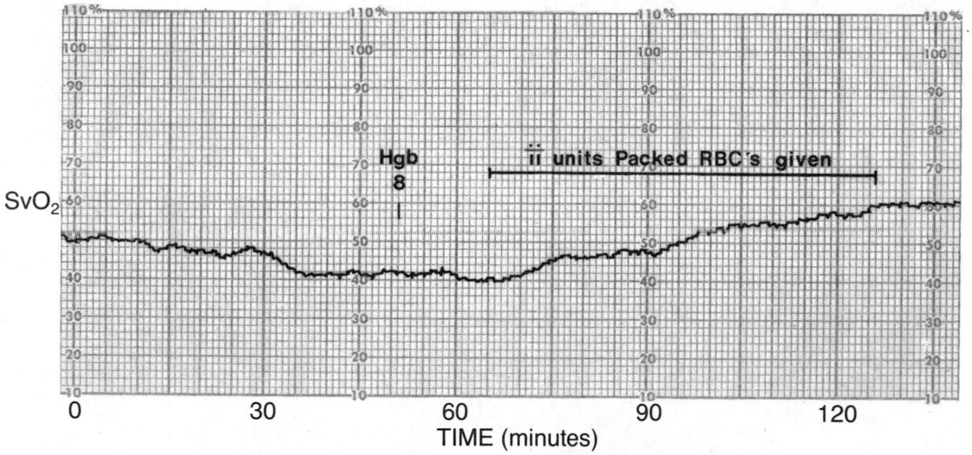

FIGURE 11–3. $S\bar{v}O_2$ as a reflection of change in hemoglobin.

the ability of the supply system, in particular cardiac output, to satisfy that demand. The clinician is prompted to investigate cardiac output as the possible cause in this instance. Once therapy to improve cardiac output is initiated, whether by preload or afterload manipulation or the use of inotropic agents, the clinician can use $S\bar{v}O_2$ to reflect the appropriateness of the therapy (Fig. 11–4). For example, a dose of dopamine that effectively reduces afterload while providing inotropic support and that improves cardiac output to the extent that O_2 supply is able to meet demand would result in a restoration of the patient's $S\bar{v}O_2$. Continuous $S\bar{v}O_2$ monitoring can provide confirmation that the assessment of the problem and the treatment were correct.[11]

The most extreme examples of depleted $S\bar{v}O_2$ can be found in those patients who have more than one reason for an inadequate oxygen supply. The patient with congestive heart failure and pulmonary edema, for example,

FIGURE 11–4. $S\bar{v}O_2$ as a reflection of change in cardiac output.

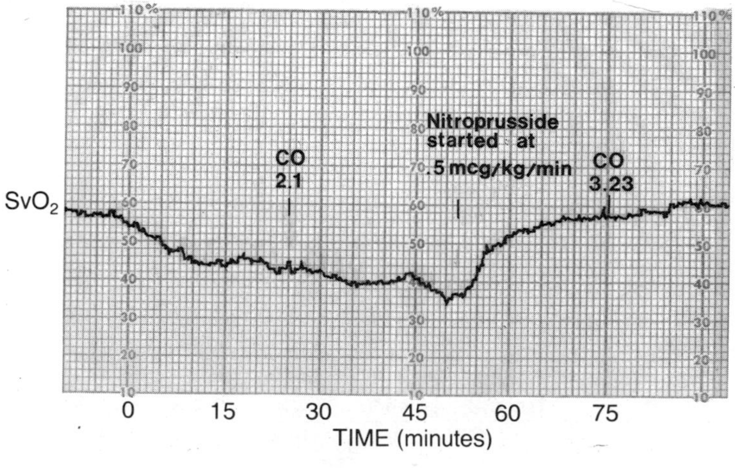

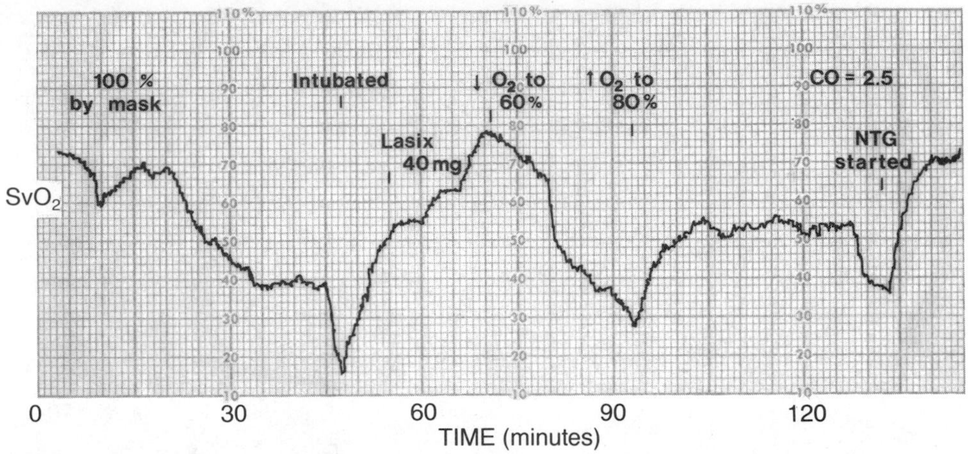

FIGURE 11–5. Wide fluctuations in $S\bar{v}O_2$ reflecting patient response to treatment for hypoxemia and pump failure.

can suffer compromise in both cardiac output and SaO_2/PaO_2 (Fig. 11–5). The deficit in oxygen supply is so great that even use of the venous oxygen reserve is not enough to satisfy tissue demands for oxygen. With oxygen consumption less than demand, anaerobic metabolism and lactic acidosis result, bringing with them further deterioration in cardiac performance.

$S\bar{v}O_2$ can be used by caregivers to individualize the level of the patient's activity according to the adequacy of the oxygen supply system (CO, Hgb, SaO_2).[11] Activities such as positioning, increased work of breathing, anxiety, shivering, or fever, which increase tissue demands for oxygen faster than the supply system can satisfy them, will be met with prompt desaturation in $S\bar{v}O_2$. Whether the patient has a marginal cardiac output, is dealing with declining hemoglobin levels, or has continued pulmonary dysfunction, the physiologic effect is the same—the patient must either increase the cardiac output to compensate, or utilize the venous oxygen reserve. Any patient with an $S\bar{v}O_2$ of less than 50% (implying a PO_2 of less than 25 mm Hg) clearly has been forced toward the latter of the two choices. Efforts to increase this patient's activity would be inappropriate in this setting. Activities such as nasogastric tube insertion, bathing, weighing, or toileting should be carried out with caution (Fig. 11–6). Measures to reduce tissue demands, such as pacing the physical activity, coaching on deep breathing exercises, providing pain medications, administering paralyzing agents, or dealing with the patient's stress, may be indicated. As the patient's oxygen supply/demand balance recovers, $S\bar{v}O_2$ can be used to pace activity according to the tolerance of the patient.

Conditions That Increase $S\bar{v}O_2$

Hemoglobin that returns to the heart with a greater than normal oxygen saturation may be an indicator that normal cell use of oxygen is impaired.

Conditions that may prohibit normal cell utilization of supplied oxygen include septicemia and cyanide toxicity.[1, 6, 8, 17] In septicemia, injury to the microvasculature with subsequent cellular hypoxia may injure the mitochondria to the extent that less oxygen is processed by the cell. Furthermore, the opening of anatomic shunts permits arterial blood to bypass the capillary. When the transported oxygen fails to be utilized at the capillary level, blood enters the venous circulation with a greater than normal content of oxygen. The phenomenon is similar in cyanide toxicity, whereby chemical blockade of the mitochondria prohibits their use of available oxygen.

A second cause of an abnormally elevated $S\bar{v}O_2$ is a leftward shift of the oxyhemoglobin dissociation curve. Hypothermia, an elevated pH, and a deficit of 2,3-diphosphoglycerate are conditions known to shift the curve to the left, thus increasing the affinity of hemoglobin for oxygen. Consequently, when cell use of oxygen results in a falling capillary PO_2, hemoglobin fails to release its store of oxygen. Hemoglobin, with its increased affinity for oxygen, returns to the heart with much of its store of oxygen still attached. Like septicemia and cyanide toxicity, the cells utilize less than the required amounts of oxygen, thus contributing to their own hypoxia and dysfunction.

SUMMARY

Assessment of hemodynamic and pulmonary function utilizing pulmonary artery catheters and arterial blood gas analyses has become standard in the care of the critically ill. The data provided, however, focus on the status of oxygen supply but not on how well the supply is meeting the demands of the tissues. Because the purpose of the cardiopulmonary system is to supply enough oxygen to meet the needs of the tissues, it is also important to assess the tissue use of oxygen. Continuous $S\bar{v}O_2$ monitoring is one technology that permits the on-going assessment of oxygen supply/demand balance. Efforts

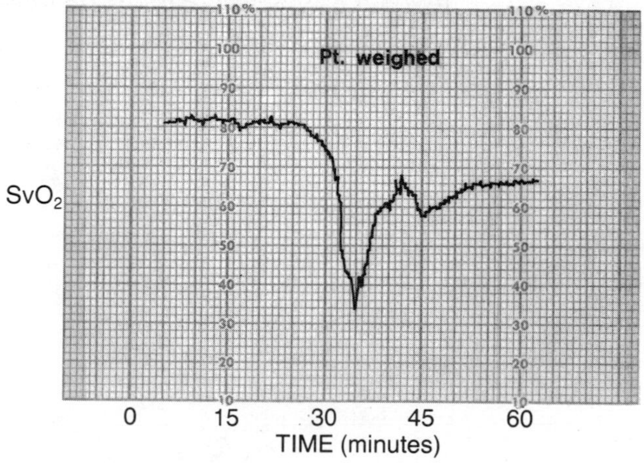

FIGURE 11–6. Effect of increased activity on one patient's $S\bar{v}O_2$.

directed toward improving supply or controlling demand, or both, may then be initiated to reverse those supply/demand imbalances that threaten the stability of the patient.

REFERENCES

1. Miller MJ: Tissue oxygenation in clinical medicine: An historical review. *Anesthesia and Analgesia* 1982; 61:527–535.
2. Comroe JH: *The Physiology of Respiration*. Chicago, Year Book Medical Publishers, 1974, pp 183–196.
3. Kandel G, Aberman A: Mixed venous oxygen saturation: Its role in the assessment of the critically ill patient. *Arch Intern Med* 1983; 143:1401.
4. Keyes JL: Blood-gases and blood-gas transport. *Heart Lung* 1974; 3:945.
5. Guyton AC: *Textbook of Medical Physiology*. Philadelphia, WB Saunders, 1981.
6. Bodai BI, Holcraft JW: Use of the pulmonary arterial catheter in the critically ill patient. *Heart Lung* 1982; 11:406–415.
7. Aberman A: Fundamentals of oxygen transport physiology in a hemodynamic monitoring context. In Schweiss JF (ed): *Continuous Measurement of Blood Oxygen Saturation in the High Risk Patient*. San Diego, Beach International, 1983, pp 13–26.
8. Divertie MG, McMichan JC: Continuous monitoring of mixed venous oxygen saturation. *Chest* 1984; 85:423.
9. Jamieson WRE, Turnbull KW, Larrien AJ, et al: Continuous monitoring of mixed venous oxygen saturation in cardiac surgery. *Can J Surg* 1982; 25:538.
10. Schmidt CR, Frank LP, Forsythe SB, et al: Continuous SvO_2 measurement of oxygen transport patterns in cardiac surgery patients. *Crit Care Med* 1984, 12:523.
11. White KM: Completing the hemodynamic picture: SvO_2. *Heart Lung* 1985; 14:272.
12. Guyton AC: The relationship of cardiac output and arterial pressure control. *Circulation* 1981; 64:1079–1088.
13. Finch CA, Lenfant C: Oxygen transport in man. *N Engl J Med* 1972; 286:407–415.
14. Shepherd AP, Granger HJ, Smith EE, et al: Local control of tissue oxygen delivery and its contribution to the regulation of cardiac output. *Am J Physiol* 1973; 225:747.
15. Cain SM: Oxygen delivery and uptake in dogs during anemic and hypoxic hypoxia. *J Appl Physiol* 1977; 42:228–234.
16. Bryan-Brown CW, Baek SM, Makabali G, et al: Consumable oxygen: Availability of oxygen in relation to oxyhemoglobin dissociation. *Crit Care Med* 1978; 1:17.
17. Folkow B, Neil E.: *Circulation*. New York, Oxford University Press, 1971, p 12.
18. Danek SJ, Lynch JP, Weg JG, et al: The dependence of oxygen uptake on oxygen delivery in the adult respiratory distress syndrome. *Am Rev Respir Dis* 1980; 122:393.

Sepsis from Invasive Hemodynamic Monitoring: Pathogenesis and Prevention

12

BONNIE WESORICK, RN, MSN

Hemodynamic monitoring is a routine and frequently essential element of care for the critically ill patient. The necessity of accessing a central or peripheral vein for pulmonary artery pressure monitoring, multiple or single vein access, or arterial catheterization is rarely questioned. The protocol of care associated with these lines, however, is in question and needs further investigation and definition. Although each kind of catheter is associated with complications, one transcends them all: *sepsis*. While those frequently involved in care of the critically ill know well the grave threat sepsis poses to these commonly debilitated, severely compromised patients, they may be insufficiently aware of the potential for and frequency of sepsis related to indwelling vascular catheters. This chapter focuses on the pathogenesis and prevention of catheter-related infection.

PERSPECTIVES

The most common cause of primary bacteremia (the presence of bacteria in the blood) is intravascular devices.[1] It is estimated that between 25 and 50 percent of nosocomial bacteremia in the ICU originates from an intravascular device. Even though technologic advances are made daily in the health care system, 30 to 50 percent of patients with septicemia are likely to die. Septicemia has no confinement. It is a complication seen in the young, the old, the debilitated, those previously strong and healthy, and the acutely or chronically ill. The mere presence of an intravascular catheter puts the patient at risk of developing bacteremia, and critically ill patients commonly have multiple indwelling vascular catheters.

DEFINITIONS AND DIAGNOSIS

Septicemia is a systemic disease produced by the presence and growth of microorganisms in the blood and portends a poor prognosis. The term *sepsis* is commonly used interchangeably with septicemia, although sepsis may be limited to the presence of bacteria and their toxins in localized tissue. Sepsis caused by indwelling vascular lines, such as those used with hemodynamic monitoring or infusion of fluids, is referred to as catheter-related sepsis (CRS).

CRS implies that the catheter or its delivery system is the primary cause of infection. Diagnosis is often difficult because the catheter's specific role in sepsis may not always be clear. For example, a positive catheter tip does not imply that the patient is septic, nor does a positive tip in a septic patient mean the catheter caused the sepsis. In order for the infectious process to be diagnosed as CRS, the following criteria should be present: The patient demonstrates some signs and symptoms of infection and has a positive catheter and blood culture with the same microorganisms; there should be no previous isolation of the microorganism from another focus; and there should be no other septic focus caused by the same microorganism as isolated from the intravascular catheter in question.

This chapter differentiates among an *infected, contaminated*, or *colonized* catheter as follows.

Colonized Catheter. A colonized catheter is one which, when cultured, shows bacterial presence or adherence. When the catheter tip culture is positive for growth of microorganisms, the practitioner must seek the cause or source, referred to as either contamination or seeding.

Contamination. This term implies that the catheter or its system is the source of the microorganisms. A contaminated catheter can then develop into a primary focus for local or systemic infection.

SEEDING. Seeding implies that the source of catheter colonization is bloodborne from another focus such as an abdominal infection. A seeded catheter can support growth of microorganisms and then reseed the blood and be as detrimental as the primary focus.

Infected Catheter. This term describes the presence of a significant number of microorganisms found on the catheter (15 colonies per agar plate per semiquantitative technique[1]). This term alone only verifies that the catheter is contaminated, not that sepsis is present or absent. However, it may be the first warning that suppurative phlebitis is beginning, a precursor to catheter-related sepsis. An infected catheter does not indicate CRS unless the patient shows septic signs and symptoms that subside after the catheter is removed or the previously listed criteria are fulfilled.

Although definition and criteria help with clarity, they are only guidelines, and the diagnosis of CRS should be considered whenever the patient has clinical signs or symptoms of sepsis, even with a negative catheter tip. For example, the catheter's delivery system may be the source of bacterial contamination. If no other cause of infection can be identified and the symptoms subside after the catheter is removed, the catheter or a component of its delivery system (tubing, stopcocks, fluid) is implicated. Monitoring the sequence of events in any infectious or septic cycle is an essential element necessary to define the catheter's role in the septic cycle as well as to differentiate between a seeded catheter and a contaminated one. For example, if the patient has had a known recent septicemia due to an *E. coli* urinary tract infection and is presently showing signs of sepsis with a positive *E. coli* intravascular catheter culture, it is likely that the catheter became seeded and colonized during the initial septic course and may now be reseeding the blood.

EPIDEMIOLOGIC FACTORS

The health care provider needs a working knowledge of the epidemiologic factors associated with CRS: associated microorganisms, clinical sources or reservoirs, modes of transmission, host status, symptomatology, or defining characteristics. These data provide the basis for the development of standards of care to prevent and identify CRS from hemodynamic monitoring equipment.

Microorganisms Associated with CRS

Microorganisms associated with CRS are not rare, exotic, or different from other infectious agents. Figure 12–1 presents an overview of the common causative microorganisms and also a pictorial depiction of the frequency with which these microorganisms are seen.

Some bacterial trends are evolving. Today, one of the major microorganisms implicated in CRS is coagulase-negative staphylococcus. Historically, all coagulase-negative staphylococci have been referred to as *Staphylococcus epidermidis*. However, recent technologic advancements have made it possible to designate more specifically staphylococci such as *S. hominis, S. capitus, S. cohnii, S. saprophyticus, S. haemolyticus, S. simulans*, and so on. The most common of the species associated with CRS is *S. epidermidis*. Although it is a normal skin inhabitant, *S. epidermidis* has evolved to become one of the major pathogenic concerns of the 1980s. In the past, blood culture reports of *S. epidermidis* were ignored and considered contaminants from skin. Today, *S. epidermidis* can no longer be considered a contaminant, especially when hemodynamic lines are being evaluated as possible sources of sepsis. Catheter materials, such as polyvinylchloride, tend to have an affinity for *S. epider-*

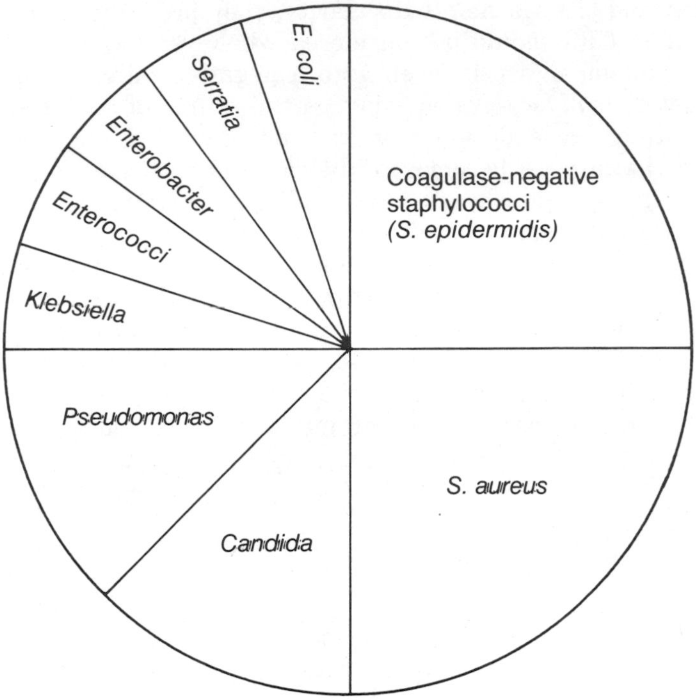

FIGURE 12–1. Bacterial pattern of line sepsis.

midis, and the catheter-adherent bacteria are additionally rendered less susceptible to phagocytosis. Catheter materials are also thrombogenic, and the thrombus may, in turn, become the nidus for bacterial proliferation. The use of systemic antibiotics may not only potentiate the overgrowth of *S. epidermidis* but may be responsible for the increase in antibiotic-resistant (especially methicillin-resistant) strains that have increased markedly in the 1980s.

Pseudomonas and *Candida* continue to be prominent causes of sepsis and occasion a high mortality rate. *Candida* is increasingly becoming another major microorganism implicated in CRS. In most cases it is associated with, but certainly not limited to, lines used for total parenteral nutrition and for patients receiving antibiotic therapy. Of the gram-negative microorganisms listed in Figure 12–1, *Klebsiella*, nonaeruginosa *Pseudomonas, Serratia*, and Enterobacteriaceae are related to sepsis associated with dextrose solutions infused through catheters. The dextrose provides a good media for growth of these bacteria.

Clinical Sources or Reservoirs of Microorganisms

For catheter-related sepsis to occur, the catheter or its delivery system must be infected. Potential modes of infection by microorganisms include:

1. Careless or traumatic insertion technique

2. Migration of microorganisms from the skin at the insertion site downward and around the catheter
3. Manipulation of the delivery system (hubs, tubing, stopcocks, transducers, particularly breaking the closed system)
4. Use of contaminated infusates
5. Hematogenous seeding of the catheter from other infected foci
6. The development of a fibrin sheath around the vascular catheter and subsequent bacterial invasion of the clot.

The two sources or reservoirs of invading microorganisms are animate and inanimate objects in the patient's environment or on or within the patient.

Animate Reservoir. The animate reservoir is the skin of the patient or another septic focus such as an abdominal wound or draining abscess. The animate reservoir also includes the skin of the health care providers, who then colonize the vascular access site or delivery system through hands-on contact. *The caregiver is the main source of bacterial contamination that causes CRS.*

Inanimate Reservoir. This source consists of the environment and fomites. Fomites are not a source of microorganisms when they come direct from the manufacturer. Inanimate objects appear to play a minor role in CRS; however, IV solutions, tubing systems, or hemodynamic monitoring equipment can be a significant source of microorganisms if manipulated or contaminated by health care providers.

Transmission of Microorganisms

Although the patient's own normal flora may be one origin of microorganisms causing CRS, the *hands of the hospital personnel appear to be the major mode of transmission of bacteria.* The skin flora of the caregiver is different from that of the patient upon entry to the hospital environment. The caregiver routinely carries a more antibiotic-resistant coagulase-negative species of staphylococci as well as a greater number of gram-negative rods such as *Pseudomonas, Klebsiella*, and *Serratia*. For this reason, an important goal in patient care is to prevent colonization of the patient or contamination of the catheter systems with the antibiotic-resistant microorganisms during the patient's hospital stay.

This may be accomplished through fastidious hand-washing technique prior to patient contact or when going from a potentially "dirty" area of the patient's body, such as a draining abdominal wound, to contact with an intravascular catheter. The use of sterile gloves provides another safeguard when any manipulation of a monitoring system catheter or tubing is considered.

Host-Related Factors

The patient's underlying illness and health status outweigh all other prognostic factors in the ultimate outcome of sepsis. In addition, the integrity

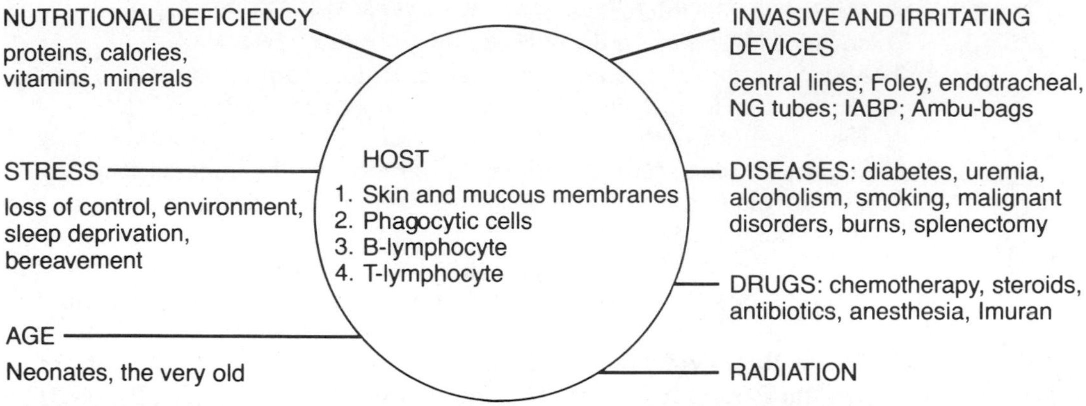

FIGURE 12–2. Factors that alter immune system and enhance risk for infection. (Used with permission from Wesorick B: Practice challenge: Potential for infection. In *Creating the Future.* California, American Association of Critical Care Nurses, 1985, p 129.)

of the immune system is critical in reducing patient vulnerability to sepsis. It is essential that the caregiver be aware of those factors that have the potential to compromise the immune system and thereby place the patient at greater risk to CRS (Fig. 12–2). Patients requiring hemodynamic monitoring often have concomitant factors that interfere with the ability of the immune system to protect against sepsis. Assessing for the presence of these factors and taking measures to alter those that can be changed, such as maintaining an adequate nutritional status and preventing sleep deprivation, will help support the patient's immune system and physical well-being.

Symptomatology/Defining Characteristics

The catheter's role as a source of sepsis is very likely unappreciated and underestimated. The patient is recognized as being septic, but the focus of the sepsis (catheter-related) may never be identified. For example, the offending catheter may be pulled because it fails to function properly before it is identified as the source of the sepsis.

One of the earliest symptoms of catheter-related sepsis is an elevated temperature. CRS from *S. epidermidis* may differ from that of other pathogens in that it is associated with a *low grade temperature*, which may be overlooked, allowing time for the bacteria to proliferate. This may lead to a more severe and prolonged septic course, such as the development of bronchopneumonia with abscess formation, before the definitive diagnosis of CRS is made. Inspection of the catheter site for signs of infection such as redness, swelling, and drainage is essential since site infection increases the risk of CRS. Other early signs specific to CRS, such as changes in mental status (irritability, confusion, lethargy, difficulty with decision making), may occur, along with a rise in glucose even before a temperature elevation is noted. Changes in cardiac output, tachycardia, tachypnea, shaking chills, diaphoresis, changes in the white blood count and platelets, along with general malaise and fatigue, may additionally alter the septic patient's clinical and laboratory picture.

PREVENTION OF CATHETER-RELATED SEPSIS

The basis for prevention of CRS lies in the health care provider's understanding of the previously outlined epidemiologic factors and also knowledge and strict practice of the standards of care relating to insertion, maintenance, and appropriate indwelling time of intravascular catheters used for hemodynamic monitoring. However, more research is needed in all areas relating to prevention of indwelling line sepsis.

Insertion

It is essential that intravascular lines be inserted under the strictest sterile technique. For central venous catheter insertion, gown, gloves, cap, and masks must be worn by the operator, and the patient insertion site should be surgically prepped and draped. All those assisting in the room should wear mask and cap. For arterial catheter placement, the operator should be masked and wearing sterile gloves.

Vascular catheters are commonly inserted into oily areas of skin, which may increase the risk of site infection. Prior to catheter insertion, the proposed area of catheter insertion should be cleansed using an antiseptic soap (such as tincture of chlorhexidine), water, and friction. Friction is essential to remove dead skin, but too much mechanical friction may abrade thin or delicate skin or cause irritation. Following soaping, the area is rinsed well with water. This cleaning function prepares the insertion site for the sterile prep by the physician and provides an added protection against infection.

The agent used for skin preparation should cause rapid microbial killing with no irritation or sensitization of the skin. The agent should additionally be compatible with and not inactivated by other substances on the skin such as alcohol, soap, or organic compounds. Acetone may increase cutaneous colonization and site inflammation. The ultimate antiseptic agent of choice that is most effective (tincture of iodine, chlorhexidine, or an iodophor) or precisely how long the skin prep should be carried out (now generally done from two to five minutes) needs further investigation. If body hair is excessive, clipping is recommended rather than shaving because shaving may produce micro-abrasions, which then become potential sites for local infection.

Percutaneous insertion is superior to cutdown because the latter causes an estimated ninefold increase in septic complications. The more traumatic the insertion, such as occurs in multiple insertion attempts, the greater the risk of infection.

When a guidewire is used for central venous catheter insertion, care must be taken to avoid advancement too far. Arrhythmias are more likely to occur, which may then distract the operator's attention from the sterile field and sterility may be violated.

Maintenance

Maintenance of vascular catheters and the hemodynamic monitoring system is usually the responsibility of the nursing service and is extremely important in the prevention of CRS. The dressing protocol is an important component of maintenance, and aseptic technique is essential. When changing the dressing, care must be taken not to contaminate the catheter insertion site with secretions, such as tracheostomy drainage, or exhalation of tracheal mist. More research is needed relating to the best type of dressing to be used and how often the dressing should be changed. The advantages between transparent and gauze dressings based on multiple studies can be noted in Table 12–1. Two important criteria that any dressing must fulfill are that it be sterile and occlusive.

The dressing change is done to cleanse and inspect the site of vascular insertion. A marked increase in catheter colonization has been noted if the site is infected. In addition, the greater the number of microorganisms found at the insertion site, the greater the chance for catheter colonization, which in turn may lead to catheter infection and CRS. Evidence of local infection, however, is not predictive of a positive catheter tip culture just as the absence of local infection is not predictive of a negative catheter tip culture.

Although controversial, a small amount of antimicrobial ointment placed at the insertion site appears to be beneficial as both a physical barrier and

TABLE 12–1. Comparison of Transparent and Gauze Dressings

Transparent	*Gauze*
ADVANTAGES	
Allows constant site visualization	Less expensive
Impervious to water and bacterial contaminants	Familiar application method
Conforms to body	Some patients prefer site covered
Secures catheter placement	Associated with less frequent colonization of skin and IV catheter tip
Oxygen and moisture permeability	
Hypo-allergenic	
Less frequent dressing changes because of site visualization	
Decreased discomfort with removal	
DISADVANTAGES	
May not adhere to diaphoretic skin	Greater nursing time for dressing changes
More expensive than gauze	Less conformity to body
Greater incidence of skin and catheter tip colonization, particularly if patient has acne, excessive perspiration, or oily skin	Site not visible
	Less stability to catheter
	Tape needed
	No bacterial or liquid barrier
	Needs more frequent dressing changes (every 48 hours for site visualization)

Used with permission from Wesorick B: Sepsis from Hemodynamic Monitoring, 1986.

bactericidal agent. The most effective agent against coagulase-negative *Staphylococcus* may determine the particular antiseptic ointment used since these bacteria constitute the major infection microorganisms in CRS. Polyantibiotic ointment appears to provide the best protection against *S. epidermidis*; however, it is not fungicidal and may promote overgrowth, particularly with *Candida*, if the patient is on systemic antibiotics. It is generally not recommended on lines used for hyperalimentation or arterial lines. Nor has povidone-iodine ointment, one of the most commonly used ointments on central venous lines, demonstrated fungicidal properties. Clearly more research is needed on the value as well as the type of ointment used.

Manipulation of the monitoring system may be one of the most significant causes of CRS because the risk of contamination of the system is increased each time it is opened by the caregiver. Repositioning an indwelling vascular catheter by withdrawal should not increase infectious complications. However, advancing a vascular catheter may introduce microorganisms into the tissue or vascular space from the nonsterile external portion of the catheter. Although much attention has focused on the possibility of bacterial migration from the skin site down and around the catheter, Sitges-Serra[2] et al found hub contamination to be the origin of the *S. epidermidis* that led to CRS. Additionally, the hub contamination appeared to be from the hands of the health care providers who manipulated the system. The hands of hospital personnel are well known to have more antibiotic-resistant gram-negative bacteria as well as more resistant *S. epidermidis* and *S. aureus* than the patient's skin flora. The internal hub is also coated with rich nutrients from IV solutions. These nutrients favor bacterial growth, as evidenced by the fact that when IV solutions leak onto the skin, the site of the leak shows a marked increase in *S. epidermidis* growth. The hub's internal environment as well as manipulation of its structures, therefore, enhances bacterial contamination and proliferation. Until more sophisticated studies are done to determine the precise origin of bacterial contaminants, the catheter insertion site may be wrongfully blamed.

Manipulation or contamination of the system can be avoided or minimized by the following measures:

- Do not break the system to change patient gowns, position the patient, or check for blood return. Gowns with arm snaps, ties, or open arm design are best used for patients with vascular catheters.
- All connection sites are potential sources of systems contamination. Whenever the lines must be manipulated (tubing change), a strict hand wash must be done prior to manipulation. Sterile gloves provide additional protection for the immune-compromised patient. An antiseptic swab is also used to cleanse the site prior to manipulation.
- Insure there is no tension on the site from the weight of tubing and keep all tubing off the floor.
- Avoid stopcocks whenever possible, and use a closed system for entry when they are necessary.
- Avoid blood stagnation in all tubing or connections.
- The use of in-line filters for infection control is controversial. The changing

of filters represents another form of manipulation and may increase risk of line contamination.
- Because solutions containing dextrose support bacterial growth, a heparinized saline solution is preferable for line irrigation.
- Multiple-dose vials for IV additions should be avoided.
- When suctioning the patient, cover the central venous site dressing with a sterile drape. This protects the site from the bacterial spray coming from the artificial airway or suction catheter during the procedure.

Catheter Indwelling Time

The duration of catheter placement is another critical factor relating to the incidence of CRS. The incidence of line sepsis increases with the length of indwelling time, rising steeply after the third or fourth day of line placement. In addition, the longer the catheter remains in place, the greater the likelihood of thrombus formation, which may then become the nidus of infection. The recommended duration of catheter placement will be discussed in a following section relating to specific types of catheters.

A readily available reference (nursing care plan, nurses' notes, progress notes) is essential for monitoring the duration of placement and known risk factors specific to the individual patient for CRS. For example, if a vascular catheter (arterial line, peripheral IV line) is inserted under emergency conditions without optimal aseptic technique, a notation in the nursing care plan alerts others to replace the line at the earliest opportunity following patient stabilization.

SPECIFIC TYPES OF VASCULAR CATHETERS

Studies have shown that a fibrin sheath develops around all catheters once in the vascular system.[3] The rate of thrombus formation relates to the catheter material. For example, polyethylene and polyurethane appear to be less thrombogenic than polyvinylchloride. For this reason, polyvinylchloride pulmonary artery catheters are now available with heparin coating, although the duration of its effectiveness is not yet known. Other factors, such as decreased cardiac output, a hypercoagulable state (cancer, fever, dehydration, acute myocardial infarction), and placement of a central venous catheter in a peripheral vein where blood flow rates are slower than in the large central veins, potentiate the formation of a thrombus. The thrombogenicity of the catheter may be an important factor in the incidence of CRS since the thrombus facilitates bacterial colonization and growth. In addition to the catheter's affinity for thrombus formation, certain catheter materials such as polyvinylchloride have adherence characteristics for coagulase-negative staphylococci. Teflon catheters seem to have the least adherence characteristics for bacteria. Development of a catheter material that will prevent thrombus formation and bacterial clumping but still have flexibility characteristics suitable for catheter insertion and flotation is a major challenge for manufacturers.

Pulmonary Artery Catheters

Use of the pulmonary artery catheter is associated with many potential complications (see Chapter 9). For example, at autopsy endocardial lesions were found in 53 percent of patients who had had a pulmonary artery catheter in place, with 7 percent having right-sided infective endocarditis.[4] The presence of these lesions was not significantly related to the length of time the catheter was left in place. The patient may be at increased risk for endocarditis if there is a primary sepsis (abdominal, pulmonary, urinary tract) during the same time period that the pulmonary artery catheter is in place.

Another significant problem associated with the pulmonary artery catheter predisposing the patient to CRS is frequent catheter manipulation. Singh[5] and Puri noted two to seven catheter manipulations of the pulmonary artery catheter following insertion. Each manipulation potentially increases the risk of CRS. The use of a plastic sleeve that covers the external portion of the pulmonary artery catheter may offer some protection when advancement of the catheter is required. However, one investigator[6] found a high level of growth under the sleeve and warned that it may give a false sense of security and may, in fact, offer little protection. How long the sleeve remains protective is uncertain because the plastic sleeve material is fragile and removing tape or dressings may disrupt its integrity.

The site used for pulmonary artery catheterization may also play a role in the incidence of CRS. The subclavian vein is preferred because it has demonstrated a lower infection rate than the jugular veins or femoral or antecubital sites. It is generally easier to maintain sterile, intact dressings, and there is less stress on the catheter due to head or extremity movement.

Removing the pulmonary artery catheter as soon as possible following hemodynamic stability reduces the likelihood of catheter-related sepsis as well as other complications. Infection rates are known to markedly increase when the catheter is left in place over four days. The critically ill patient, however, may require pulmonary artery pressure monitoring for longer than 72 to 96 hours. In this circumstance, the catheter should be changed no less frequently than every four to five days, although there is controversy regarding the best protocol in this situation: a new venipuncture site and catheter or replacing a new catheter through the original venous site over a guidewire. The controversy is rooted in the issue related to the etiology of CRS; two theories as to how the catheter becomes colonized have been discussed.

The Site as the Primary Source of Infection. Advocates of this theory recommend changing the catheter and site every three to four days.

The Catheter as the Primary Source of Growth of Microorganisms. Advocates of this belief recommend changing the catheter routinely over a guidewire to remove a potentially infected, colonized, or thrombotic catheter if the site is showing no signs of infection and the patient is showing no signs of CRS. Utilization of the same site, if clean, avoids insertional risks associated with new sites (pneumothorax, laceration of an artery, and so on). When the catheter is changed over a guidewire using the same site, the removed catheter tip is cultured. If the tip is positive and the patient is showing signs and symptoms of sepsis, a new venipuncture site and catheter may be required; however, the underlying cause of catheter colonization or infection must be determined, ie, seeding from another infected site. One authority noted that catheter tip colonization increases after four days and suggested changing or removing the existing catheter over a guidewire in septic patients after three days to prevent catheter seeding.[7]

Intra-arterial Lines

The results of several studies[8–10] indicate that arterial lines are associated with a higher rate of sepsis than previously thought. One research found arterial site contamination to be twice as common as pulmonary artery site contamination.[9] The incidence of infection may be decreased by preventing any pooling of blood at the site because blood enhances the growth of *Enterobacter, Klebsiella, Pseudomonas, E. coli* and *Candida*, all common arterial contaminants. Likewise, drawing blood from the intra-arterial catheter increases the risk of infection. Maintaining a closed system for arterial blood withdrawal by using a hep-lock cap on the stopcock may reduce the risk of contamination. Whereas changing the pressure tubing routinely has been advocated to prevent CRS, changing the pressure tubing down to the site opens the system and manipulating the catheter hub increases the risk of line colonization and infection. Usually, the connecting and irrigating tubing are changed every 48 hours. However, more research is needed to determine how often the monitoring system need be changed.

Likewise, the best dressing for the arterial cannulation site needs further research. Maki[1] found higher colonization and septic rates when a transparent dressing was used. He theorized that the small amount of blood that pools at the site of the catheter entrance into the skin enhanced the growth of bacteria. A sterile procedure using a 2 × 2 gauze and iodophor ointment, which is changed every 24 hours so that the site can be inspected and cleansed, seems to be the most advantageous. The presence of phlebitis or site infection markedly increases the risk of septicemia so, if noted, the line should be removed.

Generally, the intra-arterial catheter should be removed as soon as possible because, as with all indwelling lines, the incidence of infection increases with indwelling time. Band and Maki[8] found a significantly increased infection rate after the catheter was in place for four days. More research is needed to determine both the safest and most cost effective time frame for the duration of an arterial catheter as well as maintenance of its monitoring and irrigation systems.

Single and Multiple Lumen Central Venous Catheters

In the past, the single lumen central venous catheter was used for monitoring central venous pressure (CVP) and the administration of fluids, medications, and total parenteral nutrition (TPN). With the introduction of the pulmonary artery catheter and triple lumen catheter, the use of a single lumen catheter for CVP monitoring has decreased markedly, although it continues to be used frequently and effectively for TPN.

The triple lumen catheter provides multiple ports with only one vascular access site. The catheter can be used for CVP monitoring, blood withdrawal, and infusion of multiple solutions (blood products, crystalloids, and drugs). The frequent manipulation of the system at the multiple hubs and its use for both blood withdrawal and delivery increase the risk of CRS. The previously stated principles related to epidemiology, management standards, and catheter material also affect single and multiple lumen catheters. However, research related to the optimal indwelling time, the use of central venous catheters in the delivery of TPN, and the best protocols of care to minimize manipulation of the line and risk of sepsis is so far inadequate to define conclusive management guidelines.

TRANSDUCERS

Transducers, transducer domes, and continuous flow systems have been associated with epidemic and endemic septicemia. Studies have indicated that changing the transducer chamber-dome along with the continuous flow and administration sets every 48 hours may reduce the rate of contamination of these devices and related septicemia.[8, 12] Other studies have reported that transducer systems, disposable and nondisposable, can safely be left in place for longer than 48 hours.[12–15] However, these latter studies did not have large enough patient populations to make valid statements for protocols. It is apparent that more research is needed to determine which protocols offer the lowest infection rate as well as cost effectiveness.

If nondisposable transducers are used, meticulous attention should be paid to cleaning and sterilizing the transducer between patient uses. The physical structure of the transducer (threads, grooves, crevices) favors accumulation and retention of blood or debris that could cause contamination of the fluid-filled system through a small defect in the transducer chamber-dome. Because the interspace between the disposable dome and nondisposable transducer is a potential entrance for infection-causing microorganisms, the interspace should be kept dry. If fluid is necessary to operate the system, avoid the use of dextrose because it provides a growth media for microorganisms. Sterile saline or water may be used according to manufacturer's instructions.

REFERENCES

1. Maki DG, Weise CE, Sarafin HW: A semiquantitative method for identifying intravenous catheter-related infection. *N Engl J Med* 1977; 296:1305–1309.
2. Sitges-Serra A, Puig P, Linares J: Hub colonization as the initial step in an outbreak of catheter-related sepsis due to coagulase-negative staphylococci during parenteral nutrition. *JPEN* 1981; 8:668–672.
3. Stillman RM, Solimon F, Garcia L, et al: Etiology of catheter-associated sepsis; Correlation with thrombogenicity. *Arch Surg* 1977; 112:1497–1499.
4. Rowley K, Clubb S, Smith W, et al: Right-sided infective endocarditis as a consequence of flow-directed pulmonary artery catheterization. *N Engl J Med* 1984; 311:1152–1157.
5. Singh S, Puri V: *Prevention of Bacterial Colonization of Pulmonary Artery Catheters*. Detroit, Mt. Carmel Research and Education Corporation, 1984.
6. Groeger J, Carlon G, Howland W: Contamination shield for pulmonary artery catheters (Abstract). *Crit Care Med* 1983; 11:230.
7. Michael L, March H, McMichan J et al: Infection of pulmonary artery catheters in critically ill patients. *JAMA* 1981; 245:1032–1036.
8. Band J, Maki D: Infections caused by arterial catheters used for hemodynamic monitoring. *Amer J Med* 1979; 67:735–741.
9. Singh S, Nelson N, Acosta I, et al: Catheter colonization and bacteremia in pulmonary and arterial catheters. *Crit Care Med* 1982; 10:736–739.
10. Puri V, Carlson R, Bander J, et al: Complications of vascular catheterization in the critically ill. *Crit Care Med* 1980; 8:495–497.
11. Maki DG: Nosocomial bacteremia: An epidemiological overview. *Amer J Med* 1981: 70:719–732.
12. Maki DG, Hassemer CA: Endemic rate of fluid contamination and related septicemia in arterial pressure monitoring. *Amer J Med* 1981; 70:733–738.
13. Shinozaki T, Deane R, Mazuran J, et al: Bacterial contamination of arterial lines. *JAMA* 1983; 249:223–225.
14. Thomas F, Burke J, Parker J, et al: The risk of infection related to radial versus femoral site, for arterial catheterization. *Crit Care Med* 1983; 11:807–811.
15. Summers M, Bass L, Beiting A: Nosocomial infection related to four methods of hemodynamic monitoring. In *Creating the Future*. California, AACCN, 1985.

SUGGESTED READING

Abbott N, Walrath J, Trump E: Infection related to physiologic monitoring: Venous and arterial catheters. *Heart Lung*, 1983; 12:28–34.

Albert R, Condie F: Handwashing patterns in medical intensive care units. *Medical Intelligence* 1981: 304:1465–1966.

Axnick KS, Yarbough M (eds.): Infection Control: An Integrated Approach. St. Louis, CV Mosby, 1984.

Band J, Maki D: Infections caused by arterial catheters used for hemodynamic monitoring. *Amer J Med* 1979; 67:735–741.

Bjornson H, Colley R, Bower R et al: Association between microorganism growth at the catheter insertion site and colonization of the catheter in patients receiving total parenteral nutrition. *Surgery* 1982; 92:722–727.

Bozzetti F: Letter to editor. *Ann Surg* 1984; 20:101–103.

Bozzetti F, Terno G, Bonfanti G, et al: Prevention and treatment of central venous catheter sepsis by exchange via a guidewire. *Ann Surg* 1983;198:48–52.

Bozzetti F, Terno G, Camerini E, et al.: Pathogenesis and predictability of central venous catheter sepsis. *Surgery*, 1982; 9:383–389.

Brendel V: Current concepts in the care of central line catheters. *National Intravenous Therapy Association* 1983; 6:272–274.

Centers for Disease Control: National Nosocomial Infections Study Report. Annual Summary 1979, Issued March 1982.

Chastre J, Cornud F, Bouchama A, et al: Thrombosis as a complication of pulmonary-artery catheterization via the internal jugular vein. *N Engl J Med* 1982; 306:278–281.

Christensen GB, Bisno AL, Paris JT, et al: Nosocomial septicemia due to multiple antibiotic resistant *Staphylococcus epidermidis*. *Ann Intern Med* 1982; 96:1–10.

Cunha B, Bett M, Gobbo P: Implications of fever in the critical care setting. *Heart Lung* 1984; 13:461–465.

Darbyshire P, Weight N, Speller D: Problems associated with indwelling central venous catheter. *Arch Dis Child* 1985; 60:129–134.

Daschner F: The transmission of infections in hospitals by staff carriers, methods of prevention and control. *Infect Control* 1985; 6:97–99.

Elliot C, Zimmerman G, Clemmer T: Complications of pulmonary artery catheterization in the care of critically ill patients. *Chest* 1979; 76:647–652.

Glister S: The effect of transparent dressing and frequency of change on complications in high risk central lines. *Nutritional Support Services* 1988; 3:40–41.

Goldenheim P, Kazemi H: Cardiopulmonary monitoring of critically ill patients. *N Engl J Med* 1984; 311:776–80.

Gore J, Matsumota A, Layden J, et al: Superior vena cava syndrome: Its association with indwelling balloon-tipped pulmonary artery catheter. *Arch Intern Med* 1984; 144:506–508.

Graeve A, Carpenter C, Schiller W: Management of central venous catheters using a wire introducer. *Am J Surg* 1981; 142:752–754.

Groeger J, Carlon G, Howland W: Contamination shield for pulmonary artery catheters (abstract). *Crit Care Med* 1983; 11:230.

Gruendendemann B, Meeker M: *Alexander's Care of the Patients in Surgery*. London, CV Mosby, 1983; pp 64–66.

Gurevich I: Infectious complications after open heart surgery. *Heart Lung*, 1984; 13:472–479.

Gurman G, Kriemerman S: Cannulation of big arteries in critically ill patients. *Crit Care Med* 1985; 13:217–220.

Haessler R: Transparent IV dressing vs. traditional dressings. *National Intravenous Therapy Association*, 1983; 6:169–170.

Hoar P, Wilson R, Mangano D, et al: Heparin bonding reduces thrombogenicity of pulmonary artery catheters. *N Engl J Med*, 1981; 305:993–995.

Horst M, Obeid F, Vij D, et al: The risk of pulmonary arterial catheterization surgery. *Gynecology Obstetrics* 1984; 159:229–32.

Jacobs M, Yeager M: Thrombotic and infectious complications of Hickman-Broviac catheters. *Arch Intern Med* 1984; 144:1597–1599.

Jarrard M, Freeman J: The effects of antibiotic ointments and antiseptics on the skin flora beneath subclavian catheter dressings during intravenous hyperalimentation. *J Surg Res* 1977; 22:521–526.

Joseph P, Marzouk J: Transparent vs. dry gauze dressings for peripheral IV site. *Hospital Infection Control* 1985; 50–51.

Larson E: Effects of handwashing agent, handwashing frequency, and clinical area of hand flora. *Am J Infect Control* 1984; 12:76–82.

Larson E: Handwashing and skin: Physiologic and bacteriologic aspects. *Infect Control* 1985; 6:14–21.

Larson E, Hargiss C, Dyk L: Effect of an expanded physical facility on nosocomial infections in a neonatal intensive care unit. *Am J Infect Control* 1985; 13:16–20.

Lengthy use of arterial catheters leads to bacteremia, study shows. *Hospital Infection Control*, 1984; 56–59.

Lichtenberg D, Kunches L, McDonough A et al: A randomized study of transparent polyurethane dressings compared to dry gauze dressings for peripheral intravenous catheter sites: Colonization rates and cost effectiveness. Original paper presented at Association for Practitioners in Infection Control, 1984.

Lowry F, Hammer S: *Staphylococcus epidermidis* infection. *Ann Intern Med* 1983; 99:834–839.

Maki DG: Nosocomial bacteremia: An epidemiologic overview. *Am J Med* 1981; 70:719–732.

Maki DG: Presentation: Critical care infection control: Quality vs. cost. Trauma Symposium, Grand Rapids, Michigan, 1984.

Maki D, Band J: A comparative study of polyantibiotic and iodophor ointments in prevention of vascular catheter-related infection. *Am J Med* 1981; 70:739–744.

Maki DG, Hassemer CA: Endemic rate of fluid contamination and related septicemia in arterial pressure monitoring. *Am J Med* 1981; 70:733–738.

Maki D, MacCormick K: Acetone "defatting" in skin antisepsis (abstract). *Crit Care Med* 1981; 9:202.

Maki D, Will L: Colonization and infection associated with transparent dressings for central venous catheters: A comparative trial. Presented to Surgical Infection Society, April 1984, and Association for Practitioners in Infection Control, June 1984.

Mangano D: Heparin bonding and long term protection against thrombogenesis. *N Engl J Med* 1982, 307:894–895.

Marrie T, Costerton JW: Scanning transmission electron microscopy of in situ bacterial colonization of intravenous and intra-arterial catheters. *J Clin Microbiol* 1984; 19:687–693.

McCredie K, Lawson M, Marts K, et al: A comparative evaluation of transparent dressings and gauze dressings for central venous catheters. Abstract presentation for American Societv for Parenteral and Enteral Nutrition, Las Vegas, Nevada, 1984.

McCue J: Improved mortality in gram-negative bacillary bacteremia. *Arch Intern Med* 1984; 145:1212–1216.

Michael L, March H, McMichan J, et al: Infection of pulmonary artery catheters in critically ill patients. *JAMA* 1981; 245:1032–1036.

Miller J, Venus B, Mathru M: Comparison of the sterility of long-term central venous catheterization using single lumen, triple lumen and pulmonary artery catheters. *Crit Care Med* 1984; 12:634–637.

Peters WR, Bush WH, McIntyre RD, et al: The development of fibrin sheath on indwelling venous catheters. *Surg Gyn Obstet* 1973; 137:43–47.

Pinilla J, Ross D, Martin T, et al: Study of the incidence of intravascular catheter infection and associated septicemia in critically ill patients. *Crit Care Med* 1983; 11:21–25.

Puri V, Carlson R, Bander J, et al: Complications of vascular catheterization in the critically ill. *Crit Care Med* 1980; 8:495–497.

Quraishi Z, McGuckin M, Blais F: Duration of handwashing in intensive care units: A descriptive study. *Am J Infect Control* 1984; 12:83–87.

Reier D, Rhame F, Vesley D: Growth of microorganisms in IV solutions containing blood. Original paper presented at Association for Practitioners in Infection Control, 1984.

Researchers claim gauze dressings are "safer" than polyurethane ones. *Hospital Infection Control* 1984; 56–57.

Rowley K, Clubb S, Smith W, et al: Right-sided infective endocarditis as a consequence of flow-directed pulmonary artery catheterization. *N Engl J Med* 1984; 311:1152–1156.

Roy R: Possible hazards from catheter sheath introducers. *Crit Care Med* 1984; 12:616.

Russel J, Joel M, Hudson RJ et al: Prospective evaluation of radial and femoral artery catheterization sites in critically ill adults. *Crit Care Med* 1983; 11:936–939.

Sattler F, Foderara J, Aber R: *Staphylococcus epidermidis* bacteremia associated with vascular catheters: An important cause of febrile morbidity in hospitalized patients. *Infect Control* 1984; 5:279–283.

Shinozaki T, Deane R, Mazuzan J et al: Bacterial contamination of arterial lines. *JAMA* 1983; 249:223–225.

Simmons B: CDC guidelines for the prevention and control of nosocomial infections, guidelines for prevention of intravascular infections. *Am J Infect Control* 1983; 11:183–199.

Singh S, Nelson N, Acosta I, et al: Catheter colonization and bacteremia in pulmonary and arterial catheters. *Crit Care Med* 1982; 10:736–739.

Singh S, Puri V: Prevention of bacterial colonization of pulmonary artery catheters. Detroit, Mt. Carmel Research and Education Corporation, 1984.

Sitges-Serra A, Puig P, Linarea J: Hub colonization as the initial step in an outbreak of catheter-related sepsis due to coagulase-negative staphylococci during parenteral nutrition. *JPEN* 1981; 8:668–672.

Stillman RM, Solimon F, Garcia L, et al: Etiology of catheter-associated sepsis; Correlation with thrombogenicity. *Arch Surg* 1977; 112:1497–1499.

Stratton C: Infection related to intravenous infusions. *Heart Lung* 1982; 11:123–137.

Summers M, Bass L, Beiting A: Nosocomial infection related to four methods of hemodynamic monitoring. In *Creating the Future.* California, AACCN, 1985.

Thomas F, Burke J, Parker J, et al: The risk of infection related to radial vs. femoral sites for arterial catheterization. *Crit Care Med* 1983; 11:807–811.

Trumbore D, Kaye D: Changing patterns of hospital-associated infections. *Infections Surgery* 1985; 1:34–41.

Weinstein RA, Kabins SA, Nathan C, et al: Gentamicin-resistant staphylococci as hospital flora: Epidemiology and resistance plasmids. *J Infect Dis* 1982; 15:374–382.

Wesorick B: Caring for the immunosuppressed oncology patient. In *Caring in a Technological Age.* California, AACCN, 1984, pp 23–25.

Wesorick B: Practice challenge: Potential for infection. In *Creating the Future.* California, AACCN, 1985, 127–130.

Pharmacologic Influences on Hemodynamic Parameters

13

KEITH W. DEANS, PHARM D

Hemodynamic monitoring has greatly refined the evaluation and management of a critically ill patient, especially one who may present with shock or cardiovascular or pulmonary disease. This has led to further understanding of the complex and inherent interactions between disease state and patient response. It would be ideal if intensive care therapy could embody a singular, all inclusive treatment modality to correct fluid balance, blood flow rates, organ function, and vessel compliance. This would allow direct cause/effect or disease/treatment monitoring. Most therapy utilizes a multifaceted approach that includes some form of medication along with supportive care. Inclusion of drug therapy is aimed at altering the disease state or patient response; either will alter hemodynamic parameters. It is rare to find a critically ill patient who is not receiving medications, as many medications form the cornerstone of accepted treatment.

Drug therapy in the monitored, critically ill patient can be characterized by several basic considerations that will uniquely affect care:

- Effective drug concentrations must be achieved rapidly, owing to the urgency of the patients' conditions. To achieve this goal, a route of drug administration must be selected to allow prompt drug absorption and distribution to target organs.
- The correct medication must be chosen initially to treat the symptoms, as rapid hemodynamic circulatory changes from incorrect, or partially correct, selections often further complicate patient status.
- Most monitored patients have some degree of circulatory dysfunction because of their underlying disease state or acute changes. This will alter the medication levels and therapeutic response of agents selected. Medication

dosage regimens must be modified to accommodate these changes.

- The clinical and hemodynamic status of monitored patients often changes rapidly, which requires adjustment of drug dosing.
- Drug toxicities are poorly tolerated in critically ill patients. Thus, avoidance of excessive drug dosing is extremely important.

Pharmacologic effects of a medication have different expressions in each particular patient and disease state. The variability of these effects is compounded when multiple medications are utilized. To be effective, hemodynamic monitoring must encompass the combined effects of disease state, patient, and therapy. By not directly considering the disease state for the moment, three aspects of medication use and hemodynamic monitoring interaction are evident:

1. Hemodynamic parameter monitoring establishes dose, efficacy, and endpoint for the medication.

2. Hemodynamic parameter monitoring establishes adverse drug–patient effects, drug–disease effects, and drug–drug effects, to allow the reinitiation of effective therapy as above.

3. Medications alter the hemodynamic monitoring parameters and precipitate either warranted or unwarranted alterations in patient care.

When disease state is considered as an added factor in monitoring, changes occur in drug effect that are usually expressed as an alteration in hemodynamic parameters. Most often this is due to disease-induced changes in drug elimination and drug levels. These complex interactions are depicted in Figure 13–1. Notice the circular relationship of drug–disease interactions that occurs when further medications are added to treat or counteract adverse drug effects.

This chapter will address changes in hemodynamic parameter monitoring predicted with specific medication use and the complex changes to be expected with various disease states.

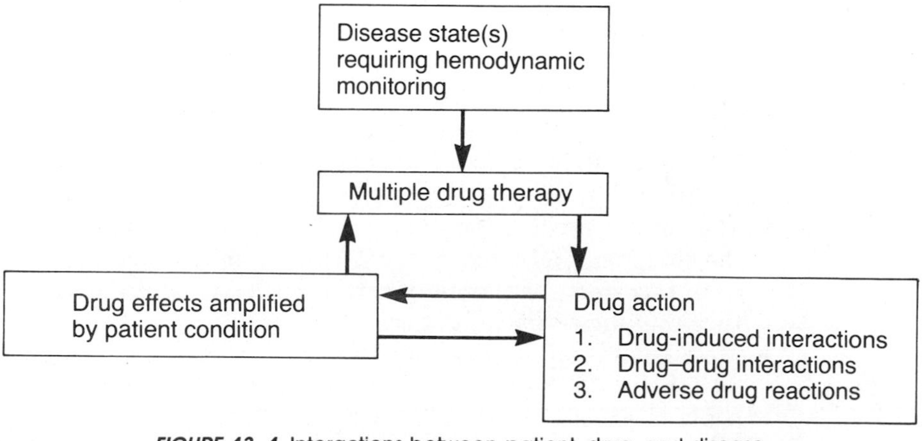

FIGURE 13–1. Interactions between patient, drug, and disease.

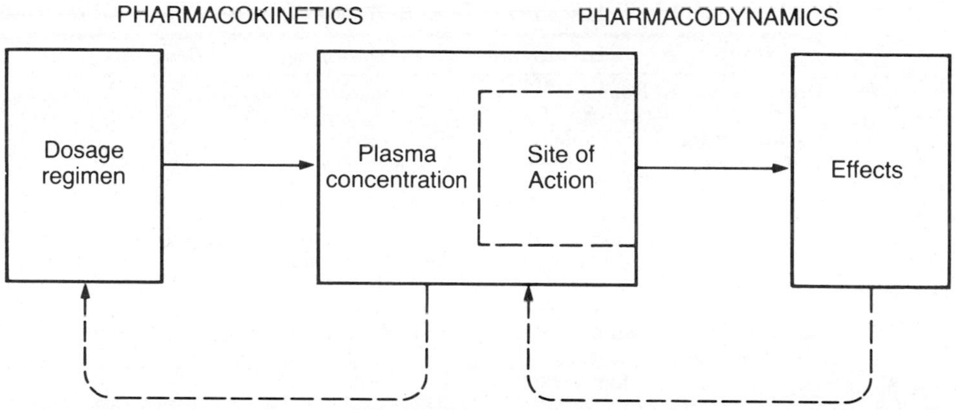

FIGURE 13–2. Interrelationship of pharmacokinetics and pharmacodynamics in a dosage regimen. Either the plasma drug concentration or the effects produced are used to modify the dosage regimen to achieve optimal therapy. (From Rowland M, Tozer TN: *Clinical Pharmacokinetics: Concepts and Applications.* Philadelphia, Lea and Febiger, 1980.)

PHARMACOKINETIC AND PHARMACODYNAMIC CONSIDERATIONS

To begin our discussion of this topic, it will be useful to define these terms; the practitioner needs to know how they interrelate with disease, medication, and patient hemodynamic response.

Pharmacokinetics. Pharmacokinetics is the relationship between route of administration, absorption, distribution within the body, and elimination and excretion for a medication. The correlation of dose, dosing interval, and serum levels achieved will be used to represent medication pharmacokinetics.

Pharmacodynamics. This term relates the mechanism of drug action to the concentration of medication at the effector (active) site and the magnitude of effects produced. This will be referred to as intensity and duration of drug effects (Fig. 13–2).

In a complex patient environment, the interaction of disease, medications, and monitoring must be evaluated together with a clearly defined clinical outcome. In terms of medication influence on hemodynamic parameters, the disease state most often alters medication pharmacokinetics, which alters the pharmacodynamic response. The various components of medication pharmacokinetics and pharmacodynamics must be considered to establish correct drug utilization.

Components of Pharmacokinetics

Route of Administration. Shock and cardiovascular and pulmonary disease most often alter the oral and intramuscular dosing routes. Peripheral blood flow is diverted away from the mesenteric vessels of the gastrointestinal

TABLE 13–1. Routes of Drug Administration for Critical Care Patients

Route	Advantage	Disadvantage	Drugs	Use
Oral	None	Slow, erratic, or no absorption	Many	None
Intramuscular, subcutaneous	Available	Slow, erratic absorption	Lidocaine	Arrhythmia prophylaxis when IV route not available
			Epinephrine	Anaphylaxis
Peripheral, intravenous	Most drugs compatible with this route	Difficult to obtain access	Most	General
Central, intravenous	Can be placed in a severely hypotensive patient	Procedural risks	Many	General
Intratracheal	Available in intubated patients	Few data available	Epinephrine, lidocaine	During cardiac arrest when IM route not available
Intracardiac	Always available	Procedural risks	Epinephrine, calcium	When no other route is available

tract and many lesser perfused muscle groups. This results in slow or poor drug absorption. In critical patients, intravenous therapy is preferred (Table 13–1).

ABSORPTION. By definition, intravenous therapy produces total absorption. Oral and intramuscular absorption rate and amount depend on the peripheral blood flow and dosage form.

DISTRIBUTION. This is dependent on the tissues and organs involved. If a medication is normally contained only within the vascular compartment, there is little change with disease states. Medications with extensive tissue distribution depend on blood flow to those tissues. In many cases, the drug level in the serum will be higher than expected because of altered distribution and poor blood flow to peripheral tissues. Changes in drug distribution with resultant changes in drug levels will readily change hemodynamic parameters.

ELIMINATION. The primary organ of elimination is the liver. As disease or drugs alter hepatic blood flow, overall metabolism and elimination will change. This usually results in decreased drug elimination, increased blood levels, and increased drug effects for a longer period of time. Changes in elimination are the most common causes of drug-induced hemodynamic alterations.

EXCRETION. This is primarily a function of the renal system. If disease or drugs alter renal blood flow, a change occurs in renal filtration, secretion, and reabsorption. This usually results in decreased drug excretion, increased drug levels, and drug effects for a longer period of time. Altered drug excretion is also a significant cause of hemodynamic alterations, which are the result of increased drug effect (Fig. 13–3). For most changes, the dose will need reduction or the dosing interval will be lengthened to maintain a normal therapeutic response and drug levels.

Components of Pharmacodynamics

MECHANISM OF ACTION. The mechanism of action and specific drug–receptor interactions will not be addressed.

CONCENTRATION OF DRUG AT THE ACTIVE SITE. This usually dictates the magnitude of drug effects observed. For most disease states, alterations in distribution, elimination, and excretion result in higher drug levels at the active site, with an increased magnitude of effect. For these considerations, reductions in drug dosage or longer dosage intervals are commonly employed to retain a standard medication intensity and duration.

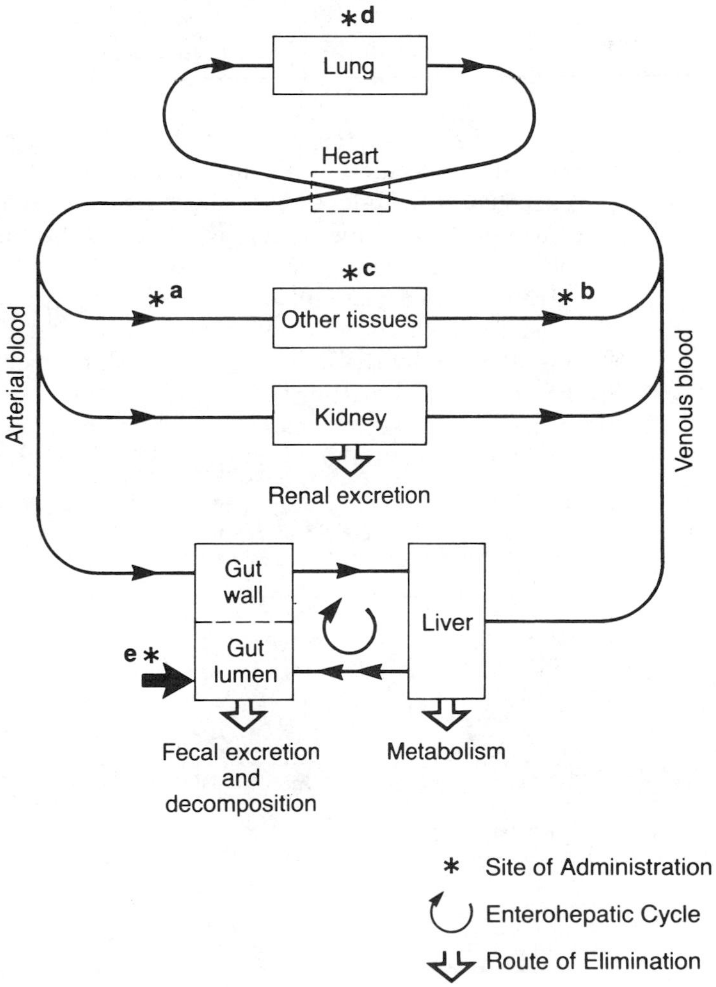

FIGURE 13–3. Once absorbed from any of the many possible sites of administration, a drug is distributed by blood to all sites within the body, including the eliminating organs. Sites of administration are *a*, artery; *b*, peripheral vein; *c*, muscle and subcutaneous tissue; *d*, lung; and *e*, gastrointestinal tract. The lines with arrows refer to the movement of drug in the blood (—➤—) or bile (—◄◄—). The absorption and disposition of virtually any drug can be followed from site of administration to site of elimination. (From Rowland M, Tozer TN: *Clinical Pharmacokinetics: Concepts and Applications.* Philadelphia, Lea and Febiger, 1980.)

CONSIDERATIONS OF DRUG ELIMINATION AND EXCRETION

Most medications presented to the body are either eliminated by the liver and associate systems or excreted by the kidneys. Both these organ systems directly depend on blood flow for their relative function and efficiency. The amount of blood flow to any organ is dependent on cardiac output and local arteriolar resistance. Should the hepatic or renal systems be presented with less blood flow per unit time, the amount of drug eliminated or excreted is reduced.

For simplicity, the term *elimination* is used to describe the hepatic action on drugs whose activity is altered by metabolic change resulting in either active or inactive compounds. The term *excretion* refers to the renal action on drugs or drug metabolites whose activity is altered by kidney filtration and removal from the body.

Hepatic Elimination

Drugs extracted by the liver are either metabolized, conjugated with another molecule to form an inactive complex that is more water-soluble, or excreted in the bile. In both shock and the majority of cardiovascular diseases, blood is shunted away from the liver to the central organs, thus reducing the effective rate of drug elimination. With pulmonary disease, changes in alveolar gas exchange, airway resistance, or respiratory rate may precipitate tissue hypoxia or changes in plasma pH. Such changes result in altered drug metabolism by the lungs and liver. Many medications will also affect hepatic blood flow and further alter hemodynamic parameters. Overall, drug dosages must be altered, or dosing intervals changed, to compensate for the altered drug levels available (Table 13–2).

TABLE 13–2. Factors That Influence Hepatic Blood Flow

	Increase	Decrease
Physiologic	Chronic respiratory problems	Acute respiratory problems
	Supine position	Upright position
		Low blood pressure
		Thermal stress
		Volume depletion
		Age over 65 years
Pathologic	Viral hepatitis	Congestive heart failure
	Uncontrolled diabetes mellitus	Cirrhosis
		Circulatory collapse
Pharmacologic	Glucagon	Propranolol
	Low-dose dopamine	High-dose dopamine
	Isoproterenol	Norepinephrine
	Albuterol	Anesthetics
	Phenobarbital	Cimetidine, ranitidine
	Clonidine	Labetalol

TABLE 13–3. Factors That Influence Renal Blood Flow

	Increase	Decrease
Physiologic	Expanded fluid volume Supine position Acetylcholine	Reduced fluid volume Vasoconstriction Age over 65 years
Pathologic	Acute volume expansion	Cardiac failure Decreased effective circulation (shock, severe dehydration, hemorrhage, hypotension) Hepatorenal syndrome
Pharmacologic	Corticosteroids Low-dose dopamine Low-dose isoproterenol Hydralazine Loop diuretics Nadolol	Nephrotoxic compounds High-dose dopamine Norepinephrine Propranolol Verapamil Indomethacin Clonidine Chlorothiazide

Renal Excretion

Drugs extracted by the kidneys are either directly excreted or first metabolized and conjugated by the liver to more water-soluble forms and then excreted. Renal blood flow influences the normal kidney functions of filtration, secretion, and reabsorption. Alteration in function by interrupted blood flow may also affect the distribution of drugs, change the excretion rate, and result in altered plasma levels. Since blood flow is also shunted away from the kidneys in shock and cardiovascular disease, the effective rate of excretion is decreased. With pulmonary disease, renal tissue oxygenation and pH balance in the tubule change, resulting in decreased filtration/secretion and altered reabsorption. Overall, medication dosages must be altered and dosing intervals changed to compensate for the altered drug levels that result (Table 13–3).

MECHANISMS OF DRUG ACTION

Effects on the Sympathetic Nervous System

Most of the agents presented in this chapter alter hemodynamic parameters through either direct or indirect activity on the sympathetic nervous system. This activity is mediated by effects on adrenergic receptors located in the heart, kidney, vessels, and other tissues. Direct activity involves action of the agent at a sympathetic adrenergic receptor. Indirect activity involves the release of endogenous sympathomimetic compounds, which then exert action at a sympathetic adrenergic receptor. Drugs may act as either agonists (stimulators) or antagonists (inhibitors) of the sympathetic receptors. Studies of the sympathetic nervous system have identified alpha, beta, and dopaminergic receptors. These are further subdivided into $alpha_1$ and $alpha_2$ receptors, $beta_1$ and $beta_2$ receptors, and subclassifications of dopaminergic receptors. Sympathomimetic agents are important modulators of cardiac, vascular, and renal functions. In general, stimulation of alpha receptors results in vascular and smooth muscle constriction, whereas beta receptor stimulation causes increased cardiac drive, plus vascular dilation and smooth muscle relaxation. Alpha adrenergic vasoconstrictive effects predominate over weaker beta vasodilation effects. The location and primary effects of adrenergic receptors that have impact on hemodynamic parameters are summarized in Table 13–4.

Response to a sympathomimetic agent requires consideration of several factors in addition to intrinsic receptor activity (agonist or antagonist) and dose. First, response is dependent on the relative proportion of receptor type and overall receptor density present in the tissue. Second, sympathomimetic agents affect reflex homeostatic mechanisms (e.g., decreased heart rate due to alpha vasoconstriction). Third, prolonged use of sympathomimetic agents decreases the response of adrenergic receptors. Stimulation or inhibition of each receptor type evokes a distinct change in hemodynamic parameters that may be predicted based on known pharmacologic actions.

Effects on the Cardiac Action Potential

Antiarrhythmic agents alter hemodynamic parameters primarily by activity on the cardiac action potential. The electrical impulse that triggers a normal cardiac contraction originates at regular intervals in the sinoatrial (SA) node due to cellular automaticity, usually at a rate of 60 to 100 beats per minute. This impulse spreads rapidly through the atria and enters the atrioventricular (AV) node, which is the only normal conduction pathway between atria and ventricles. Impulse propagation then proceeds through the His-Purkinje system and spreads to all parts of the ventricles. A synchronous

TABLE 13–4. Classification, Location, and Primary Action of Adrenergic Receptors

Receptor	*Location*	*Primary Action*
ALPHA-ADRENERGIC		
$alpha_1$	Vascular smooth muscle	
	Arterioles and venules	Constriction
$alpha_2$	Presynaptic nerve terminals	Feedback inhibition of catecholamine release
BETA-ADRENERGIC		
$beta_1$	Heart (myocardium)	Increased contractility
	SA node	Increased heart rate
	AV node	Increased automaticity
$beta_2$	Vascular smooth muscle	
	Arterioles and venules	
	Pulmonary, bronchial smooth muscle	Dilation
		Relaxation
DOPAMINERGIC	Vascular smooth muscle (renal, coronary, mesenteric)	Dilation

TABLE 13–5. Classification and Action of Antiarrhythmic Agents

Class	Electrophysiologic Effect	Agents
I	Depresses phase 0; depresses either phase 4 or prolongs effective refractory periods	Lidocaine, quinidine, procainamide, phenytoin
II	Blocks beta receptors	Propranolol, labetalol
III	Prolongs effective refractory period, action potential duration	Bretylium, amiodarone
IV	Blocks calcium channels	Verapamil

contraction of ventricular muscle results in hemodynamically effective cardiac output. Arrhythmias deviate from this normal progression and result from disturbances in impulse formation, disturbances in impulse conduction, or both.

The objectives of antiarrhythmia therapy are to reduce cardiac pacemaker activity and modify impaired conduction pathways. Major mechanisms for accomplishing these objectives are 1) sodium channel blockage; 2) calcium channel blockade; 3) prolongation of effective refractory period or action potential duration; and 4) blockade of sympathetic effects in the heart. Agents are divided into four basic classes of activity based on these mechanisms (Table 13–5).

Antiarrhythmia agents decrease automaticity, conduction, and excitability in cardiac cells. This is done by selectively blocking the sodium or calcium channels of depolarized cells specifically during Phase 0 (depolarization) or Phase 2 (plateau prior to repolarization). In cells with abnormal pacemaker automaticity, agents reduce the Phase 4 slope (from resting potential to threshold potential) by blocking either sodium or calcium channels. This reduces the ratio of sodium or calcium permeability to potassium permeability and slows pacemaker discharge rates. In addition some agents may increase the threshold potential to make it less likely that a discharge will occur. Beta-adrenergic receptor blocking agents indirectly alter the Phase 4 automaticity slope by blocking the positive chronotropic actions of norepinephrine in the heart. The site of action of the antiarrhythmia agents in relation to the cardiac action potential is shown in Figure 13–4.

By these mechanisms, antiarrhythmia agents can suppress abnormal automaticity and conduction in depolarized cells, which renders them electrically silent while minimally affecting electrical activity in normal polarized portions of the heart. The overall effects of these agents are similar in regard to hemodynamic parameters, as all will decrease, or have no effective change on, cardiac output through alteration of heart rate, rhythm, or stroke volume.

Other Effects

The remaining agents generally have effects by 1) direct vasodilation of vascular smooth muscle in arterioles, venules, or both; 2) blockade of vascular vasoconstriction; and 3) reduction of effective vascular volume. Homeostatic

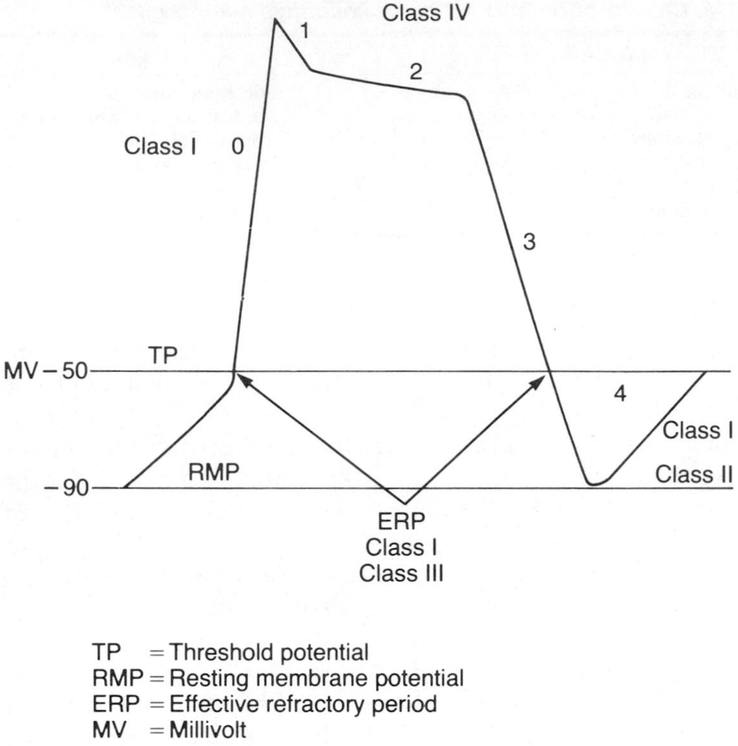

FIGURE 13–4. Primary sites of action potential effect for antiarrhythmic agents.

mechanisms are often involved with these actions, making it difficult to predict overall effects on patient hemodynamic parameters.

INTRAVENOUS MEDICATIONS COMMONLY EMPLOYED IN MONITORED PATIENTS

The medications described here are commonly used in the critical care area and monitored patients. Described for each agent is activity, available IV preparations, dosage, elimination, general monitoring parameters, and any specific cautions with drug use or important drug-disease interactions. This listing is not all-inclusive, but all the medications presented alter hemodynamic parameters directly or interact in the patient to cause indirect hemodynamic alterations. A summary of the expected change in hemodynamic parameters with these medications appears in Table 13–6.

Vasodilating Agents

Nitroglycerine. Nitrates possess peripheral hemodynamic effects, primarily a reduction of preload, but also a slight reduction of afterload. Because of afterload reduction at higher doses, reflex tachycardia, as well as increased stroke volume, results in increased cardiac output.

PREPARATIONS: Tridil, Nitrostat, Nitro-Bid; 0.5 mg/ml, 0.8 mg/ml, 5 mg/ml.

DOSING. Continuous infusion beginning at 0.06 to 0.1 μg/kg/min (average 5 μg/min), with increases of the above dose every 5 minutes until blood or wedge pressure response is obtained. Dosage increments may be increased to 10 μg/min if required.

ELIMINATION. Hepatic metabolism. Half-life is 2 to 4 minutes.

MONITOR. BP, HR, PWP.

Nitroprusside. Nitroprusside is a direct-acting dilator of vascular smooth muscle, both in veins and arteries of the systemic, coronary, pulmonary, and renal circulations. Decreased preload results in reflex tachycardia, and decreased afterload results in increased stroke volume.

PREPARATIONS. Nipride, Nitropress and others; 25 mg/ml, 10 mg/ml.

DOSING. Continuous infusion, begin at 0.5 to 2 μg/kg/min and titrate for BP effect. Increase to maximum of 10 μg/kg/min.

ELIMINATION. Nitroprusside is degraded by electron donation from oxyhemoglobin. Breakdown results in free cyanide ions, some of which react with

TABLE 13–6. Effect on Hemodynamic Parameters of Common Intravenous Medications for Monitored Patients

	HR	*MAP*	*PAP*	*PWP*	*CVP*	*SVR*	*SV*	*CO*
Vasodilating Agents								
Nitroglycerin	↑	↓	↓	↓	0/↓	↓	↑	↑
Nitroprusside	↑	↓	↓	0/↓	0/↓	↓	↑	↑
Hydralazine	↑	↓	↓	0/↓	0/↓	↓		↑
Phentolamine	↓	↓	↓	↓	↓	↓	↑	↑
Vasopressor Agents								
Phenylephrine	0/↓	↑	↑	↑	↑	↑		↓
Metaraminol	0/↑	↑	↑	↑	↑	↑		↑/↓
Mixed Activity Agents								
Epinephrine	↑	↑	↑	↑	↑	↑/↓		↑
Norepinephrine	0/↑	↑	↑	↑	↑	↑		↑/↓
Ephedrine	↑	0/↑	0/↑	0/↑	0/↑	↑		↑
Dopamine	0/↑	0/↑	0/↑	0/↑	0/↑	↑		↑
Inotropic Agents								
Dobutamine	0/↑	0/↑	0	0	0/↑	0/↑		↑
Isoproterenol	↑	0/↑	0/↑	0/↓	0/↓	0/↓	↑	↑
Amrinone	0	↓	↓	↓	0/↓	↓	↑	↑
Digoxin	↓						↑	↑
Antiarrhythmic Agents								
Lidocaine	0	0/↓	0/↓	0	0	0/↓		0/↑
Quinidine	0/↓	↑	0/↓	0/↓	0/↑	0		↓
Procainamide	0	↓	0/↓	0/↓	0/↑	0		↓
Propranolol	↓	↓	0/↓	0/↓	0/↓	0		↓
Labetalol	↓	↓	↓	↓	↓	↓		↓
Bretylium	↑/↓	0	0	0	0	0		0
Verapamil	↑/↓	0/↓	0/↓	0/↓	0/↓	↓		↑/↓

KEY: 0, Little or no change; ↑, increase; ↓, decrease.

CO, cardiac output; CVP, central venous pressure; HR, heart rate; MAP, mean arterial pressure; PAP, pulmonary artery pressure; PWP, pulmonary capillary wedge pressure; SV, stroke volume; SVR, systemic vascular resistance.

free hemoglobin; other ions react with thiosulfate in the liver to form thiocyanate. Thiosulfate is available only in low quantities, so it is very possible for nitroprusside to cause cyanide toxicity.

MONITORING. HR, PWP, BP. Cyanide toxicity: metabolic acidosis, base deficit over 8, serum cyanide (CN) or thiocyanate (SCN) levels.

CAUTIONS. Careful use is indicated, with monitoring in a patient with decreased liver and renal function, or one severely debilitated. Use should not exceed 48 hours. Protect agent from direct light.

Hydralazine. This is a direct-acting dilator of vascular smooth muscle. The primary effect is on arterial resistance, with minor effects on venous resistance. Pulmonary and renal vascular resistance also decreases. There is some reflex tachycardia secondary to afterload reduction.

PREPARATIONS. Apresoline, 20 mg/ml.

DOSING. Intermittent infusion or injection of 5 to 20 mg.

ELIMINATION. Hydralazine is metabolized in the liver. The duration of action is 3 to 6 hours.

MONITORING. BP, HR, liver function. Measurement of antinuclear antibody titers gives an early indication of drug-induced systemic lupus erythematosus syndromes (SLE) that commonly occurs with continued drug dosing.

CAUTIONS. Dose must be reduced with liver dysfunction or poor cardiac output states.

Phentolamine. Phentolamine is an alpha adrenergic blocking agent that causes peripheral vasodilatation by relaxation of vascular smooth muscle. It also stimulates cardiac beta adrenergic receptors, which results in increased heart rate and cardiac output.

PREPARATIONS. Regitine; 5 mg.

DOSING. A bolus of 0.06 to 0.1 mg/kg (average, 5 mg) is followed by an infusion of 3 to 8 μg/kg/min; titrate for effects.

ELIMINATION. Not determined.

MONITORING. HR, BP, CO, ECG.

CAUTIONS. Cardiac arrhythmias and infarction have been reported when used in patients with heart failure or coronary artery disease.

Diazoxide. Diazoxide reduces peripheral vascular resistance by direct effects on arteriole smooth muscle. The degree of response is determined by the degree of vasoconstriction present; best effects occur with malignant hypertension. Rapid IV push administration is required for maximal vasodilatation. Sustained use will cause both sodium and fluid retention, which worsens congestive failure. Inhibition of pancreatic insulin release increases blood glucose levels.

PREPARATIONS. Hyperstat, 15 mg/ml.

DOSING. Initial dose of 1 to 3 mg/kg (75 to 150 mg) administered IV and undiluted over 30 seconds or less. Repeat with 1 to 3 mg/kg every 5 to 15 minutes to sustain decreased blood pressure.

ELIMINATION. Diazoxide is both metabolized in the liver to inactive forms and excreted unchanged by the kidneys. Drug half-life is 28 hours, so some effects are cumulative.

MONITORING. HR, BP, ECG, PWP, renal function, serum glucose.

CAUTIONS. Injection solution is light-sensitive (protect from light); do not use the solution if it is darkened. Dosage must be reduced in renal dysfunction. Diabetic ketoacidosis often develops with decreased renal function. Extravasation causes local tissue necrosis.

Vasopressor Agents

Phenylephrine. Phenylephrine is a sympathomimetic amine that acts by stimulation of alpha adrenergic receptors in the peripheral vasculature to increase both systolic and diastolic blood pressure. It produces an indirect effect by release of norepinephrine. Minimal cardiac beta stimulation occurs at high doses. Blood flow to peripheral organ and coronary and pulmonary vessels is reduced owing to general vascular constriction.

PREPARATIONS. Neo-Synephrine, 10 mg/ml.

DOSING. Begin with an infusion of 1.5 to 3.0 μg/kg/min and reduce to 0.5 to 1 μg/kg/min after blood pressure stabilizes; titrate to desired effect.

ELIMINATION. Phenylephrine is eliminated by tissue uptake and hepatic metabolism.

MONITORING. HR, BP, CO, PWP, renal function, acid-base balance.

CAUTIONS: Reflex bradycardia, decreased stroke volume and increased cardiac work may induce or exacerbate heart failure.

Metaraminol. Metaraminol is a synthetic catecholamine with predominately alpha adrenergic direct stimulation that causes general vascular constriction. Direct $beta_1$ adrenergic effects also cause cardiac stimulation, but no pulmonary or peripheral vasodilation effects. Metaraminol has an indirect effect of releasing norepinephrine.

PREPARATIONS. Aramine, 10 mg/ml.

DOSING. A bolus dose of 0.5 to 5 mg, followed by an infusion of 2 mg/kg at a rate to maintain blood pressure.

ELIMINATION. The drug is eliminated by tissue uptake and renal excretion of unchanged drug. Effects last 15 to 30 minutes.

MONITORING. HR, BP, renal function, acid-base balance.

CAUTIONS. When metaraminol is used for prolonged periods, it depletes norepinephrine stores at sympathetic nerve endings and may predispose the patient to tachyphylaxis. In addition, secondary vasodilation and a capillary leak syndrome may predispose to hypovolemia.

Mixed Activity Agents (Vasopressor and Inotropic)

Epinephrine. This drug is a catecholamine with alpha and beta adrenergic stimulation effects, primarily beta at low doses and alpha at higher doses. Beta effects cause general vessel dilation and cardiac stimulation whereas alpha effects primarily cause vasoconstriction.

PREPARATIONS. Adrenalin and others; 1 mg/ml (1:1000) and 0.1 mg/ml (1:10,000).

DOSING. Infusion or bolus of 1 to 2 μg/min (beta effects); 2 to 10 μg/min (mixed alpha and beta effects); 10 to 20 μg/min (alpha effects). Dosage is adjusted for effects, not altered for disease states.

ELIMINATION. The drug is eliminated by cellular reuptake and general peripheral tissue metabolism. Duration of action is 1 to 2 minutes.

MONITORING. HR, BP, CO, PWP.

CAUTIONS. Local tissue necrosis may result if extravasation occurs.

Norepinephrine. This is a catecholamine with predominant alpha and some beta adrenergic stimulation. It causes direct cardiac stimulation and constriction of all arterial vascular beds.

PREPARATIONS. Levophed, 1 mg/ml

DOSING. Begin with an infusion of 0.1 to 0.2 μg/kg/min; titrate for effect. Maintenance dose is generally reduced to 0.04 to 0.08 μg/kg/min. Administer the smallest effective dose for the shortest possible time.

ELIMINATION. It is eliminated by cellular reuptake and general peripheral tissue metabolism. Duration of action is 1 to 2 minutes.

MONITORING. HR, BP, CO.

CAUTIONS. Care should be taken to avoid extravasation as local tissue necrosis may result. Addition of 5 to 10 mg of phentolamine to each liter of norepinephrine infusion may prevent tissue sloughing, without altering the pressor effect. Discard solution if a brown color or precipitation occurs.

Ephedrine. Ephedrine is a sympathomimetic agent that directly stimulates both alpha and beta adrenergic receptors and indirectly causes release of norepinephrine. It causes arteriolar constriction and stimulation of the cardiac muscle. A resultant increase in cardiac irritability may precipitate ventricular arrhythmias.

PREPARATIONS. Ephedrine, 25 and 50 mg/ml.

DOSING. Usual dose is 25 to 50 mg by SC, IM, or slow IV every 3 to 4 hours as necessary.

ELIMINATION. The primary route is excretion of the unchanged drug by the kidneys; the amount is dependent on urine pH. Small amounts are metabolized in the liver. The half-life is 3 to 6 hours.

MONITORING. HR, BP, ECG, PWP, renal function.

CAUTIONS. Dosage should be reduced for renal dysfunction. Do not use in cardiogenic, hemorrhagic, or traumatic shock. Discard solutions if they are colored or have a precipitate.

Dopamine. Dopamine is a catecholamine with alpha- and beta-type adrenergic stimulation. Beta effects with cardiac stimulation and increased renal perfusion are evident at doses to 10 μg/kg/min; higher doses result in predominantly alpha stimulation and vasoconstriction.

PREPARATIONS. Intropin and others; 40 mg/ml, 80 mg/ml, 160 mg/ml.

DOSING. Begin with 1 to 2 μg/kg/min infusion; titrate for desired effects to a maximum dose of 50 μg/kg/min.

ELIMINATION. Dopamine is metabolized in the plasma and tissues. Duration of effect is approximately 2 minutes.

MONITORING. HR, BP, ECG, PWP, CO, urine output.

CAUTIONS. At high doses, dopamine alters perfusion to organs of elimination and affects other drugs. Severely impaired peripheral perfusion may result from high doses given over extended periods. Care should be taken to avoid extravasation as local tissue necrosis may result.

Inotropic Agents

Dobutamine. Dobutamine is a synthetic catecholamine that primarily has beta adrenergic effects and results in myocardial stimulation. An increase in cardiac output is due to increased myocardial contractility and stroke volume.

PREPARATIONS. Dobutrex, 12.5 mg/ml.

DOSING. Begin with infusion of 2 μg/kg/min; titrate for effect to a maximum dose of 20 μg/kg/min.

ELIMINATION. The drug is metabolized in the liver and other tissues. Duration of effects is approximately 2 minutes.

MONITORING. HR, BP, CO, PWP, ECG.

CAUTIONS. Increased heart rate and ectopic beats are dose-related problems.

Isoproterenol. Isoproterenol is a synthetic catecholamine with beta adrenergic stimulation. It is a potent cardiac stimulant that causes dilation of most vascular smooth muscle and increased cardiac output.

PREPARATION. Isuprel and others; 0.05 mg/ml, 0.2 mg/ml.

DOSING. Although a bolus of 0.2 to 0.6 μg/kg may be given in extreme cases, it is best to begin with a 0.01 to 0.1 μg/kg/min infusion and titrate for effect.

ELIMINATION. It is eliminated primarily by tissue uptake and peripheral tissue metabolism, also some direct conjugation.

MONITORING. HR, BP, PWP, ECG, urine output.

CAUTIONS. Cardiac rhythm disturbances often occur with IV use, especially with patient in cardiogenic shock. Isoproterenol is generally contraindicated in patients having coronary artery disease because of the tremendous increase in myocardial oxygen consumption associated with its use.

Amrinone. This is a bipyridine derivative with positive inotropic effects that increases myocardial contractility, cardiac output, and stroke volume. There is also some vasodilatory action.

PREPARATIONS. Inocor, 25 mg/ml.

DOSING. A bolus loading of 0.5 to 1.5 mg/kg over 2 or 3 minutes is followed by an infusion of 5 to 10 μg/kg/min. Total dose should not exceed 12 mg/kg/day, although some continued response is observed with increasing doses.

ELIMINATION. It is primarily metabolized and conjugated in the liver, with a variable amount excreted in the urine unchanged.

MONITORING. HR, BP, CO, PWP, ECG, drug fever, thrombocytopenia, renal function.

CAUTIONS. Reduce dose for decreased hepatic perfusion or renal function.

Digoxin. Digoxin is a cardiac glycoside that possesses positive inotropic effects. This results in increased myocardial contractility, cardiac output, and stroke volume.

PREPARATIONS. Lanoxin; 0.1 mg/ml, 0.25 mg/ml.

DOSING. A loading dose of 7 to 14 μg/kg is given in 2 or 3 slow bolus injections. Follow with maintenance injections of 2 to 5 μg/kg daily and adjust dose for proper serum levels.

ELIMINATION. It is mainly excreted in the urine as unchanged drug; there is a variable amount of metabolism. The half-life is 36 hours with normal renal function, up to 18 days in anephric patients.

MONITORING. HR, ECG, CO, digoxin levels, renal function.

CAUTIONS. Cardiac arrhythmias are common signs of overdose or drug accumulation; reduce dose proportional to renal function.

Antiarrhythmia Agents

Lidocaine. Lidocaine controls ventricular arrhythmias by suppressing both Purkinje system automaticity and spontaneous depolarization of the ventricles. At therapeutic concentrations, little activity occurs at the SA or AV nodes. There is a variable effect on the effective refractory period and action potential duration. Lidocaine may slightly decrease blood pressure, myocardial contractility, and cardiac output.

PREPARATIONS. Xylocaine and others; 2, 4, and 8 mg/ml for infusion, 10, 20, 40, 100, and 200 mg/ml for injection.

DOSING. Initiate with a loading dose of 1 mg/kg, followed by an infusion of 20 to 50 μg/kg/min. Titrate for effect slowly, as the duration of effect is 10 to 40 minutes.

ELIMINATION. Elimination is by hepatic metabolism; it is very dependent on hepatic blood flow and hepatocellular activity. Active metabolites are excreted by the kidneys.

MONITORING. ECG, serum levels, hepatic and renal function. Toxicity often presents with CNS symptoms of blurred vision, paresthesias, and seizures.

CAUTIONS. Monitor carefully in patients with decreased cardiac output or hepatic and renal dysfunction, and with drugs that alter hepatic function or blood flow.

Quinidine. Quinidine decreases the myocardial depolarization rate and action potential amplitude by altering sodium conductance during Phase 0 of the action potential. It depresses myocardial contractility and causes a decrease in vascular resistance by direct vasodilation and indirect alpha adrenergic blockade.

PREPARATIONS. Only quinidine gluconate should be used for IV therapy, 80 mg/ml.

DOSING. An initial dose of 5 to 8 mg/kg may be given over 30 to 60 min, followed by an infusion of 0.2 to 0.4 mg/kg/hr.

ELIMINATION. Elimination is primarily by hepatic metabolism, with some renal excretion of unchanged drug.

MONITORING. BP, ECG, serum levels.

CAUTIONS. Cumulative doses greater than 10 mg/kg when initiating therapy may precipitate arrhythmias or vascular collapse in sensitive patients.

Procainamide. It decreases the Phase 0 amplitude and depolarization speed of the action potential; it depresses Phase 4 depolarization. Other effects are similar to those of quinidine.

PREPARATIONS. Pronestyl, 100 mg/ml, 500 mg/ml.

DOSING. A bolus dose of 5 to 15 mg/kg is given at 20 mg/min, followed by an infusion of 1.5 to 3 mg/kg/hr.

ELIMINATION. Sixty percent of the dose is hepatically metabolized to an active form, *N*-acetyl procainamide (NAPA). Some degradation by plasma cholinesterase occurs; the remainder is excreted unchanged in the urine. NAPA is eliminated by renal excretion.

MONITORING. BP must be closely monitored; also HR, ECG, serum levels, and hepatic and renal function. Long-term monitoring should include antinuclear antibodies as an early indication of systemic lupus erythematosus–like syndrome.

CAUTIONS. Procainamide and NAPA cause significant problems when both hepatic and renal function are reduced.

Propranolol. This is a nonspecific beta adrenergic antagonist that prevents catecholamine-induced cardiac stimulation. Direct membrane effects decrease the maximum rate of conduction and depolarization. This decreases heart rate and myocardial contractility.

PREPARATIONS. Inderal, 1 mg/ml.

DOSING. A bolus of 0.2 to 0.3 mg/kg is given over 2 to 5 minutes, followed by an infusion of 0.5 to 2 mg/min. Adjust for effect.

ELIMINATION. Elimination is by hepatic metabolism.

MONITORING. HR, BP, CO. Serum levels are usually not of value.

CAUTIONS. Do not use propranolol if patient has heart block, bradycardia, or hypotension. It is extremely sensitive to changes in hepatic blood flow and enzyme activity. This agent decreases the metabolism (and increases levels) of many other medications.

Labetalol. Labetalol is a beta adrenergic blocking agent (similar in this aspect to propranolol), but with additional alpha adrenergic blocking properties. There is a reduction in catecholamine-induced cardiac stimulation and a reduction in blood pressure by decreased peripheral vascular resistance. Labetalol is useful in hypertensive crisis, severe angina, and atrial arrhythmias.

PREPARATIONS. Trandate, Normodyne; 5 mg/ml.

DOSING. A bolus dose of 1 to 2 mg/kg, or increments of 20 mg to a total of 2 mg/kg, are followed by an infusion of 0.5 to 1 mg/kg/hr and titrated for effect. Due to a long half-life, infusion should be increased slowly after observing effects.

ELIMINATION. It is metabolized in the liver, with metabolites excreted in the urine and bile. A small amount is excreted unchanged in the urine. Half-life is 5 to 8 hours.

MONITORING. HR, BP, CO.

CAUTIONS. Dosage reduction is required for hepatic dysfunction or reduced hepatic blood flow states. The drug may worsen heart failure.

Bretylium. Bretylium is an adrenergic blocking agent that has actions on the sympathetic nervous system and ventricular myocardium. A transient release of norepinephrine is followed by blockade of neuronal uptake, so overall release is inhibited. Ventricular tachycardia and fibrillation suppression result from adrenergic blockade.

PREPARATIONS. Bretylol, 50 mg/ml.

DOSING. A bolus of 5 to 10 mg/kg is given over 1 to 2 minutes, followed by an infusion of 1 to 2 mg/min, or 5 to 10 mg/kg every 6 hours.

ELIMINATION. Elimination is by renal excretion of unchanged drug that is related to renal function and urine output.

MONITORING. BP, ECG, renal function.

CAUTIONS. Orthostatic hypotension is common after dosing. Dosage must be reduced with decreased renal function and urine output.

Amiodarone. Amiodarone has both alpha- and beta-antiadrenergic effects; vasodilation due to alpha effects may offset negative chronotropic activity due to beta antagonist effects. This agent is extremely effective in both refractory ventricular and supraventricular arrhythmias, but this usefulness is balanced by serious adverse effects.

PREPARATIONS. Cardarone, injection.

DOSING. An initial IV loading dose of 5 to 10 mg/kg is given over 5 to 30 minutes, followed by continuous infusion of 10 to 20 mg/kg given over 24 hours for 3 to 7 days. Intravenous therapy should be via a central venous catheter. Continued oral dosing of 200 to 600 mg/day maintains suppression.

ELIMINATION. It is extensively metabolized in the liver. Dosing adjustments should be considered in hepatic dysfunction, but guidelines are not available.

MONITORING. Hypotension is the main complication of IV therapy; also monitor HR, CO, ECG, and hepatic enzymes. This agent increases the serum levels of other antiarrhythmics and digoxin; if present, these agents must be carefully monitored with both clinical assessment and serum levels. Because of a long drug half-life (9 to 50 days), monitoring is prolonged.

CAUTIONS. Use with calcium antagonists and beta antagonists may result in sinus arrest or AV block. Adverse effects include serious pulmonary fibrosis, ocular keratopathy, heart failure, peripheral neuropathies, and elevation of hepatic enzymes.

Verapamil. Verapamil is a calcium-channel blocking agent that inhibits the transmembrane influx of calcium ions in the myocardium and vascular smooth muscle, which in turn inhibits the contractile process, relaxes smooth muscle to dilate arteries, reduces resting heart rate, and slows AV conduction.

PREPARATIONS. Calan, Isoptin; 2.5 mg/ml.

DOSING. A bolus of 0.075 to 0.15 mg/kg is given over 2 minutes, followed by an infusion of 0.8 to 1 μg/kg/min.

ELIMINATION. It is eliminated by hepatic metabolism and is very dependent on hepatic function and blood flow.

MONITORING. HR, BP, ECG, hepatic function.

CAUTIONS. Do not use if patient is bradycardic or hypotensive. Dose should be reduced with decreased hepatic blood flow or function.

Other Agents

Theophylline. Theophylline is primarily used for its ability to relax bronchial smooth muscle, but it also stimulates the central nervous system, produces diuresis, stimulates cardiac muscle, and decreases peripheral vascular resistance.

PREPARATIONS. Many preparations are available of theophylline and its salt form, aminophylline.

DOSING. Usually begun with a loading dose of 4 to 5 mg/kg (with no recent theophylline use), followed by a continuous infusion of 0.2 to 0.9 mg/kg/hr.

ELIMINATION. It is metabolized by the liver.

MONITORING. HR, BP, CO, ECG, serum levels, hepatic function.

CAUTIONS. Vomiting, seizures, and cardiac arrhythmias are common at high serum levels (greater than 25 mg per liter).

Cimetidine. Cimetidine is a histamine receptor blocking agent that reduces gastric acid secretion from the parietal cells. Cimetidine inhibits hepatic microsomal enzyme function and reduces blood flow through the liver. This results in increased levels of medications with hepatic elimination.

PREPARATIONS. Tagamet, 150 mg/ml.

DOSING. A rapid IV injection or intermittent infusion of 20 to 50 mg/kg is generally given every 6 hours.

ELIMINATION. There are approximately equal amounts of hepatic metabolism and renal excretion of unchanged drug. Dosage interval should be increased with renal or hepatic dysfunction. Creatinine clearances below 30 ml/min have a recommended dosing interval of 12 hours.

MONITORING. Careful monitoring of drug levels and hemodynamic effects of medications with hepatic elimination.

Furosemide. This is high-output diuretic that inhibits reabsorption of electrolytes in the ascending limb of the loop of Henle. It also decreases reabsorption of sodium and increases potassium excretion in the distal renal tubule. Due to renal vasodilatory effects and increased renal blood flow, drugs eliminated by renal excretion may have decreased serum levels.

PREPARATIONS. Lasix, 10 mg/ml, and others.

DOSING. An IV injection or intermittent infusion of 0.5 to 2 mg/kg is given one to four times daily, with dosage increases of 0.25 to 0.5 mg/kg added as required.

ELIMINATION. It is eliminated by hepatic metabolism and renal excretion. Dosage should be reduced with hepatic and renal dysfunction, as duration of drug effects will be altered.

MONITORING. This agent alters levels of agents that are excreted renally. Monitor drug levels and hemodynamic effects of medications with renal elimination.

DISCUSSION

In many situations with monitored patients, a rapidly changing clinical status does not permit measurements of drug concentrations in the blood, even if such levels are available. Decisions on drug dosing must be made on the basis of patient status and hemodynamic values. Table 13–6 lists the expected hemodynamic changes induced by individual agents. It may be helpful in predicting dosage requirements or adjustments for subsequent therapeutic agents used in combination. When one or two therapeutic agents are utilized, drug dose modification can be anticipated from the known hemodynamic and pharmacokinetic effects of these agents. For the complex drug therapy situation, decisions on medication use and dosage are made on the basis of pharmacokinetic-pharmacodynamic aspects of a particular drug. These are considered with the patient's hemodynamic status, other medications already in use, and how the three factors (hemodynamics-pharmacokinetics-medications) interact.

Table 13–7 lists common vasoactive medications and their general indications and dosages. Because of short duration of activity and multiple sites of elimination, dosages of these agents are titrated for a specific effect. Their therapeutic effects may change the pharmacologic effects of other medications already in use. Table 13–8 lists other medications that are commonly employed in monitored patients. This list is not all-inclusive, but includes important medications for which research is sufficient to make dosing recommendations. The agents are longer acting, have significant drug and disease interactions, and will further alter patient hemodynamic monitoring.

TABLE 13–7. Vasoactive Agent Dosages and Uses

Drug	*Indication*	*Dose*	*Monitoring*
Epinephrine	Cardiac arrest	IV: 0.5–1.0 mg over 1 min IT: 1 mg	Heart rate and blood pressure; local tissue necrosis if drug extravasation occurs
	Hypotension	5–10 μg/min IV, titrate for effect	
Norepinephrine	Hypotension	4–8 μg/min IV, titrate for effect	Heart rate and blood pressure
Dopamine	Circulatory failure	1–2 μg/kg/min IV, titrate for effect up to a maximum of 50 μg/kg/min	Heart rate and blood pressure; cardiac output; renal function
Dobutamine	Circulatory failure	2–2.5 μg/kg/min IV, titrate for effect to a maximum of 20 μg/kg/min	Heart rate and blood pressure; cardiac output
Isoproterenol	Bradycardia, AV heart block	0.01 μg/kg IV bolus; 0.5 μg/min IV, titrate for effect	Heart rate and blood pressure

TABLE 13–8. Therapeutic Concentrations and Dosage Adjustments of Common Intravenous Medications for Monitored Patients

Drug	Therapeutic Concentration	Patient State	Loading Dose	Maintenance Dose
Lidocaine	1.5–5.0 μg/ml	DCP* absent	100–150 mg IV bolus	2 mg/min
		DCP present	40–75 mg IV bolus	1 mg/min
		MI,† DCP absent	150–250 mg IV as multiple boluses	3 mg/min
		MI, DCP present	100–200 mg IV as multiple boluses	1.5–2 mg/min
Quinidine	2–5 μg/ml	DCP absent	5–8 mg/kg (gluconate) over 30–60 minutes	0.2–0.4 mg/kg/min
		DCP present	3.5–6 mg/kg as above	0.1–0.3 mg/kg/min
Procainamide	4–10 μg/ml PA 10–30 μg/ml PA plus NAPA	DCP absent	17 mg/kg IV at a rate of 20 mg/min	2–3 mg/kg/hr IV
		DCP present	13 mg/kg IV at a rate of 20 mg/min	1–1.5 mg/kg/hr IV
Propranolol	50–100 ng/ml	DCP absent	0.2–0.3 mg/kg over 2–5 min	0.5–2 mg/min IV for effect
		DCP present	0.08–0.15 mg/kg over 2–5 min	0.125–1 mg/min IV for effect
Bretylium	not established	DCP absent	5–10 mg/kg over 10 min to max of 40 mg/kg	1–2 mg/min
		DCP present	5–10 mg/kg over 10 min to max of 30 mg/kg	0.5–1.5 mg/min
Verapamil	100–300 ng/ml	DCP absent	0.075–0.15 mg/kg IV bolus over 2 min	0.8–1 μg/kg/min IV
		DCP present	0.075–0.15 mg/kg IV bolus over 3 min	0.5 μg/kg/min IV
Digoxin	0.9–2.5 ng/ml	DCP absent	7–14 μg/kg IV in 2 or 3 doses, 6 hr apart	2–5 μg/kg/day IV
		DCP present	same	1–3 μg/kg/day IV
Amrinone	not established	DCP absent	0.5–1.5 mg/kg over 2 or 3 min	5–10 μg/kg/min, total dose not to exceed 10–12 mg/kg/day
		DCP present	same	4–7 μg/kg/min
Theophylline	10–20 μg/ml	DCP absent	5 mg/kg IV over 30 min, less if already on med	0.5–0.9 mg/kg/hr IV
		DCP present	same	0.2–0.6 mg/kg/hr IV
Cimetidine	0.5–4 μg/ml	DCP absent	5–8 mg/kg IV push	20–40 mg/kg/day over 24 hr
		DCP present	same	10–25 mg/kg/day over 24 hr
Furosemide	not established	DCP absent	0.5–4 mg/kg IV push	6 mg/kg/day infused over 24 hr
		DCP present	same	2–4 mg/kg/day infused over 24 hr
Morphine	50–150 ng/ml	DCP absent	4–12 mg IV	40–95 mg/hr
		DCP present	same	25–50 mg/hr
Phenytoin	10–20 μg/ml	DCP absent	15 mg/kg IV at a rate of 50 mg/min or less	3–7 mg/kg/day
		DCP present	same	2–5 mg/kg/day
Phenobarbital	15–45 μg/ml	DCP absent	15 mg/kg IV at a rate of 50 mg/min or less	2–6 mg/kg/day
		DCP present	same	1–4 mg/kg/day
Heparin	PTT‡ 1.2–2.0 times baseline value	DCP absent	70–100 units/kg	25 units/kg/hr
		DCP present	same	15–20 units/kg/hr

*Decreased cardiovascular and/or pulmonary function.
†Myocardial infarction.
‡Partial thromboplastin time.

Most of the agents listed have toxic effects that will indirectly alter hemodynamics and induce symptoms that could necessitate further drug therapy for control. Guidelines are given for initial and maintenance dosing, plus the generally accepted therapeutic drug concentrations required for efficacious activity.

CONSIDERATIONS FOR MEDICATION USE

For most patients requiring hemodynamic monitoring, it is necessary to rapidly achieve therapeutic drug concentrations and to adjust drug dosages as the clinical and hemodynamic status changes. Those patients with shock or cardiovascular or pulmonary diseases often have major organ dysfunction that may alter both drug pharmacokinetics and pharmacodynamics. Cardiovascular failure causes sympathetic mediated vasoconstriction in most tissues, sparing only the heart, brain, and lungs owing to autoregulation inherent to the vascular beds of these organs. In low perfusion states, blood flow to the peripheral tissues is reduced, with a redistribution of the available cardiac output to provide a greater proportional flow to the brain and heart. This results in slowed drug absorption and tissue distribution, with a higher initial drug concentration in the blood. Initial loading doses of many parenteral medications should be reduced to prevent cardiac, central nervous system, and pulmonary toxicity. These toxicities markedly alter predicted patient hemodynamic parameters.

Drug administration is a particular problem in patients with shock or other low perfusion states. Compensatory peripheral vasoconstriction due to autoregulation renders oral, intramuscular, and subcutaneous administration unacceptable because of variable drug absorption and distribution problems. As mentioned earlier, these routes must be used cautiously with cardiotoxic or vasoactive medications since the effective drug volume is much smaller with vasoconstriction, and the effective central drug levels will be increased. The route of administration chosen, therefore, will greatly influence resultant hemodynamic effects.

Maintenance drug dosing in monitored patients with shock or cardiovascular or pulmonary disease is a particular problem that results in a major portion of drug-induced hemodynamic alterations. Hepatic elimination may be impaired by reduced hepatic blood flow or hepatocellular dysfunction. Renal elimination and excretion may be impaired by reduced renal blood flow or tubular dysfunction. Changes in these primary drug elimination pathways result in increased drug levels and a much longer duration of effect. The maintenance dose of many medications employed in monitored patients, therefore, must be reduced to avoid serious adverse effects and hemodynamic alterations.

Vasoactive agents, such as catecholamines, have short biologic activity because of general tissue elimination and do not exhibit major effect or duration changes. Other vasoactive, inotropic, and antiarrhythmic agents require specific hepatic or renal elimination pathways, which typically have decreased function. These medications are of particular concern with hemodynamic monitoring. Finally, medications without inherent cardiovascular activity may affect the intensity and duration of cardiovascular drugs and thus cause hemodynamic alterations.

SUMMARY

Patient hemodynamic monitoring has added refinement and increased knowledge to critical care health delivery. It is particularly valuable, when the patient is receiving medications that affect cardiovascular function, to indicate needed changes in pharmacologic interventions or to monitor increased or decreased drug effects. The patient most at need for this therapy, however, is also the most likely to develop complications. Health care professionals need to be aware of the complex interrelationship of disease, medication therapy, and patient response. Hemodynamic monitoring is the best indicator of this relationship.

SUGGESTED READINGS

Benet LZ, Massoud N, Gambertoglio JG: *Pharmacokinetic Basis for Drug Treatment.* New York, Raven Press, 1984.

Benowitz NL, Meister W: Pharmacokinetics in patients with cardiac failure. *Clin Pharmacokinet* 1976; 1:389–405.

Brown JE, Shand DG: Therapeutic drug monitoring of antiarrhythmic agents. *Clin Pharmacokinet* 1982; 7:125–148.

Cadwallader DE: *Biopharmaceutics and Drug Interactions.* New York, Raven Press, 1983.

Daily EK, Schroeder JS: *Techniques in Bedside Hemodynamic Monitoring.* St. Louis, CV Mosby, 1985.

Duchin KL, Schrier RW: Interrelationship between renal hemodynamic, drug kinetics, and drug action. *Clin Pharmacokinet* 1978; 3:58–71.

Eskridge RA: The management of septic shock. *Drug Intell Clin Pharm* 1983; 17:92–99.

Feely J, Wade D, McAllister CB, et al: Effect of hypotension on liver blood flow and lidocaine disposition. *N Engl J Med* 1982; 307:866–869.

George, CF: Drug kinetics and hepatic blood flow. *Clin Pharmacokinet* 1979; 4:433–448.

Goodman LS, Gilman AG, Gilman A (eds): *The Pharmacologic Basis of Therapeutics.* New York, Macmillan, 1980.

Houston MC, Thompson WL, Robertson D: Shock: Diagnosis and management. *Arch Intern Med* 1984; 144:1433–1439.

Kaplan JA (ed): *Cardiac Anesthesia*, vols I and II. New York, Grune and Stratton, 1983.

Kuhn GJ, White BC, Swetnam RE, et al: Peripheral vs central circulation times during CPR: A pilot study. *Ann Emerg Med* 1981; 10:417–419.

McEvoy GK (ed): *American Hospital Formulary Service: Drug Information 1985.* American Society of Hospital Pharmacists, 1985.

Patak RV, Lifschitz MD, Stein JH: Acute renal failure: Clinical aspects and pathophysiology. *Cardiovasc Med* 1979; 4:19–38.

Pentel R, Benowitz N: Pharmacokinetic and pharmacodynamic considerations in drug therapy of cardiac emergencies. *Clin Pharmacokinet* 1984; 9:273–308.

Redding JS, Asuncion JS, Pearson JW: Effective routes of drug administration during cardiac arrest. *Anesthesiol Analges* 1967; 46:253–258.

Richardson PD, Withrington PG: Liver blood flow: Intrinsic and nervous control of liver blood flow. *Gastroenterology* 1981; 81:159–173.

Richardson PD, Withrington PG: Liver blood flow: Effects of drugs and hormones on liver blood flow. *Gastroenterology* 1981; 81:356–375.

Rowland M, Tozer TN: *Clinical Pharmacokinetics: Concepts and Applications*. Philadelphia, Lea and Febiger, 1980.

Schumer W: Hypovolemic shock. *JAMA* 1979; 240:615–621.

Shine KI, Kuhn M, Young LS, et al: Aspects of the management of shock. *Ann Intern Med* 1980; 93:723–734.

Weil MH, Shubin H, Carlson R: Treatment of circulatory shock. *JAMA* 1975; 231:1280–1286.

White RD, McIntyre KM: Cardiovascular Pharmacology: Parts I and II. In *Textbook of Advanced Cardiac Life Support*. American Heart Association, 1981.

Monitoring the Patient in Shock

14

Shock, a widespread abnormality in cell metabolism secondary to an insult, is not a specific disease with a single cause. A uniform hemodynamic and pathophysiologic description of the patient in shock, therefore, is not possible. The causes, pathophysiology, hemodynamic profile, clinical presentation, and treatment of shock are discussed separately with each etiologic subset.

In general, shock is a syndrome (collection of symptoms) that reflects the body's attempt to adapt to an insult and preserve its most vital functions. The insult may be traumatic, hemorrhagic, septic, neurogenic, embolic, allergic, or cardiogenic. The consistent common denominator in all forms of shock is widespread abnormal cell metabolism that results in a diminution of the life-generating forces within the cell. Depending on the magnitude of the insult and progression of shock as more cells and tissue beds become involved, major organ dysfunction may threaten the person's life. In most forms of shock, cell dysfunction is due to inadequate capillary (nutrient) blood flow. Additionally, shock may be due to biochemical factors that adversely affect the cell's oxygen uptake or utilization.

CELLULAR AND BIOCHEMICAL ALTERATIONS IN SHOCK

When cells metabolize in an oxygen-enriched environment, the *aerobic metabolism* of the one mole of glucose produces carbon dioxide (which is ultimately exhaled), water (which is added to the body's water pool), and 38 moles of adenosine triphosphate (ATP). This high-energy compound must be generated in adequate amounts to maintain normal cell and organ function and to sustain life. Considerable amounts of the energy produced by the cell drive a cell membrane pump that maintains an ionic gradient across the cell wall. Intracellular sodium and potassium levels are approximately 10 mEq/liter and 140 mEq/liter respectively, whereas extracellular sodium and potassium levels are 140 mEq/liter and 4 mEq/liter. This ionic gradient is important in determining cell size and shape as well as energy production and cell function.

When deprived of oxygen, the cell is forced into an alternate pathway of metabolism. *Anaerobic metabolism* results in lactic acid production. As large areas of tissue metabolize anaerobically, blood lactate levels rise, with concomitant decreases in serum bicarbonate and body base. Lactacidemia is a feature common to all forms of shock, and the severity of shock can be related to the amount of lactic acid produced. In addition, anaerobic metabolism results in an approximate twentyfold decrease in energy production. The energy-deficient sodium-potassium pump allows a potassium leak from the intracellular to the extracellular space. As sodium followed by water enters the cells, the cells swell and become irregular in shape. Swelling of the capillary endothelial cells may further compromise nutrient flow by narrowing the capillary lumen. The clefts that form between cells allow a transudation of fluid from the vascular spaces to tissue spaces (third space losses). Ultimately, damage to the cell is followed by lysosomal rupture, and the subsequent release of potent digestive enzymes autolyses the cell. These enzymes are most active in an acid environment that increases the destructive potential to neighboring tissue. The hypoxic sequence of cellular events is illustrated in Figure 14–1.

In addition, a number of hormonal and biochemical substances released locally and systemically have varying effects on cell and organ function. These include products of the complement cascade, the kinin system, the coagulation mechanism, the sympathoadrenal system, the renin-angiotensin axis, and the ACTH-endorphin systems. These systems are biologically designed to protect the person through initiation of the inflammatory response; redistribute blood flow to organs necessary for immediate survival; increase phagocytosis, preventing blood loss, and so on. However, the ongoing activation of these systems may eventually result in a metabolic phenomenon that

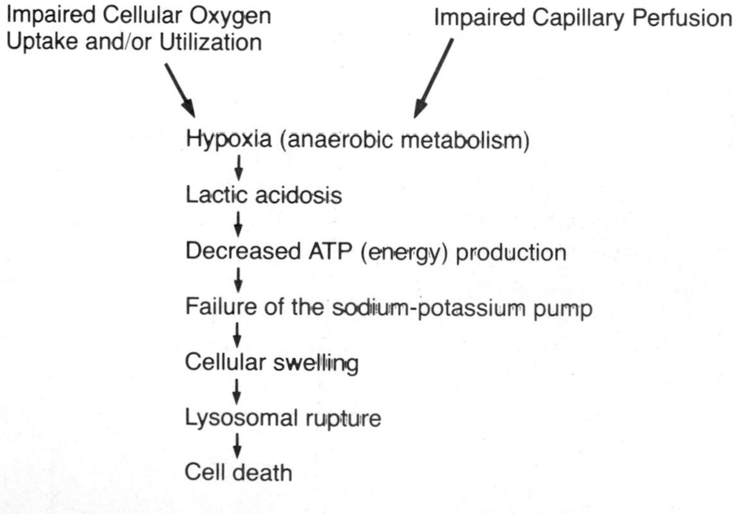

FIGURE 14–1. The hypoxic sequence in cellular events in shock.

is associated with progressive deterioration and destruction of organ systems, and ultimately the patient's death. The clinical expressions of this phenomenon include the adult respiratory distress syndrome (ARDS), disseminated intravascular coagulation (DIC), immune system suppression, a hypermetabolic state, and multiple system organ failure. The severity of this phenomenon is a function of individual patient response, the severity of the insult, and the duration of shock. This underscores the importance of early recognition of the shock process and aggressive type-specific management.

In summary, shock cannot be simplistically thought of as a purely physical defect, ie, hypotension or poor capillary perfusion. Rather, it is an extremely complex altered physiologic state that is variably tolerated, depending on the magnitude of the initiating insult, the presence or absence of preexisting disease, and individual physiologic characteristics.

GENERAL MANAGEMENT PRINCIPLES

The goals in the management of shock are to correct the primary problem and to institute measures that maximize cell oxygen availability and decrease tissue oxygen demands. Therapeutic measures include the following.

- Insure an adequate airway and ventilation. Maintenance of an adequate tidal volume or ventilatory rate or both may require ventilatory assistance. This may considerably decrease oxygen demand by eliminating the work of breathing, particularly when breathing has been difficult.
- Administer oxygen to maintain a PaO_2 of at least 80 to 100 mm Hg.
- Restore intravascular volume without fluid overloading. Insertion of two large-bore *peripheral* vascular catheters away from areas of trauma facilitates rapid administration of fluid. The rate of fluid infusion is guided by patient response as assessed by changes in hemodynamic parameters, heart rate, urine output, mentation, skin temperature, color, and so on. The means of obtaining the hemodynamic parameters, the associated pitfalls, and assessment of the patient's hemodynamic response to volume repletion are discussed below.

Arterial Pressure Monitoring

The auscultatory and palpation methods of obtaining an arterial pressure in patients with reduced cuff pressures, dulled sensorium, and cool, clammy skin may give grossly inaccurate readings. In patients with insufficient pulsatile flow (decreased stroke volume) or alterations in the vessel wall (vasoconstriction), the vascular vibrations under the cuff may be too weak to be heard or palpated. Cohn[1] demonstrated an average 33.1 mm Hg difference between the intra-arterial and cuff pressures in patients with low stroke volume and high peripheral vascular resistance; more commonly, the cuff pressure underestimated the true intra-arterial pressure. In shock states, therefore, an intra-arterial line is recommended for accurate monitoring of arterial pressure. Another important advantage of the intra-arterial line is that it provides access to arterial blood for blood gas analysis and other laboratory measurements.

Central Venous Pressure Monitoring (CVP)

The CVP measures pressure in the superior vena cava or right atrium and is used to monitor blood volume and the heart's competency to accept the fluids administered. Normal values are 3 to 11 cm H_2O. Some investigators believe that 12 to 15 cm H_2O is the end point for fluid administration.[2] However, isolated values are not as meaningful as are patient and pressure responses to fluid challenge. Rapid increases in CVP that do not decrease toward normal values within 10 minutes indicate fluid overload. Because several factors influence CVP, it may not correlate with fluid needs or left ventricular function in the critically ill patient. For example:

- Increases in pulmonary vascular resistance secondary to sepsis, hypoxemia, acidemia, pulmonary embolism, or respiratory failure, through its effect on right ventricular function, may produce normal or high CVP readings despite volume depletion and decreased left ventricular filling volume.
- The use of vasopressors produces venoconstriction, thus increasing venous return to the heart. If the patient is receiving vasopressors, therefore, the CVP may be misleadingly high in the presence of intravascular volume depletion.
- Normally the CVP tends to move in the same direction as the pulmonary artery wedge pressure (PWP). However, it is the last value to change in left ventricular dysfunction. By the time blood dams up in the back of the failing left ventricle to the CVP catheter tip in the right atrium or superior vena cava, pulmonary vascular congestion and/or edema are well established. Therefore, the use of the pulmonary artery catheter is recommended in patients older than 50 years with preexisting cardiopulmonary disease or in those who have severe, multiple system dysfunction.

The Pulmonary Artery Catheter

The pulmonary artery catheter provides a means of assessing pulmonary vascular resistance, intravascular fluid volume, and left heart function. Additionally, it provides a more accurate means of evaluating the hemodynamic effects of fluid resuscitation in patients with acute myocardial infarction, preexisting myocardial dysfunction, respiratory failure, or sepsis. It is the most invasive tool for assessing hemodynamic status and therefore has the highest attendant risks. Risk must always be carefully weighed against anticipated benefit after the patient's needs have been carefully evaluated.

The protocol for fluid challenge in hypovolemia utilizing the pulmonary artery catheter varies from institution to institution. The rationale and method proposed by Weil using the 3:7 rule is presented here.[3]

The Rationale of the 3:7 Rule. The pulmonary artery diastolic pressure (PAd) or PWP may not indicate hypovolemia following massive blood or fluid loss in patients having limited cardiac reserve. Therefore, PAd and PWP *responses* to fluid challenges are used as a guide to volume replacement.

Significant reductions in intravascular volume reduce venous return to the heart which, in turn, reduces cardiac output and arterial pressure. This may produce critical reductions in coronary blood flow, particularly in patients with coronary artery disease. A poorly perfused myocardium is less compliant (stiff) and contractile, thus increasing left ventricular end-diastolic pressure, PWP, and PAd. The restoration of intravascular volume improves cardiac output, arterial pressure, coronary blood flow, and thus ventricular contractility and compliance are returned to normal. The left ventricular end-diastolic pressure, PWP, and PAd may then decline. In summary, the PWP and PAd are not affected by intravascular volume alone but also by the relationship between the volume of blood that is delivered to the heart, its competency to receive and pump it out, and ventricular compliance.

The Method of Fluid Challenge Using the 3:7 Rule. Crystalloids (normal saline or Ringer's lactate solutions) or colloid (5% albumin) is systemically administered in measured boluses. Because only an estimated one third of infused crystalloids remains in the vascular space after 20 minutes of infusion, overall greater volumes of crystalloid replacement may be anticipated. Fluids are infused through an IV route other than the pulmonary artery catheter used for monitoring.

1. Obtain measurements of the PAd or PWP during a 10 minute observation period.
   a. If the PAd or PWP is less than 11 mm Hg, fluid is infused at a rate of 20 ml/min over a 10 minute period.
   b. If the PAd or PWP is 11 to 18 mm Hg, fluid is infused at a rate of 10 ml/min over a 10 minute period.
   c. If the PAd or PWP is greater than 18 mm Hg, fluids are infused at a rate of 5 ml/min over a 10 minute period.
2. If during infusion the PAd or PWP increases at any time by greater than 7 mm Hg above the preinfusion pressure and remains at that level for more than 1 minute, the fluid infusion is discontinued.
3. If the PAd or PWP increases by more than 3 mm Hg but less than 7 mm Hg, infusion is discontinued after 10 minutes. It is common for the PAd or PWP to fall to within ± 3 mm Hg of the preinfusion pressure. If this occurs, additional fluid boluses are administered over the next 10 minutes.
4. The fluid challenges are repeated until the pressure values increase to greater than 7 mm Hg or continue greater than 3 mm Hg during any given 10 minute period. In each instance, the pressure measurements immediately preceding the fluid challenge serve as the reference measurement.

Once the fluid loss is arrested, several liters of fluid may be required to restore an adequate perfusion status.

- Correct acid-base abnormalities. With restoration of adequate tissue perfusion and oxygenation, the metabolic acidosis commonly seen in shock states tends to self-correct. Decreases in myocardial contractility, however, may occur if the arterial pH is decreased below 7.20, perpetuating the shock process. Therefore, the administration of sodium bicarbonate should be considered if the arterial pH is less than 7.15 to 7.20.
- Attempt to keep the patient's temperature normal. Conservation of the patient's body heat (a form of energy) is accomplished by blanketing. Hypothermia due to heat loss, administration of room temperature IV fluid or cold blood, lying in wet linen, and so on, may produce additional physiologic abnormalities (conduction defects, bradycardia, arrhythmias, decreased coagulability, leftward shift of the oxyhemoglobin dissociation curve) and, if accompanied by shivering, increased oxygen consumption and carbon dioxide production. All may adversely affect the resuscitation attempt.
- Provide inotropic support for the heart if evidence of heart failure is present, ie, elevation of the PWP, low cardiac output, gallop rhythm, increasing tachypnea and dyspnea, crackles or wheezes in the lungs, and so on.
- Maintain recumbency with 30 degree elevation of the legs for shock in which hypovolemia is a suspected factor. When the most physiologically beneficial position is in question, as in pulmonary edema complicating cardiogenic shock, a good principle to remember is that most patients spontaneously assume a position of comfort that is most physiologically advantageous for them.

CLASSIFICATION

For the purpose of this discussion, shock is classified into six categories: hypovolemic, septic, anaphylactic, neurogenic, cardiogenic, and other. The discussion of specific types of shock that follows focuses on the anticipated direction of pathophysiologic, hemodynamic, clinical changes, and laboratory rather than absolute values (Table 14–1). However, in the individual patient co-existing disease and/or complicating factors may alter or even reverse the anticipated direction of change.

Hypovolemic Shock

Hypovolemic shock is due to a critical reduction in circulating intravascular volume, which leads to inadequate tissue perfusion and ischemic hypoxia. An associated interstitial volume deficit may also be present. Hypovolemia is the most common cause of shock and frequently complicates other forms of shock.

TABLE 14–1. Guidelines to Anticipated Hemodynamic Changes in Several Types of Shock

Disorder	Arterial Pressure	Pulse Pressure	Systemic Vascular Resistance	Pulmonary Vascular Resistance	Central Venous Pressure	Pulmonary Artery Pressure	Pulmonary Wedge Pressure	Cardiac Output	SvO_2
HYPOVOLEMIC									
Compensated	~	↓	↑	~	↓	↓	↓	~↓	↓
Decompensated	↓	↓	↑	↑	↓	↑~↓	↓	↓	↓
SEPTIC*									
Hyperdynamic	~↓	↓~↑	↓	~↑	↓~	↑~↓	~↓	↑	~↑
Hypodynamic	↓	↓	↑~↓	~↑	↓~↑	↑~↓	↑~↓	↓	↓~↑
ANAPHYLACTIC	↓	↓	↓	~↑	↓	↓	↓	↓	↓
NEUROGENIC	↓	↓	↓	~↑	↓	↓	↓	~↓	↓
CARDIOGENIC	↓	↓	↑~	↑	~↑	↑	↑	↓	↓

*The hemodynamic profiles of hyperdynamic and particularly hypodynamic septic shock are quite variable.
KEY: ↑, increase; ↓, decrease; ~, no change.

CAUSES

Intravascular volume depletion may result from blood loss, third space fluid shifts, or dehydration (Table 14–2).

PATHOPHYSIOLOGY

The pathophysiologic response, hemodynamic profile, and clinical presentation relate to the amount of volume lost, the rapidity of volume loss, and the length of time the volume loss continues. Initially, the person may maintain mean arterial pressure and remain "compensated." With continued or massive volume loss, "decompensation" ensues, accompanied by a decrease in mean arterial pressure.

COMPENSATED SHOCK

Typically, an approximate 20 to 25 percent intravascular volume deficit occurs. This represents approximately 1000 to 1200 ml for a 70 kg man.[4] Due to the loss in intravascular volume, venous return to the heart and ventricular filling volumes are reduced. As a result, ventricular performance falls below normal. To compensate for the decrease in stroke volume and maintain arterial pressure, there is a sympathetic nervous system–mediated increase

TABLE 14–2. Causes of Hypovolemic Shock

Blood Loss	Third Space Fluid Shifts	Dehydration
Frank wound hemorrhage	Soft tissue trauma (swelling)	Vomiting and/or diarrhea
Bleeding at fracture sites	Sepsis	Diuretic therapy
GI bleeding	Peritonitis	Excessive sweating
Hemothorax	Ascites	Diabetes mellitus or insipidus
Retroperitoneal bleeding	Intestinal obstruction	
	Burn injuries	

in systemic vascular resistance (arterial pressure is determined by systemic vascular resistance and stroke volume). Precapillary and postcapillary sphincters constrict. Venous tone increases, which displaces blood from the high volume venous bed centrally to core organs. These responses serve to (1) maintain arterial pressure and shunt blood centrally to maintain perfusion pressure and flow to the brain and myocardium; and (2) decrease capillary hydrostatic pressure while colloid osmotic pressure remains unchanged. This favors fluid movement from the tissue to the intravascular space to restore plasma volume. If 1400 ml of intravascular fluid are lost in 1 hour, approximately 400 to 600 ml might move from the tissue space to the intravascular space, thus offsetting the intravascular volume deficit.

Although this stage might be well tolerated initially, prolonged perfusion deficits to bowel, kidney, and skeletal muscle lead to organ dysfunction and promote biochemical changes that may sustain the shock syndrome.

Hemodynamic Profile (see Table 14–1). ARTERIAL PRESSURE. Peripheral vasoconstriction maintains or elevates the diastolic pressure. The systolic pressure may be maintained at normal or near normal levels; however, the pulse pressure narrows, reflecting the decrease in stroke volume.

The use of isolated "numbers" as a guide to hemodynamic status and tissue perfusion may be very misleading, ie, using a systolic pressure of 90 to 100 mm Hg as a cut-off point for the diagnosis of shock. The systolic pressure driving blood to core organs may be 90 to 100 mm Hg or higher. However, large tissue beds may be receiving minimal blood flow because of local vasoconstriction. The interrelationship of hemodynamic values, their relationship to the clinical presentation, and changes in response to treatment provide more meaningful assessment tools. The *arterial pressure waveform* appears damped owing to the narrowed pulse pressure. There may also be cyclic variations in amplitude that relate to changes in intraventricular volume and stroke volume within the respiratory cycle (pulsus paradoxus). Ordinarily, the inspiratory fall and expiratory rise in left ventricular filling volume do not produce significant changes in stroke volume and arterial pressure. With hypovolemia, the relatively small expiratory increase in left ventricular filling volume (steep portion of the ventricular function curve) may be associated with a large increase in stroke volume, which is reflected in the momentary widening pulse pressure.

SYSTEMIC VASCULAR RESISTANCE. This parameter is elevated from generalized peripheral vasoconstriction.

PULMONARY VASCULAR RESISTANCE. This value is generally within normal limits.

CVP OR RIGHT ATRIAL PRESSURE. These values are decreased owing to the decrease in venous return to the heart. However, compensatory venoconstriction and/or myocardial dysfunction may produce a value that is misleadingly high relative to the amount of volume lost.

PULMONARY ARTERY AND WEDGE PRESSURES. These values are decreased and reflect the reduction in pulmonary intravascular and left ventricular filling volumes. The contour of the pulmonary artery waveform is unchanged.

CARDIAC OUTPUT. This parameter may be maintained in the normal range by sympathetic nervous system stimulation or may be slightly decreased.

MIXED VENOUS OXYGEN SATURATION ($S\bar{v}O_2$). This value is decreased secondary to hypoperfusion of large areas of tissue and/or anemia if hemorrhage is the cause of hypovolemia.

Clinical Presentations. MENTATION. The patient is typically fully alert, lucid, and mildly anxious. Frequently the patient will complain of thirst.

CUTANEOUS. The complexion is pale and the extremities may be cool and clammy. However, the trunk is warm and dry.

CAPILLARY BLANCH TEST. This assessment technique is performed by depressing the patient's fingernail, thus squeezing blood from the underlying capillary bed. Normally, the color returns in less than 2 seconds upon release of pressure. Because of poor peripheral capillary perfusion in compensated shock, the return to color takes longer (positive test).

HEART RATE AND PERIPHERAL PULSES. As compensatory measure to maintain cardiac output and tissue perfusion in the presence of a decreasing stroke volume, the heart rate increases above 100 beats per minute. However, if the patient has been taking calcium channel or beta blocking agents, the heart rate may be deceptively low relative to the amount of fluid lost. The volume of the pulse is small.

NECK VEINS. The external jugular veins will be collapsed and nonvisible with the patient in the supine position.

RESPIRATORY RATE AND CHARACTER OF BREATHING. The patient is typically tachypneic, with a rate of 20 to 30 breaths per minute. Ventilatory movements are commonly visible.

URINE OUTPUT. Urine flow rates may be decreased to 20 to 30 ml/hour. Because sodium and water are being reabsorbed by the kidney, urine sodium is low and the specific gravity is greater than 1.025.

ACID/BASE. A base deficit below -5 mEq of HCO_3 per liter reflects poor tissue perfusion, anaerobic metabolism, and lactic acid production. An increase in serum lactate is a grim indicator of the hypoxic insult being borne by many cells despite apparent hemodynamic stability. Some cells are being traumatized by hypoxic insult, whereas others may be dying. Nevertheless, the arterial pH may be maintained within normal limits by the compensatory respiratory alkalosis or may even be in the alkalemic range (greater than 7.45) because trauma and stress are very potent stimuli to ventilation and may override the metabolic effects of shock.

DECOMPENSATED SHOCK

Decompensated shock usually accompanies an acute intravascular volume loss greater than 30 percent. In a 70 kg man, this represents a loss greater than 1500 ml.[4] When compensatory mechanisms are maximized and fluid losses continue, the systolic pressure falls. Thus, a falling systolic pressure does not represent the onset of shock but rather a level of shock in which compensatory mechanisms are exhausted. Blood flow to extensive tissue beds is shut down and perfusion to core organs may be severely compromised.

Hemodynamic Profile (see Table 14–1). ARTERIAL PRESSURE. The "numbers" are now in a conventionally unacceptable range—that is, a significant drop in arterial pressure in a patient who is known to be previously hypertensive or a systolic pressure less than 90 to 100 mm Hg in a previously normotensive patient. The pulse pressure is narrowed, the rate of rise of the arterial pressure waveform is slowed, and the waveform appears damped (Fig. 14–2).

SYSTEMIC VASCULAR RESISTANCE. This value continues to be increased relative to the amount of compensatory vasoconstriction present.

PULMONARY VASCULAR RESISTANCE. Hypoxemia and acidemia, which accompany decompensated shock, have potent pulmonary vasoconstrictor effects. Therefore, the degree of increase in pulmonary vascular resistance relates to the severity of shock; marked increases portend a poor prognosis.

CVP OR RIGHT ATRIAL PRESSURE. Progressive intravascular volume losses produce grater decrements in right atrial pressure and CVP. The lowest values seen in patients with acute hemorrhage are in the range of −8 to −10 mm Hg.

PULMONARY ARTERY AND WEDGE PRESSURES. These values remain low. The rate of rise of the upstroke of the pulmonary artery waveform may be slowed and the narrowed pulse pressure reflects a decreased right ventricular stroke volume. If increased pulmonary vascular resistance accompanies hypovolemic shock, the pulmonary artery systolic and diastolic pressures increase while the PWP remains low (widening of the PAd-PWP gradient.) The PWP waveform may also appear damped.

CARDIAC OUTPUT. This value is decreased and may fall progressively, secondary to continued fluid loss, which reduces ventricular filling volume. Myocardial depression secondary to poor coronary blood flow and/or chemical substances released from ischemic tissue (myocardial depressant factor) may additionally depress cardiac function.

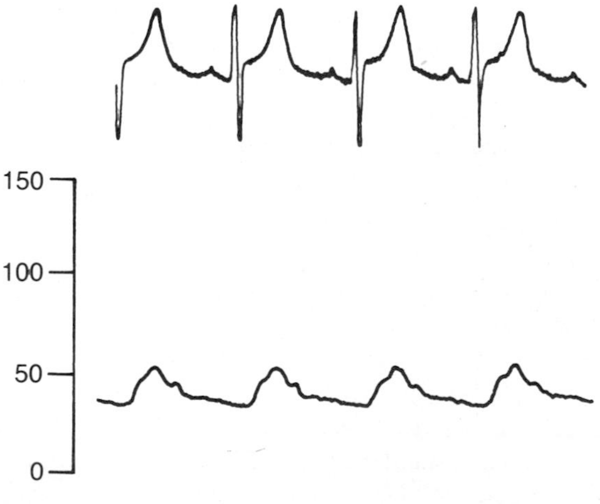

FIGURE 14–2. Arterial pressure tracing from a 50-year-old man in hemorrhagic shock. Note the damped-appearing waveform, slowed rate of rise of the upstroke, and narrow pulse pressure.

MIXED VENOUS OXYGEN SATURATION ($S\bar{v}O_2$). Values are decreased below normal due to capillary hypoperfusion and/or decreased arterial oxygen content (hypoxemia or anemia that frequently accompanies hemorrhage).

Clinical Presentation. MENTATION. The decompensated state is characterized by increasing anxiety, confusion, and/or changes in affect, which may progress to obtundation, stupor, and coma.

CUTANEOUS. The skin is pale with waxen mucous membranes and nail beds. Patients in decompensated shock typically have ashen, gray, haggard faces. The skin is cool to touch over most of the body.

CAPILLARY BLANCH TEST. The test is positive at the nail bed, and compression of skin over the chest may additionally show poor capillary refilling.

HEART RATE AND PERIPHERAL PULSES. Pulses are weak and thready, with rates greater than 120 beats per minute.

NECK VEINS. The neck, as well as peripheral veins, are collapsed.

RESPIRATORY RATE AND CHARACTER OF BREATHING. Tachypnea, in the range of 30 to 40 breaths per minute, is common. Failure to hyperventilate in shock indicates that disease, drugs, or trauma has altered or blunted the normal ventilatory response to shock. Because the patient is at risk for respiratory failure, the source of the problem must be identified rapidly and corrected.

URINE OUTPUT. Urine flow rates may fall to less than 15 ml/hour.

ACID/BASE. The accumulation of lactic acid overrides the respiratory alkalosis and a metabolic acidosis (pH less than 7.35) prevails.

TREATMENT

The goals of treatment are to eliminate the primary problem and provide patient support. Steps are taken to: 1) insure adequate ventilation and oxygenation; 2) identify and stop the source of fluid loss; and 3) restore intravascular volume. The type of fluid lost generally determines the fluid used for replacement. For example, when dehydration is the cause of hypovolemic shock, electrolyte solution is the fluid of choice. Suggested therapy by the American College of Surgeons[4] for hemorrhagic volume loss less than 1000 to 1250 ml is 3 ml of crystalloid (Ringer's lactate, normal saline) for every 1 ml of estimated volume lost. This ratio is used because within 20 minutes after administration, two thirds of infused crystalloid fluids transudate into the tissue space. When blood products or synthetic colloid solutions such as hetastarch (Hespan) or rheomacrodex (Dextran) are used to restore volume, 1 ml of solution is used for every estimated 1 ml of shed blood.

Crystalloid plus blood component therapy or blood component therapy alone is recommended for volume losses greater than 1500 ml.[4]

Septic Shock

Septic shock is shock associated with any infectious disease.

CAUSES

The infecting agents may be viruses, spirochetes, parasites, rickettsia, fungi, or gram-negative or gram-positive bacteria. Despite the fact that gram-negative bacilli such as *Escherichia coli, Pseudomonas aeruginosa* and *Klebsiella* species are the most common causes of hospital infection and septic shock, the fact that *Staphylococcus epidermidis* is frequently the cause of vascular line sepsis (see Chapter 12) serves as a reminder of the clinical importance of septic shock unrelated to gram-negative bacteria.

Predisposing Factors. Patients who have a primary infection, who are immune compromised, and who have experienced invasive procedures or organ damage are at high risk for septicemia (Table 14–3).

PATHOPHYSIOLOGY

In septicemia (the presence and growth of microorganisms in the blood), high circulating levels of bacterial toxins systemically activate a number of metabolic pathways. These activated systems result in the release of numerous and varied biochemical mediators that interact to produce the pathophysiologic events that characterize the septic shock syndrome. Fundamentally, these physiologic events represent various aspects of the normal immune response such as complement, kinin, coagulation and fibrinolytic systems activation. In septicemia, however, systemic unregulated and amplified immune system activation occurs, resulting in profound changes in cardiovascular, pulmonary, and hemostatic function.

The signs and symptoms of septicemia do not differ significantly with differences in infecting microorganisms. Shock (defined as abnormal cell metabolism secondary to an insult) associated with septicemia is classified into hyperdynamic and hypodynamic cardiovascular phases (Fig. 14–3).

TABLE 14–3. Factors Predisposing to Septicemia

Inadequate Immune Response	*Primary Infections*	*Iatrogenic Sources*
Granulocytopenia	Pneumonia	Indwelling vascular catheters
Diabetes mellitus	Urinary tract infection, especially following instrumentation	Indwelling urinary catheters
Liver disease	Female genital tract	Instrumentation of the urinary tract
Neoplasms	Cholecystitis	Extensive major abdominal or pelvic surgery
Neonates	Peritonitis	
The elderly (over 60 years of age)	Abscess	
Alcoholics		
Renal failure		
Pregnancy		
Protein-calorie malnutrition		
Massive trauma/shock states		

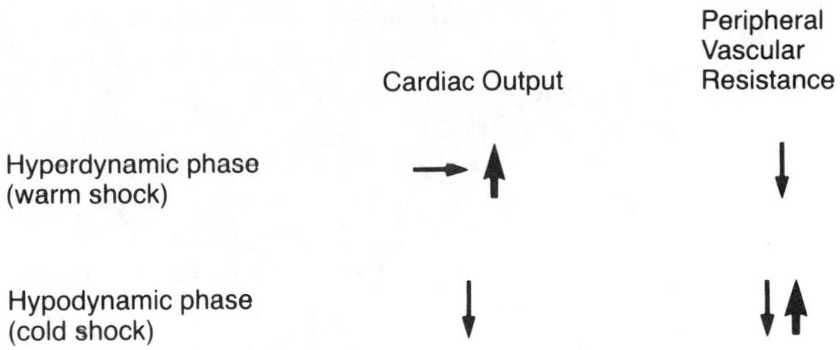

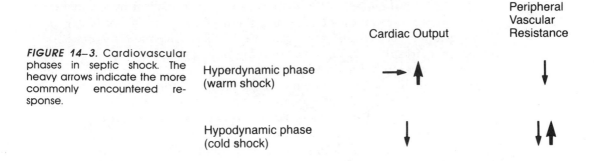

FIGURE 14–3. Cardiovascular phases in septic shock. The heavy arrows indicate the more commonly encountered response.

The Hyperdynamic Phase (Warm Shock)

This phase is characterized by a normal-to-high cardiac output and decreased systemic vascular resistance (systemic vasodilator reaction). Hypovolemia also plays a critical role in septic shock. The hypovolemia has two components; (1) Biochemical mediator-induced systemic vasodilation results in a relative hypovolemia. That is, the intravascular volume is decreased relative to the size of the expanded vascular compartment; and (2) Biochemical mediator-induced systemic vascular permeability allows a functional loss of fluid from the vascular to the tissue spaces that can exceed 200 ml/hour (third space losses). Total body water may be normal or increased if the patient is receiving replacement fluids; however, the fluid is being shifted into nonfunctional areas.

The sympathetic nervous system–induced increase in cardiac output serves as a compensatory mechanism to maintain arterial pressure. The increased cardiac output, however, may not be effectively distributed throughout all body tissue. In septicemia, blood flow through mediator-induced vasodilated areas may exceed local tissue needs, and the unused oxygen is returned to the cardiopulmonary unit. In other areas, flow may be inadequate to meet local tissue needs. Anatomic shunts (vascular channels that open from arterioles to venules and divert blood from the capillary bed) have also been described. Additionally, the cells may have difficulty in extracting and utilizing available oxygen secondary to mitochondrial injury and/or abnormalities in red blood cell function that favors retention of oxygen by hemoglobin.

At the same time, there is systemic and simultaneous activation of the clotting and fibrinolytic systems. This is the pathophysiologic description of disseminated intravascular coagulation (DIC). The clots that form are typically at the capillary level, which further compromises effective distribution of blood to the nutrient beds. Systemic and accelerated consumption of coagulation factors, in conjunction with accelerated fibrinolytic activity and production of fibrin-split products (potent inhibitors to clotting), predisposes to hemorrhage. If hemorrhage complicates DIC, the hypovolemic component of septic shock is compounded.

Increased pulmonary vascular resistance, as measured by a widening of the pulmonary artery diastolic to pulmonary artery wedge pressure (PAd-PWP) gradient occurs in some patients with septicemia and predicts an increased mortality. The mechanisms for pulmonary hypertension are not known; however, proposed mechanisms include pulmonary vascular plugging by microthrombi and/or pulmonary vasoconstriction mediated by components and products of the immune system.

Hemodynamic Profile (see Table 14–1). ARTERIAL PRESSURE. This parameter may be in the near-normal range or slightly decreased. There may be an orthostatic fall in blood pressure (fall in systolic pressure greater than 10 mm Hg on rising). The contour of the waveform is unchanged and may show a steep upstroke.

SYSTEMIC VASCULAR RESISTANCE. Values are below normal secondary to generalized vasodilation.

PULMONARY VASCULAR RESISTANCE. This value may be in the normal range or elevated.

CVP OR RIGHT ATRIAL PRESSURE. Values may be decreased secondary to intravascular volume loss and the expanded size of the vascular bed. The values obtained, however, may not accurately reflect intravascular volume status if right ventricular filling volumes and pressures are altered secondary to changes in pulmonary vascular resistance.

PULMONARY ARTERY AND WEDGE PRESSURES. These values tend to be decreased secondary to third space losses and vasodilation. However, an increase in PA systolic and diastolic pressure with a widening of the PAd-PWP gradient accompanies increases in pulmonary vascular tone. The contour of the waveforms is unchanged.

CARDIAC OUTPUT. Because of the hyperdynamic cardiovascular state, cardiac output is normal or elevated. The cardioadaptive response to septicemia may increase heart work to a level similar to that of heavy exercise. In contrast to the exercise performed in health, this level of heart work is maintained for days or weeks as the body is progressively weakened and damaged by sepsis.

MIXED VENOUS OXYGEN SATURATION ($S\bar{v}O_2$). This value may be above normal reflecting the abnormality in oxygen uptake and/or utilization at the cellular level.

Clinical Presentation. MENTATION. Patients frequently complain of malaise and "not feeling well." The patient may additionally present with confusion, restlessness, intellectual impairment, or delirium, which may be consistently maintained or may alternate with periods of apparently normal mental function.

CUTANEOUS. The skin is warm to the touch. Because hyperdynamic sepsis represents a vasodilator reaction, the warm skin may also be flushed. The complexion of some septic patients appears sallow rather than pink.

HEART RATE AND CHARACTER OF PULSE. The patient is tachycardic with a bounding pulse.

RESPIRATORY RATE AND CHARACTER OF BREATHING. The respiratory rate is increased with visible ventilatory movements. Hyperventilation, inappropriate to any apparent physiologic need, may be one of the first indications that the patient is septic.

URINE OUTPUT. If intravascular volume is not being placed at a rate equal to losses, the urine output will decrease.

ACID/BASE. Respiratory alkalosis secondary to the inappropriate hyperventilation is typical of early sepsis.

BODY TEMPERATURE. Fever may be accompanied by shaking chills. The elderly or severely debilitated patient may fail to increase body temperature in response to infection. Rather, the patient may become hypothermic, which predicts poor prognosis.

The hyperdynamic phase may last from hours to weeks, depending on the amount and virulence of infecting agents contaminating the blood, host resistance and constitution, and cardiovascular reserve. A critical determinant of the patient's ability to maintain the hyperdynamic state is the ability of the heart to increase and maintain cardiac output commensurate to the expanding size of the vascular bed, fluid losses, and metabolic need.

THE HYPODYNAMIC PHASE (COLD SHOCK)

This phase is characterized by a falling cardiac output and increased systemic vascular resistance. When the heart can no longer increase or maintain cardiac output at a level to compensate for the vasodilator reaction and/or intravascular volume losses, hypotension ensues. Cardiac decompensation may occur because:

- Preexisting cardiovascular disease has limited cardiac reserve.
- Intravascular volume losses decrease preload below a critical level. At this time volume loading may restore ventricular performance to a level necessary for normalization of arterial pressure. In such a case, the hyperdynamic state may be reestablished.
- As the duration of septicemia increases, myocardial performance progressively deteriorates. With progressive deterioration in the inotropic state of the myocardium, volume loading produces no significant increase in ventricular performance (Fig. 14–4).

The reasons for the progressive myocardial deterioration are not known; the presence of a myocardial depressant factor has been suggested, and myocardial performance returns to normal in patients surviving the septic episode.

Vascular resistance may remain reduced in the hypodynamic phase. When hypovolemia and cardiac depression are present, however, vasoconstriction may increase systemic vascular resistance, producing the clinical picture of "cold shock." The hypodynamic phase is associated with profound changes in tissue perfusion that result in multiple system dysfunction.

Hemodynamic Profile (see Table 14–1). ARTERIAL PRESSURE. Hypotension may occur over a period of hours or precipitously. The accompanying waveform may show a slow rate of rise and appears damped.

SYSTEMIC VASCULAR RESISTANCE. Vascular resistance may remain reduced or vasoconstriction may occur in response to hypotension.

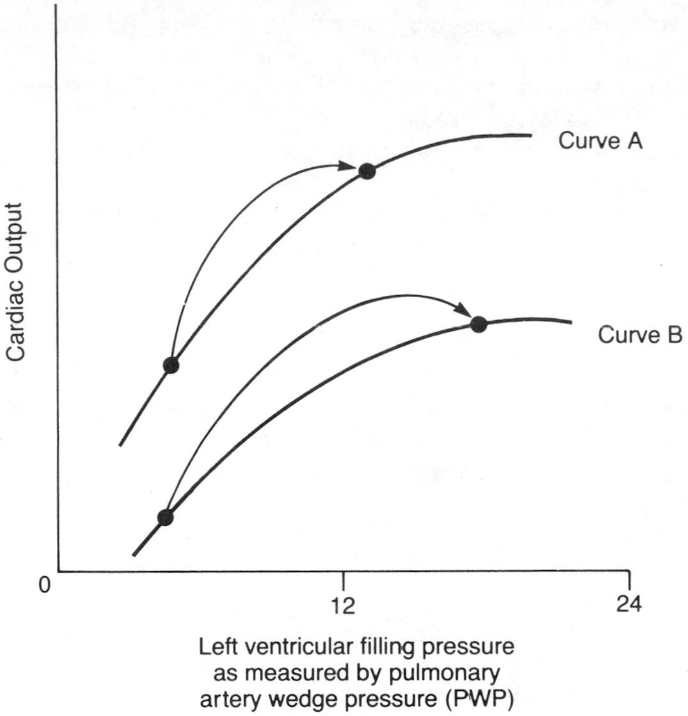

FIGURE 14–4. Deterioration of myocardial performance from septic shock. In Curve A, the patient is in septic shock without myocardial depression. The decrease in cardiac output is the result of low ventricular filling volume/pressure. Volume loading restores heart function back to normal.

In Curve B, the patient is volume depleted but also has myocardial depression. Volume loading fails to restore cardiac performance to an acceptable level.

PULMONARY VASCULAR RESISTANCE. This value may be in the normal range but is more likely to be elevated.

CVP OR RIGHT ATRIAL PRESSURE. Values are decreased if volume replacement has not been adequate. On the other hand, changes in pulmonary vascular resistance or ventricular failure may elevate these values.

PULMONARY ARTERY AND WEDGE PRESSURES. These measurements are likewise low if volume replacement has not been adequate. Simultaneous elevations in pulmonary artery pressures and PWP accompany myocardial dysfunction and ventricular failure. Widening of the PAd-PWP gradient relates to increased pulmonary vascular resistance.

CARDIAC OUTPUT. Typically, this value falls progressively.

MIXED VENOUS OXYGEN SATURATION ($S\bar{v}O_2$). At this stage of disease, this value is variably affected. Due to the abnormal cellular uptake and/or utilization of oxygen, the mixed venous oxygen saturation may remain increased. However, perfusion failure secondary to cardiovascular dysfunction may decrease mixed venous oxygen saturation. It is possible, therefore, for the mixed venous oxygen saturation to be increased or decreased (depending on which defect predominates) or in the normal range. This does not reflect a physiologic norm but more likely is due to two physiologic derangements oppositely influencing this value.

Clinical Presentation. MENTATION. The level of consciousness falls and may end in stupor or coma. The rate of deterioration relates to the rate of cardiovascular deterioration which, as stated earlier, may be abrupt or gradual.

CUTANEOUS. The skin is typically cold, clammy, and pale with peripheral mottling and cyanosis.

HEART RATE AND CHARACTER OF PULSE. Tachycardia continues, but the pulse becomes weak and thready or may be imperceptible peripherally.

NECK VEINS. The external jugular veins are not visible while the patient is in the supine position, and the visible veins are collapsed.

RESPIRATORY RATE AND CHARACTER OF BREATHING. The patient remains tachypneic but ventilatory movements may become shallow. Altered breathing patterns, such as Cheyne-Stokes, may also be present late in the septic course.

URINE OUTPUT. Urine flow rates may be greatly reduced to the point of anuria.

ACID/BASE. The rapid accumulation of lactic acid overrides the effects of hyperventilation, and metabolic acidosis prevails. Ineffective ventilatory movements or patterns may produce a combined respiratory and metabolic acidosis.

TREATMENT

The goals of treatment are identification and elimination of the septic focus, effective antibiotic therapy, and patient support. Measures include:

1. Maintenance of adequate ventilation and oxygenation.
2. Culture and sensitivities of blood, urine, wound drainage, indwelling catheters and all possible sites of infection.
3. Fluid replacement to restore intravascular volume and ventricular filling pressures to levels that will maximize cardiac output.
4. Correction of acid-base abnormalities.
5. IV administration of broad spectrum antibiotics. This assures more rapid onset of action and predictable blood levels than oral or IM administration. Selection of antibiotics is based on the pathogens known to be prevalent in the observed site of infection, the gram-stain smears, and the antibiotic sensitivity patterns of flora endogenous to the hospital. Typically, an aminoglycoside (gentamicin is the most commonly chosen) or a cephalosporin is used. High doses of an antipseudomonas penicillin such as carbenicillin are added if the patient is granulocytopenic. In the presence of abdominal or gynecologic infection in which *Bacteroides fragilis* is a likely pathogen, clindamycin is combined with gentamicin. For all other patients, gentamicin and a cephalosporin such as cefazolin are preferred agents.[5, 6]
6. Removal of the septic focus. This may require incision and drainage of an abscess, debridement of necrotic or grossly infected tissue, or simple removal of an infected vascular catheter. The importance of this measure cannot be overemphasized because sepsis will continue to ravage the patient until the septic source is eradicated.
7. Cooling measures for temperatures of 102°F (38.5°C).

8. Administration of massive doses of glucocorticoids to counter the inflammatory effects of the disease. This treatment is controversial. If used, methylprednisolone (Solu-Medrol), 30 mg/kg of body weight, is given slowly (over 15 minutes) as a single bolus at the onset of shock and is repeated in 4 hours if no beneficial response is noted with the first dose.

Anaphylactic Shock

Anaphylactic shock relates to circulatory failure and biochemical abnormalities secondary to a systemic allergic reaction to an antigenic substance. Anaphylactic reactions are particularly common in the hospital environment.

Causes

A large and varied number of substances are capable of producing anaphylactic reactions. These include anesthetic and analgesic agents, foods, drugs, blood products, diagnostic agents, and venoms (Table 14–4).

Anaphylactic reactions occur more commonly in individuals with a history of multiple allergies. These people seem to have a genetically acquired in-

TABLE 14–4. Agents Commonly Causing Anaphylaxis

Antibiotics	***Foods***
Penicillin and penicillin analogs	Eggs
Aminoglycosides	Dairy products
Cephalosporins	Nuts
Tetracyclines	Legumes
Amphotericin B	Shellfish
Nonsteroidal Anti-inflammatory Agents	Citrus fruit
Salicylates	Chocolate
Colchicine	Grains
Ibuprofen	***Dextrans***
Venoms	Rheomacrodex, 40, 70
Bees	***Narcotic Analgesics/Anesthetics***
Wasps	Thiopental
Hornets	Morphine
Yellowjackets	Codeine
Fire ants	Meprobamate
Snakes	***Extracts Used in Desensitization***
Spiders	***Blood and Blood Products***
Local Anesthetics	Gamma globulin
Xylocaine (lidocaine)	Plasma
Procaine	Whole blood
Diagnostic Agents	***Miscellaneous Drugs***
Iodinized radiocontrast material	Protamine
Hormones	Iodides
Insulin	Thiazide diuretics
ACTH	Parenteral iron
Vasopressin	Heparin
Pollens	
Ragweed	
Grass	

ability to control the immune mechanism under certain stimuli. Anaphylactic reactions may also occur in people with no allergic history.

Pathophysiology

Exposure to an antigenic agent results in the production of IgE (immunoglobulin E) antibodies. When exposure to the antigen is repeated, the antigen combines with IgE antibodies and activates surface receptors on basophil and mast cells. This initiates a sequence of biochemical events that leads to the release of mediator substances into the extracellular fluid. These mediator substances include histamine, prostaglandins, kinins, slow-reacting substances of anaphylaxis (SRS-A), complement fragments, and components of the coagulation cascade.

Some substances, such as iodinized radiocontrast agents, may directly activate the surface receptors of mast cells and basophils and require no prior exposure for the anaphylactic reaction to occur.

Systemic and massive mediator substance release produces a systemic permeability defect that results in massive third space fluid losses, an arteriolar dilator reaction and bronchoconstriction. Initially, cardiac output increases secondary to the decrease in systemic vascular resistance. However, with the development of the shock syndrome, myocardial function deteriorates.

Hypovolemia plays a critical role in hypotension and cardiovascular collapse in anaphylactic shock and has two components: 1) dilatation of the vascular bed, which results in a relative hypovolemia; and 2) increased capillary permeability, which results in the functional loss of intravascular volume into the tissue spaces.

Systemic activation of the coagulation cascade may result in coagulopathies seen in some patients.

Although the hemodynamic and clinical responses may vary with individuals, the response pattern in a particular individual to a specific substance tends to repeat. The severity and rate of progression of the reaction depends on the amount of the antigenic material ingested, the route of ingestion and the allergic potential of the antigen to the individual.

Hemodynamic Profile

(See Table 14–1)

Arterial Pressure. Systolic and diastolic pressures fall due to vasodilation and intravascular fluid loss. This fall may occur dramatically and precipitously.

Systemic Vascular Resistance. Systemic vasodilation results in a generalized decrease in vascular resistance.

Pulmonary Vascular Resistance. This value may be in the normal range or elevated.

CVP, Pulmonary Artery and Wedge Pressures. Loss of intravascular volume (third space shifts) and expansion of the size of the vascular bed reduce these values.

Cardiac Output. Initially, cardiac output may be increased as a result of decreased afterload but then rapidly falls due to the reduction in ventricular filling volume and coronary underperfusion.

Mixed Venous Oxygen Saturation ($S\bar{v}O_2$). Levels fall below normal due to the low perfusion state and/or hypoxemia.

Clinical Presentation

Mentation. The patient is typically restless, obtunded, and may have a sense of impending doom.

Cutaneous. The complexion is variably affected. Because anaphylaxis represents a vasodilator reaction, the skin may be flushed and warm; however, with profound circulatory collapse, the skin is typically ashen. There may also be considerable swelling of subcutaneous and mucous tissue. The skin may itch and there may be hives.

Heart Rate and Character of Pulse. The rapid rate, low volume pulse is often irregular due to significant ectopic activity.

Airway Response. Two patterns of airway response may occur; a patient may have both, neither, or only one.

1. Upper airway obstruction due to edema of the larynx, epiglottis and/or vocal cords. Sensations of tightness in the throat or a lump in the throat that cannot be cleared with coughing occur with lesser degrees of airways obstruction or edema. With 70 percent or greater obstruction of the upper airway, an inspiratory crowing noise (stridor) and dyspnea may precede death by suffocation.

2. Lower airway obstruction due to diffuse bronchoconstriction. This is characterized by wheezing and a profound expiratory effort. Suprasternal, substernal, intercostal, and supraclavicular retractions may be noted as the patient forces a rapid inspiration in order to provide more time for the difficult exhalation. The intercostal spaces may bulge on exhalation.

Pulmonary Response. The patient may show clinical evidence of pulmonary edema. Pulmonary edema fluid with albumin concentrations close to or identical to those of plasma may be suctioned from the airways. Because this occurs in the presence of a low PWP, a pulmonary capillary permeability defect is likely present (see Chapter 15, ARDS). An associated increase in pulmonary vascular resistance, reflected in an increased PAd-PWP gradient, may be present.

Gastrointestinal Response. The patient may experience nausea, vomiting, abdominal cramping, or diarrhea.

Treatment

Treatment of anaphylactic shock involves the following measures.

Provision of an adequate airway, ventilation and oxygenation are critical priorities. Upper airway obstruction may require intubation or emergency tracheotomy. Bronchospasm may be treated with theophylline (aminophylline) 5 to 6 mg/kg injected slowly over a 15 to 30 minute period. Rapid injection may worsen the tachycardia and ectopic activity, produce seizures, or induce vomiting.

For mild anaphylactic reactions, aqueous epinephrine 1:1000 is given 0.3 to 0.5 ml IM or subcutaneously. The dose may be repeated at 5 to 10 minute intervals. For severe reactions, 3 to 5 ml of the 1:10,000 aqueous solution is administered IV.

A tourniquet should be placed above the site of introduction to the antigen when applicable. This may reduce the systemic absorption of the antigen.

Rapid correction of hypovolemia is undertaken with a crystalloid or albumin titrated to maintain an adequate perfusion pressure. This may require massive amounts of fluid, such as 2 to 3 liters over a 15 minute period.

If hypotensive, the patient is placed in a supine position with 30 degree elevation of the legs.

Persistent hypotension may require vasopressors.

Neurogenic Shock

Neurogenic shock is shock initiated by damage to and/or dysfunction of the sympathetic nervous system.

Causes

Neurogenic shock may be produced by spinal cord damage or pharmacologic blockade of the sympathetic nervous system at the level of T-6 or higher. Hypotension due to brain damage or head injury does not occur unless damage is to the brainstem or death is imminent. Typically, the arterial systolic pressure increases with increases in intracranial pressure associated with head injury. If a patient with head injury develops hypotension, another cause of hypotension (as hemothorax, hemoperitoneum) must be identified and treated.

Pathophysiology

The neurons of the sympathetic nervous system located in the thoracolumbar portion of the spinal cord depend on stimulation from the brain for maintenance of vasoconstrictive and cardioaccelerator reflexes. High spinal cord damage or pharmacologic blockade (spinal anesthesia) interrupts central vasoconstrictor and cardioaccelerator impulses. The loss of sympathetic nervous system control of arterioles produces a massive vasodilator reaction with pooling of blood in the peripheral circulation. This creates a relative hypovolemia, a decrease in venous return to the heart, and a consequent decrease in cardiac output. Bradycardia may worsen hemodynamics. The higher the level of damage to the cord, the greater the anticipated decrease in arterial pressure and heart rate.

HEMODYNAMIC PROFILE

(See Table 14–1)

Arterial Pressure. The systolic, diastolic, and pulse pressures are reduced. If the patient is maintained in the supine position, the systolic pressure may not fall below 100 mm Hg. However, patients with high spinal cord dysfunction are very sensitive to position changes, and profound falls in blood pressure may occur if the upper part of the body is elevated.

Systemic Vascular Resistance. Massive vasodilation occurs owing to the loss of sympathetic nervous system control of resistance vessels (arterioles), and systemic vascular resistance falls.

CVP, Pulmonary Artery, and Wedge Pressures. These values tend to be decreased owing to the relative hypovolemia.

Cardiac Output. This parameter may remain within normal values or may be decreased because of the inappropriate bradycardia and/or decreased ventricular filling volume.

Mixed Venous Oxygen Saturation ($S\bar{v}O_2$). This value falls secondary to generalized poor capillary blood flow.

CLINICAL PRESENTATION

Mentation. Changes in mentation (confusion, lethargy, stupor) accompany falls in arterial pressure.

Cutaneous. The complexion is typically warm, pink, and dry, reflecting the vasodilated state.

Heart Rate and Character of Pulse. Bradycardia, due to the loss of sympathetic nervous system influence of the heart, commonly accompanies neurogenic shock. The pulse may be of normal or low volume.

Respiratory Response. Injuries of the cervical spine may be associated with upper airway obstruction if the atonic tongue falls back and occludes the oropharynx. In cervical spinal cord lesions, paralysis of the intercostal and abdominal muscles often occurs, making ventilation entirely dependent on the diaphragm. In this circumstance, the patient may exhibit "paradoxical respirations"; the thorax collapses with inspiration as the diaphragm descends and expands with expiration as the diaphragm ascends. With high cervical spine lesions, the patient may be entirely apneic.

Temperature Regulation. The body temperature of patients with cervical spinal cord lesions tends to be that of their environment (poikilothermia). Loss of the ability to sweat and passive dilation of the cutaneous vascular bed impairs these aspects of the normal thermoregulatory mechanism.

TREATMENT

Treatment of neurogenic shock involves the following steps:

- Adequate arterial oxygenation must be maintained. This may require insertion of an artificial airway and/or ventilatory support.

- Crystalloid (electrolyte) solution should be infused at a rate sufficient to maintain a systolic pressure above 100 mm Hg. Elevation of the legs may restore acceptable arterial pressure.
- Sinus bradycardia secondary to cervical spinal cord injury usually does not require therapy. However, if the heart rate falls below 40 beats per minute or if nodal or ventricular escape rhythms predominate, atropine 0.5 to 1.0 mg may be given IV.

Cardiogenic Shock

Cardiogenic shock (pump failure, generator failure) exists when the heart is unable to maintain a cardiac output sufficient to meet the metabolic needs of major organ systems. The resulting major organ dysfunction begets more deleterious physiologic changes and a rapid, progressive, downward clinical course ensues. Cardiogenic shock is the most severe form of heart failure and is associated with a mortality rate of 80 to 100%.

As in all forms of shock, clinical and/or laboratory indications of systemic underperfusion should be used to define shock rather than numerical values such as arterial pressure and cardiac output because:

—The arterial pressure obtained by auscultation and palpation tends to be unreliable in low perfusion states.

—The individual tolerance to hypotension is variable.

—Large areas of tissue may be underperfused despite a "normal" arterial pressure.

—Cardiogenic shock may occur in association with a normal or elevated cardiac output. This is seen clinically when disorders such as anemia, sepsis, hyperthyroidism or multiple arteriovenous fistulae require an increased cardiac output, but the heart is unable to mount or maintain a cardiac output commensurate with the body's increased needs. Hence, an anemic patient who normally requires a cardiac output of 10 liters/minute to maintain adequate tissue oxygenation may exhibit signs of shock if cardiovascular disease limits cardiac output to 6 liters/minute.

CAUSES

Cardiogenic shock is commonly seen in the end stage of many forms of heart disease. Factors that may acutely produce profound heart failure and shock include:

Tachyarrhythmias. Normal hearts generally tolerate rapid heart rates well. Tachycardias, however, may produce a shock syndrome in patients with preexisting deficiencies in cardiac performance by the following mechanisms:

—A rapid heart rate reduces ventricular filling time and preload. Patients with myocardial dysfunction are dependent on an adequate ventricular filling volume. A relatively small increase in heart rate may produce a critical decrease in preload and stroke volume in the preload-dependent heart.

—Increased heart rates result in increased myocardial oxygen demand and a concomitant decrease in coronary perfusion (diastolic) time. Ventricular dysfunction is particularly likely to occur if the patient has coronary artery disease as the force of myocardial contraction diminishes in direct proportion to the myocardial oxygenation deficit. As a result of the factors that worsen the ischemic process, tachyarrhythmias ravage the ischemic-prone heart.

—Ventricular arrhythmias may produce distorted ventricular contractions that result in inefficient chamber emptying. The loss of the atrial kick may additionally impair ventricular performance by reducing preload. In fact, any arrhythmia that results in asynchrony between atria and ventricles may significantly reduce cardiac output in patients with abnormal ventricular function.

Bradyarrhythmias. Shock may result when the heart rate falls in a circumstance where stroke volume cannot increase to maintain cardiac output. This may be seen in hypovolemia or in patients with fibrotic or ischemic heart disease.

Substances or Factors That Depress Myocardial Function. These include acidemia, severe hypoxemia; hypoglycemia; septicemia; hyperkalemia; hyponatremia; hypocalcemia; and/or drugs such as beta or calcium channel blockers, quinidine, and procainamide.

Mechanical Defects. Rupture of the intraventricular septum, grossly abnormal valve function, a large intracardiac ball-valve thrombus, or rupture of the free wall of the left ventricle all produce shock because of severely reduced forward blood flow.

Following Major Surgery (Particularly Cardiac Surgery) or Trauma. The associated hemodynamic and metabolic changes may predispose to pump dysfunction.

Acute Myocardial Infarction (AMI). Shock is estimated to occur in 10 to 15 percent of patients who enter the hospital with myocardial infarction. Destruction or dysfunction of the right or more commonly left ventricle is the most common cause of cardiogenic shock. For this reason, this discussion will be limited to AMI shock.

Pathophysiology

Cardiogenic shock represents progressive hemodynamic and metabolic deterioration. The initiating event, acute myocardial infarction, is a dynamic process involving progressive myocardial necrosis extending outward from the subendocardium into the surrounding metabolically unstable ischemic zones. Factors that determine the severity and rate of progression of events include:

1. the amount of coronary artery obstruction;
2. the amount of tissue normally perfused by the occluded vessel;
3. the interplay of myocardial oxygen supply and demand; and
4. the adequacy of the preexisting collateral coronary circulation.

The ischemic areas of myocardium suffer abnormalities in compliance (increased wall stiffness) and contractility relative to the severity of oxygen deprivation.

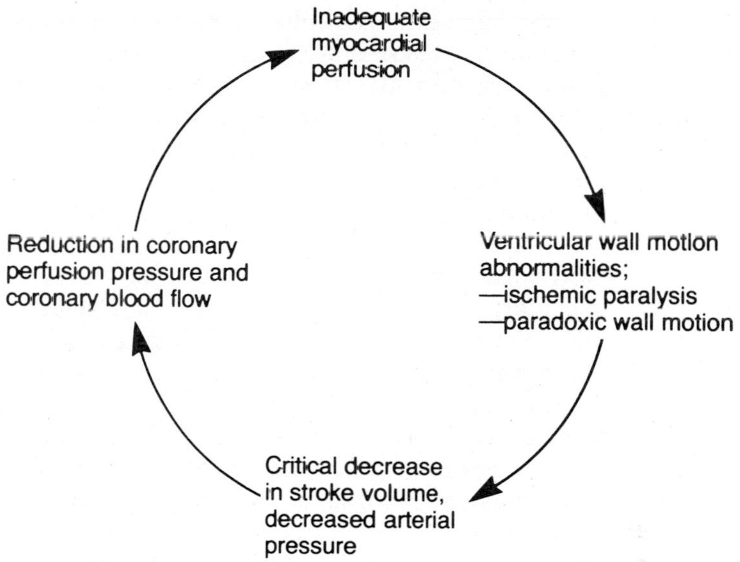

FIGURE 14 5. The self-perpetuating vicious cycle of progressive myocardial damage and dysfunction in A.M.I. shock.

The central, severely oxygen-deprived area ceases to contract whereas the more peripherally located jeopardized areas may weakly contract. In addition, the area of ischemic paralysis may bulge outward while the uninvolved myocardium contracts in systole. (See Chapter 16, Ischemic Heart Disease, Hemodynamic Effects.) Loss of functional myocardium and paradoxical wall motion seriously interferes with ventricular emptying. When the decreasing cardiac output reaches a critical level, arterial pressure and effective perfusion of major organs falls. In the presence of coronary artery disease, coronary blood flow is critically dependent on coronary perfusion pressure (aortic diastolic pressure minus central venous pressure). Therefore, a decrease in mean arterial pressure causes an abrupt and often severe fall in coronary blood flow. This predisposes to more ischemic myocardial dysfunction and damage, thus establishing the vicious cycle illustrated in Figure 14–5.

Inadequate coronary and systemic blood flow forces anaerobic metabolism and its resulting deleterious lactic acidosis. There is also a tremendous sympathetic nervous system (stress) response reflected metabolically by increases in plasma levels of glucose and free fatty acids.

Hemodynamic Effect

During an acute ischemic attack, the myocardium experiences a decrease in power and compliance. This has two important hemodynamic implications:

1. The decrease in power results in a decrease in cardiac output. Typically this is associated with compensatory peripheral vascular constriction, which attempts to maintain mean arterial pressure. However, the increased systemic vascular resistance is a double-edged sword. Arterial pressure may be sup-

ported but peripheral blood flow is reduced. In addition, the more difficult it becomes for blood to flow out of the arterial circulation into the capillary bed, the more difficult it becomes for the left ventricle to eject blood into the arterial circulation—particularly in a diseased state. Therefore, stroke volume and cardiac output may be further reduced.

Some patients with AMI develop abnormal vascular reflexes so that systemic vascular resistance may increase only slightly or may actually decrease. In these individuals, blood pressure may be severely decreased although cardiac output may not be markedly reduced. This response has been attributed to the activation of left ventricular stretch receptors that are more numerous in the left ventricular inferior wall. The hypotension and bradycardia due to stimulation of these vagal receptors are seen more commonly in inferior wall infarcts.

2. The decrease in myocardial compliance alters the ventricular volume/pressure relationship. In other words, for any given ventricular filling (end-diastolic) volume, the filling pressure as reflected by PWP will be higher than it would normally be. Because intraventricular end-diastolic volume, not pressure, determines ventricular performance by the Starling mechanism, a reduction in cardiac output may occur with minimal or no change in PWP.

Hemodynamic Profile

(See Table 14–1)

Arterial Pressure. A systolic pressure of less than 80 to 90 mm Hg is characteristic of, but not prerequisite to, cardiogenic shock. A patient known to be previously hypertensive typically has a significant fall in arterial pressure. The *arterial waveform* appears damped with a slowed rate of rise, reflecting the decreased stroke volume and force of ejection.

Systemic Vascular Resistance. The sympathetic nervous system response may increase systemic vascular resistance to greater than 2000 dynes/sec/cm^{-5}. As mentioned previously, in some patients systemic vascular resistance may increase only slightly or may be in the low normal range.

Pulmonary Vascular Resistance. This value may increase due to hypoxemia and acidemia. The increase in pulmonary vascular resistance may be worsened by complicating pulmonary edema.

CVP or Right Atrial Pressure. These values will be elevated with ischemic involvement of the right ventricle. In the clinical context of isolated left ventricle involvement, this value will be elevated only if left ventricular failure is reflected back to the right heart.

Pulmonary Artery and Wedge Pressures. In health, the left ventricular filling pressure is slightly higher than the right, 4 to 12 mm Hg and 0 to 8 mm Hg respectively. In ischemic disease, a disparity in right and left ventricular function occurs altering the normal pressure relationship. Because ischemic disease more commonly involves the left ventricle, the PWP is commonly elevated. Pulmonary artery and then right ventricular pressures may ultimately increase as blood is dammed up in the vascular and cardiac structures proximal to the failing left ventricle.

When right ventricular dysfunction predominates, the right ventricle may become unable to maintain adequate pulmonary blood flow and left ventricular filling. The pulmonary artery and PWP pressures may then fall below normal values. The decrease in left ventricular filling volume may then produce a decrease in left ventricular performance by the Starling mechanism. In addition, the elevated right ventricular filling pressure matched against a normal or decreased left ventricular filling pressure alters the normal right and left ventricular end diastolic pressure relationship. The intraventricular septum is shifted toward the lower pressure left ventricle and alters its internal shape and renders it less compliant. This distorts the normal left ventricular volume/pressure relationship and also adversely affects left ventricular function.

Cardiac Output. The decreased isovolumetric and ejection phases of systole and decreased stroke volume result in a fall in cardiac output.

Mixed Venous Oxygen Saturation ($S\bar{v}O_2$). This value falls relative to the severity of pump failure as the patient depletes the venous oxygen reserve in an attempt to maintain tissue oxygen needs. This value may be additionally compromised if arterial oxygen content is reduced by hypoxemia, which commonly occurs in conjunction with cardiogenic shock.

Clinical Presentation

Overall, the patient appears gravely ill. This is commonly accompanied subjectively by a sense of impending doom.

Mentation. Depending on the severity of perfusion failure and individual cerebral responses to hypoperfusion, the patient may be restless, apprehensive, confused, irritable, obtunded, or stuporous.

Cutaneous. The skin is typically pale, cool, and clammy, with peripheral cyanosis. If the patient fails to vasoconstrict appropriately in response to the decrease in cardiac output, the complexion may appear ruddy.

Heart Rate and Character of Pulse. The heart rate is commonly greater than 90 beats per minute and may, in part, compensate for the decreased stroke volume. If a bradyarrhythmia complicates AMI (sinus bradycardia, junctional rhythm, heart block) the hemodynamics may be significantly worsened. Disturbances in rhythm (premature atrial beats, atrial fibrillation, premature ventricular beats, ventricular tachycardia) frequently complicate cardiogenic shock. The peripheral pulses are typically weak and thready.

Heart Sounds. The heart sounds are weak and muffled due to the decreased force of ventricular contraction (S_1) and possible decreased closing (diastolic) pressure in the aorta (S_2). An atrial and ventricular gallop are invariably present but may be barely audible.

Palpation of the Precordium. It may be difficult to perceive the precordial movements because of the weakened ventricular contractions. If cardiac failure has developed acutely in a patient with a previously normal heart, the apex beat is likely to occupy the normal location or be only slightly displaced leftward. With more long-standing failure (several days), the apex beat of the dilated heart will be displaced downward and to the left. Wall motion abnormalities and the atrial and ventricular gallop may not be perceptible.

Neck Veins. The external jugular veins will be visibly distended with primary right ventricular involvement or right ventricular failure secondary to primary left ventricular dysfunction.

Respiratory Rate and Character of Breathing. Irregularities in the breathing pattern may be present with the rapid, shallow breathing that is typical. If pulmonary edema is present, the patient will also complain of dyspnea. The overall increased work of breathing, which is augmented by pulmonary edema, diverts additional blood flow to the respiratory muscles, thus further impairing perfusion of other body tissue and vital organs.

Lung Sounds. In the absence of pulmonary edema with alveolar flooding, the lungs are clear to auscultation.

Urine Output. A small volume, concentrated urine is produced. Urine flow rates are usually less than 30 ml/hour. Diuretic therapy invalidates urine output and specific gravity as an assessment tool.

Acid Base. Metabolic acidosis, hypoxemia, and hypocapnia are present. The severity of these abnormalities relates to the severity of shock.

TREATMENT

Goals in the management of AMI shock are to:

1. Improve myocardial oxygen supply by increasing aortic pressure and coronary blood flow, and insure adequate arterial oxygenation.
2. Decrease myocardial oxygen requirements by decreasing heart work.
3. Increase cardiac output and peripheral perfusion.

The following measures are directed toward these goals:

Maintain adequate ventilation and an arterial PO_2 greater than 80 mm Hg.

Relieve pain and provide rest for the patient. Morphine titrated in small doses at frequent intervals is generally regarded as the drug of choice in treating AMI pain. Morphine analgesia reduces sympathetic nervous system stimulation, thereby reducing the potential for arrhythmias as well as myocardial and systemic oxygen requirements; diminishes diaphoresis and fluid losses; reduces preload, which may relieve pulmonary vascular congestion if present; induces a sense of well-being, which allows the patient rest; and, on a purely humanitarian basis, relieves suffering.

Control rhythm disturbances. Conduction disturbances may be managed with pacing or atropine. Antiarrhythmic agents for the treatment of ectopic arrhythmias are to be used cautiously because of their potential myocardial depressive effect.

Make therapeutic adjustments in ventricular filling pressure. Hypovolemia secondary to nausea, vomiting, diuretic therapy, third space losses, and/or diaphoresis may complicate AMI shock. Because preload is an important determinant of ventricular performance, ventricular filling pressure may have to be increased by fluid challenge to levels that optimize myocardial performance.

In the presence of cardiac disease, the filling pressures required to normalize cardiac output are typically greater than the upper normal limit for the involved ventricle. For example, in patients with acute myocardial infarction, a left ventricular filling pressure (PWP) of 15 to 18 mm Hg may be required to increase cardiac output and restore arterial pressure to acceptable levels. With right ventricular impairment, a filling pressure as high as 10 to 15 mm Hg may be required to normalize the output of the right ventricle and left ventricular filling.

On the other hand, when the left ventricular filling pressure exceeds 20 to 22 mm Hg or if pulmonary edema is present, diuretics, phlebotomy, or venodilator agents may be required to lower preload to a level most beneficial for the individual patient.

Make pharmacologic adjustments of peripheral vascular resistance. Low perfusion states are commonly accompanied by compensatory increases in peripheral vascular resistance. Pharmacologic agents that dilate the systemic arteries ease left ventricular unloading. Thus, tissue perfusion is improved and myocardial oxygen consumption is decreased. When used for ventricular failure, the increase in stroke volume may offset the vasodilator effects on the arterial pressure and mean arterial pressure may remain unchanged. The application of this form of therapy is limited by a systolic pressure less than 90 mm Hg.

Conversely, the patient with severe hypotension may require treatment with pharmacologic agents that increase systemic peripheral vascular resistance; these agents are commonly also inotropes. Although agents that increase systemic vascular resistance may further reduce peripheral perfusion, as well as stroke volume, by increasing ventricular outflow resistance, the maintenance of a central aortic pressure compatible with adequate coronary and cerebral perfusion is of paramount importance for the immediate support of life.

Provide inotropic support of the heart. Agents that improve cardiac output by increasing myocardial contractility may have the undesirable effects of increasing automaticity, myocardial oxygen requirements, and peripheral vascular resistance. The concomitant use of a vasodilator agent, such as nitroprusside (Nipride) may offset the vasoconstrictive effect of the commonly used inotropes, thereby further increasing cardiac output and peripheral blood flow. Table 14–5 lists vasoactive agents that additionally have inotropic effects.

Digitalis, a relatively weak inotrope, is generally not used in shock. The metabolic and oxygenation abnormalities associated with shock predispose to potentially lethal digitalis-induced arrhythmias.

The preceding discussion of pharmacologic management of cardiogenic shock indicates that any anticipated benefit may also carry a risk. For example, if ventricular impedance is lowered by the use of vasodilators, coronary perfusion pressure may drop below a critical level, worsening the ischemic process. If arterial pressure is raised with vasoconstrictors to improve

TABLE 14–5. Vasoactive Agents with Inotropic Effects

Inotropic agents that have a vasoconstrictor effect on the peripheral vasculature
Epinephrine (Adrenalin)
Norepinephrine (Levophed)
Metaraminol (Aramine)
Dopamine (Intropin)—at doses usually greater than 20 μg/kg/min
Digitalis
Inotropic agents that have a vasodilator effect on the peripheral vasculature
Isoproterenol (Isuprel)
Dobutamine (Dobutrex)
Dopamine (Intropin)—at low-to-moderate dose
Amrinone (Inocor)

Adapted from Cohn JN: Recognition and management of shock and acute pump failure. In Hurst JW, et al (eds): *The Heart.* New York, McGraw-Hill, 1982, p. 470.)

coronary perfusion pressure, peripheral blood flow may be sacrificed and the increased afterload may increase myocardial oxygen requirements sufficient to worsen ischemia. The specific hemodynamic pattern dictates the clinical approach while the clinical and monitored responses of the patient are closely observed to determine if the overall pharmacologic effect is beneficial or harmful.

Institute therapy with the intra-aortic balloon pump (balloon counterpulsation). The principle of counterpulsation is that a mechanical device causes intra-aortic pressure to rapidly fall synchronously with ventricular systole and rise rapidly simultaneous with ventricular diastole. The intra-aortic balloon pump is a mechanical counterpulsation device that benefits the patient in cardiogenic shock by reducing afterload as well as increasing coronary and systemic perfusion. The balloon pump console uses the *R*-wave of the ECG for automatic timing.

For balloon counterpulsation, a catheter is advanced up the aorta until the tip of the catheter lies just distal to the left subclavian artery. A sausage-shaped balloon of 30 to 40 ml inflation volume is located at the distal end of the catheter so that, when in place, the inflated balloon fills the thoracic aorta. The bottom of the balloon lies just above the renal arteries.

DIASTOLE. Inflation of the balloon occurs immediately following closure of the aortic valve and is maintained until just prior to the onset of ventricular systole (Fig. 14–6*B*). The period of balloon inflation relates to the crest of the *T*-wave to the *R*-wave on the ECG. Balloon inflation raises aortic root diastolic pressure and displaces a volume of blood equal to 25 to 75 percent of its inflation volume. This is approximately 10 to 30 ml for a 40 ml balloon. A portion of the balloon-displaced blood perfuses the cerebral and coronary circulations. As 75 to 80 percent of coronary perfusion occurs in diastole, this "thrust" of blood from balloon displacement into the coronary arteries improves perfusion to the normal as well as the jeopardized areas of myocardium. Forward displacement of blood improves renal, mesenteric, and general systemic perfusion.

SYSTOLE. Deflation of the balloon occurs at the end of isovolumetric contraction (just prior to opening of the aortic valve) and is maintained until the onset of diastole (Fig. 14–6*A*). This period coincides with the R-wave to the crest of the T-wave on the ECG.

Because balloon inflation reduces aortic blood volume, balloon deflation causes pressure in the aorta to be less than normal just prior to ventricular systole (the presystolic dip). The left ventricle therefore encounters less resistance in opening the aortic valve and emptying into the systemic circulation. This improves left ventricular performance (increasing stroke volume) and decreases myocardial work and myocardial oxygen consumption. Preload usually decreases secondary to improved left ventricular emptying. Overall, myocardial oxygen supply and demand are brought into more favorable balance and the ischemic process is relieved. With improvement in systemic perfusion, organs regain their special function: kidneys make urine, cerebration improves, intestinal motility returns, etc.

Frequently, initiation of intra-aortic balloon pumping is followed quickly by marked clinical improvement and reversal of the shock process. Sometimes, however, the patient who appears to be stable deteriorates as balloon pumping is discontinued or expires suddenly during or following balloon counterpulsation. In these circumstances, it is assumed that massive permanent cardiac damage had occurred prior to institution of balloon pumping. For this reason,

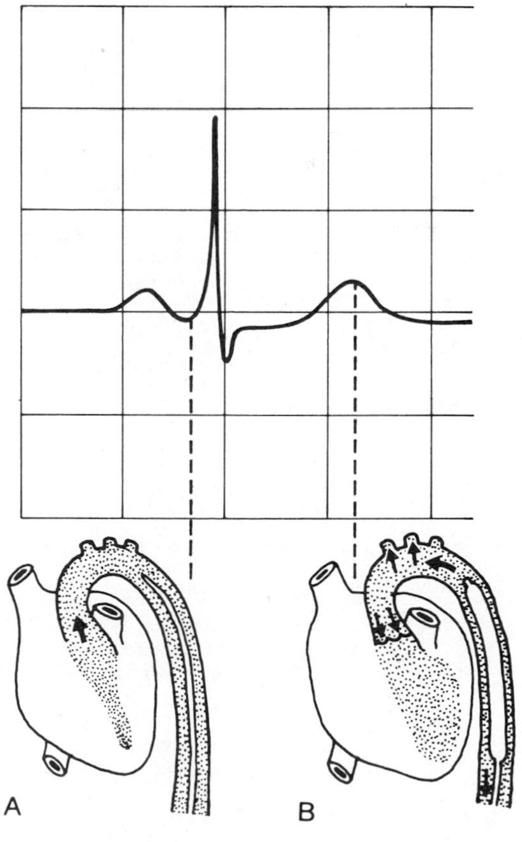

FIGURE 14–6. Schematic presentation of the ECG and mechanical sequence of balloon counterpulsation.

A. *Systole.* Deflation of the balloon coincides with the *R*-wave. The resulting decrease in aortic pressure reduces impedance to left ventricular ejection.

B. *Diastole.* The balloon inflates with closure of the aortic valve which corresponds to the crest of the *T*-wave on the ECG. Balloon inflation increases pressure in the aorta, thus increasing coronary and systemic perfusion.

it is recommended that the intra-aortic balloon pump be instituted early in the acute ischemic episode before severe, massive damage occurs. Indeed, the use of the intra-aortic balloon pump in the management of cardiogenic shock is most successful when applied early in acute unstable myocardial infarction, preferably before hemodynamic deterioration is apparent. In addition, it is felt that surgical correction of anatomic defects, such as ventricular septal rupture or coronary revascularization in conjunction with balloon pumping, offers the greatest long-term benefit for the patient.

Other Categories of Shock

Shock may also occur in association with a wide variety of physiologic abnormalities. For example, hypoglycemia and drug overdose are associated with a shocklike syndrome. It is well beyond the scope of this text to present a discussion of the numerous other causes of shock. In each, the precipitating event has to be identified and hemodynamic expression determined and then treated accordingly.

REFERENCES

1. Cohn JN: Blood pressure measurements in shock. *JAMA* 1967; 199:972–976.
2. Wilson RF: Shock. In *Principles and Techniques of Critical Care.* Vol. I. Kalamazoo, MI, The Upjohn Company, 1976, pp 26–27.
3. Weil MH: Principles of fluid challenge for routine treatment of shock. In Weil HM, Daluz PL (eds): *Critical Care Medicine Manual.* New York, Springer-Verlag, 1978.
4. Shock. In *Advanced Trauma Life Support.* The American College of Surgeons, 1981.
5. Gardner P, Provine HT: General management of the septic patient. In *Manual of Acute Bacterial Infections,* Ed. 2. Boston, Little, Brown, 1984, pp 170–173.
6. Glew RH, Blacklow NR: Approach to fever and use of antibiotics in the treatment of the intensive care patient. In Rippe JM, Irwin RS, Alpert JS (eds): *Intensive Care Medicine.* Boston, Little, Brown, 1985, pp 630–636.

SUGGESTED READING

General Reference

Abboud FM: Shock. In Wyngaarden JB, Smith LH (eds): *Textbook of Medicine*, Ed. 7. Philadelphia, WB Saunders, 1985.

Ayers SM, Giannelli S, Mueller HS: Shock. In *Care of the Critically Ill.* E. Norwalk, CT, Appleton-Century-Crofts, 1974.

Guyton AC: Circulatory shock and physiology of its treatment. In *Textbook of Medical Physiology*, Ed. 7. Philadelphia, WB Saunders, 1986.

Hale DJ, et al: Circulatory collapse in shock. In Dietzman RH, Lillehei RC: *Practice of Medicine.* Medical Dept Loose Leaf Service. Vol. 6, New York, Harper and Row, 1979, pp 1–21.

Rainey TG: Pharmacology of colloids and crystalloids. In Charnow B (ed): *The Pharmacologic Approach to the Critically Ill Patient.* Baltimore, Williams & Wilkins, 1983.

Rice V: Shock; A clinical syndrome. Parts I, II, III. *Crit Care Nurse,* March, April, May-June, July-August, 1981.

Shoemaker WB: Pathophysiology and therapy of shock syndromes. In Shoemaker WB, Thompson WL, Holbrook PR (eds): *Textbook of Critical Care,* Philadelphia, WB Saunders, 1984.

Sibband WJ: Shock. In Sibbald WJ (ed): *Synopsis of Critical Care,* ed. 2. Baltimore, Williams and Wilkins, 1984.

Virgilio RW: Assessment and therapy of the shock syndrome. In Sproul CW, Mullanney PJ (eds): *Emergency Care; Assessment and Intervention.* St. Louis, CV Mosby, 1974.

Weil MH: Proposed classification of shock states with special reference to distributive defects. In Hinshaw LB, Cox BG, (eds): *The Fundamental Mechanisms of Shock.* New York, Plenum Press, 1972.

Wilson RF: Shock. In *Principles and Techniques of Critical Care.* Vol. 1. Kalamazoo, MI, The Upjohn Company, 1976.

Hypovolemic Shock

Rackow ED, Falk JL, Fein A, et al: Fluid resuscitation in circulatory shock: A comparison of the cardiorespiratory effects of albumin, hetastarch, and saline solutions in patients with hypovolemic and septic shock. *Crit Care Med* 1983; 11:839.

Shamji FM, Todd TRJ: Hypovolemic Shock. In *Crit Care Clin* 1985; 1:609–629.

Walt AJ, Peltier LF, Pruitt BA, et al: Blood and fluid replacement in shock. In ACS Committee on Trauma: *Early Care of the Injured Patient,* ed. 3. Philadelphia, WB Saunders, 1982.

Zamora BO: Management of hemorrhagic shock. *Hosp Med* 1979; 15:6–29.

Septic Shock

Austin TW: Septicemia. In Sibbald WJ (ed): *Synopsis of Critical Care,* ed. 2. Baltimore, Williams and Wilkins, 1984.

Darovic GO: Septic shock. In Carolan JM (ed): *Shock, A Nursing Guide.* Oradell, NJ, Medical Economics Books, 1984.

Hinshaw L: Overview of endotoxin shock. In Cowley RA, Trumb BF (eds): *Pathophysiology of Shock, Anoxia and Ischemia.* Baltimore, Williams and Wilkins, 1982.

Jacoby I: Septic shock. In Rippe JM, Irwin RS, Alpert JS, et al: *Intensive Care Medicine.* Boston, Little, Brown, 1985.

McCabe WR: Gram negative bacteremia. *Adv Intern Med* 1974; 19:135–158.

Parrillo JE: Septic shock; Clinical manifestations, pathogenesis, hemodynamics and management in a critical care unit. In Parillo JE, Ayres Sm (eds): *Major Issues in Critical Care Medicine.* Baltimore, Williams and Wilkins, 1984.

Rice V: The clinical continuum of septic shock. *Crit Care Nurse* Sept/Oct, 1984.

Robinson JA, Klondnycky ML, Loeb HS, et al: Endotoxin, prekallikrein, complement and systemic vascular resistance. *Amer J Med* 1975; 59:61–67.

Sheagren JN: Shock syndromes related to sepsis. In Wyngaarden JG, Smith LH (eds): *Textbook of Medicine,* ed. 17. Philadelphia, WB Saunders, 1985.

Wilson RF, Thal AP, Kindling PH, et al: Hemodynamic measurements in septic shock. *Arch Surg* 1965; 91:121–129.

Anaphylactic Shock

Giansiracusa DF, Upchurch KS: Anaphylactic and anaphylactoid reactions. In Rippe JM, Irwin RS, Alpert JS, et al (eds): *Intensive Care Medicine.* Boston, Little, Brown, 1985.

Haupt MT, Carlson RW: Anaphylactic and anaphylactoid reactions. In Shoemaker WB, Thompson WL, Holbrook PR (eds): Philadelphia, WB Saunders, 1984.

Lichtenstein LM: Anaphylaxis. In Wyngaarden JB, Smith LH (eds): *Textbook of Medicine.* Philadelphia, WB Saunders, 1985.

Neurogenic Shock

Albin MS: Acute cervical spinal injury. *Crit Care Clin* 1985; 1:267–284.

Franco LM: Neurogenic shock. In Carolan JM (ed): *Shock; A Nursing Guide.* Oradell, NJ, Medical Economics Books, 1984.

Tyson GS: Acute care of the spinal-cord injured patient. *Critical Care Quarterly*, 1979.

Cardiogenic Shock

Balooki H: *Clinical Application of Intra-Aortic Balloon Pump,* ed. 2. New York, Futura Publishing, 1984.

Chatterjee K: Myocardial Infarction Shock. *Crit Care Clin* 1985; 1:563–590.

Cohn JN: Recognition and management of shock and acute pump failure. In Hurst JW: *The Heart*, ed. 5. New York, McGraw-Hill, 1982.

Donut WE, Weiner BH: Syndromes of left ventricular failure. In Rippe JM, Irwin RS, Alpert JS, et al (eds): *Intensive Care Medicine.* Boston, Little, Brown, 1985.

Mueller HS: Cardiogenic shock. In Parillo JE, Ayres SM (eds): *Major Issues in Critical Care Medicine.* Baltimore, Williams and Wilkins, 1984.

Quall SJ: *Comprehensive Intra-Aortic Balloon Pumping.* St. Louis, CV Mosby, 1984.

Sobel BE: Cardiac and noncardiac forms of acute circulatory failure (shock). In Braunwald E (ed): *Heart Disease, A Textbook of Cardiovascular Medicine.* Philadelphia, WB Saunders, 1984.

Monitoring the Patient with Pulmonary Disease

15

The only functions of the respiratory system are to transfer oxygen from the atmosphere to blood and then to cells, and to transfer carbon dioxide from cells to blood to atmosphere. The system fails when these functions are not performed adequately to meet the metabolic needs of the body. Clinically, this may be defined by a PaO_2 of less than 50 mm Hg and a $PaCO_2$ of greater than 50 mm Hg while the patient is at rest and breathing room air at sea level. Although both abnormalities in blood gases have deleterious physiologic effects, they may be the "steady state" in a patient with chronic pulmonary disease. In these patients, acute respiratory failure is defined as an abrupt deterioration in the previous steady state.

Acute respiratory failure is one of the most common life-threatening problems in hospitals and is present in the majority of ICU patients. It may occur as a primary disorder or may complicate other disease conditions.

Some forms of respiratory failure are associated with destruction or obstruction of the pulmonary vascular bed. Owing to the large capacity and distensibility of the pulmonary vessels, an increase in pulmonary vascular resistance (reflected in increased pulmonary artery systolic and diastolic pressure) typically does not occur until the cross-sectional area of the pulmonary vascular bed is reduced by more than 50 per cent. Hypoxemia and acidemia frequently accompany respiratory failure and have potent constrictor effects on the pulmonary vasculature (see Pulmonary Blood Flows and Pressures in Chapter 2), which also increases pulmonary artery pressure.

A normal right ventricle is able to eject adequately into the pulmonary circulation until the mean pulmonary artery pressure exceeds 35 to 45 mm Hg. Beyond this point, the right ventricle is acutely unable to generate a systolic pressure sufficient to provide adequate forward flow to the pulmonary circuit and left ventricle. Thus, left ventricular filling volume falls and left ventricular performance is likewise reduced by the Starling effect. Stroke volume decreases as ventricular end-diastolic volume falls, and vice versa. Further, as a result of an enlarged right ventricular filling volume, the ventricular septum may bulge toward the left ventricle, altering its normal internal shape (Fig. 15–1). This change in intraventricular geometry may additionally compromise left ventricular performance and alter the normal left ventricular filling volume/pressure relationship. Therefore, acute

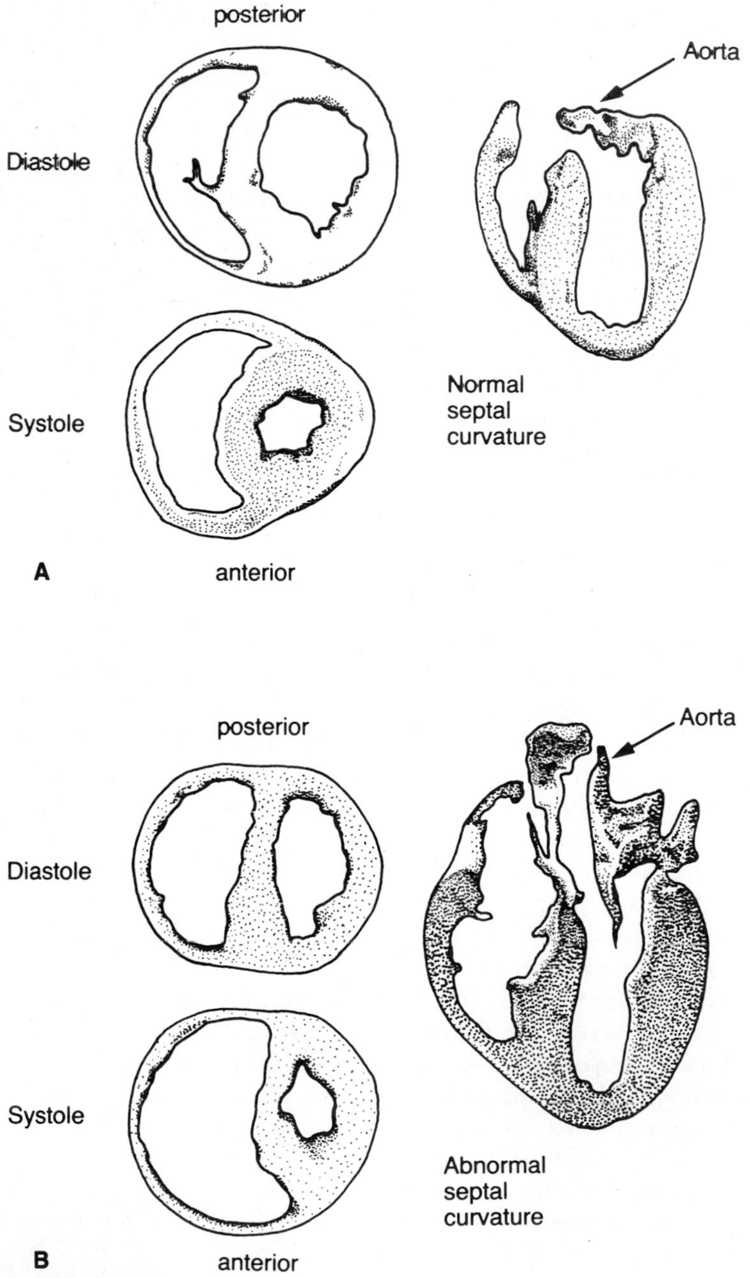

FIGURE 15–1. *A.* The normal septal curvature in the cross-sectional and longitudinal views in systole and diastole. The intraventricular septum is normally curved toward the right ventricle. *B.* With distention of the failing right ventricle, the septum is deviated toward the left ventricle and may additionally encroach on the left ventricular outflow tract. (Adapted from Weber KT, Janicki JS, Shroff SG, et al: The cardiopulmonary unit. The body's gas transport system. *Clin Chest Med* 1983; 4:101–110.)

changes in the pulmonary vessels induced by hypoxemia, acidemia, or obstruction may have profoundly adverse effects on cardiovascular function and hemodynamics. This defines cor pulmonale (pulmonary heart disease), which is cardiac dysfunction or structural change that results from pulmonary hypertension caused by disease of the lung.

The gradual increase in pulmonary artery pressure seen in chronic disease is accompanied by a corresponding increase in right ventricular size. Under these circumstances, the gradually stressed and hypertrophied right ventricle may be capable of increasing systolic pressure to levels as high as 70 to 90 mm Hg to force blood through the chronically altered pulmonary circulation (chronic cor pulmonale). Given any additional hemodynamic burden, such as acute pulmonary embolism or pulmonary infection, however, the right ventricle may suddenly fail.

Causes of acute respiratory failure commonly seen in the acute care setting are discussed in this chapter. Although the inciting events may differ, the aforementioned principles relating to cor pulmonale apply to all.

PULMONARY EMBOLISM

A pulmonary embolism is a plug that has impacted in the pulmonary circulation. The occlusive plug may be a tumor, air, amniotic fluid, a septic or fat embolism, or a foreign body such as a broken portion of a vascular catheter. More than 90% of pulmonary emboli are blood clots that originate in the deep veins of the iliofemoral system or the legs.

A *massive pulmonary embolism* involves the main pulmonary trunk, the right or left main pulmonary artery, or two or more lobar branches. The term *submassive pulmonary embolism* relates to circumstances involving lesser degrees of vascular obstruction.

Incidence

Pulmonary embolism is perhaps the most common pulmonary complication in hospitalized patients and the most commonly undiagnosed serious acute illness. It is estimated to be the third most common cause of death in the United States; in many cases the correct cause of death is ascertained on the autopsy table. The estimated annual incidence of pulmonary embolism in the United States is approximately 630,000. Of these patients, approximately 11% die within the first hour. Of the initial survivors, an estimated 71% are not correctly diagnosed, and of these, 30% die. Of the 29% initial survivors who are correctly diagnosed, only 8% die.[1] This underscores the importance of early and correct diagnosis and appropriate therapy.

Evidence suggests that the incidence of pulmonary embolism is increasing. The proposed reasons for the apparent increase are a generally larger and sicker patient population, prolongation of life in patients with metastatic disease, greater use of oral contraceptives, a larger elderly population, and an increased recognition of pulmonary embolism.

Predisposing Factors

Over a hundred years ago, Virchow delineated the following three most important factors that favor clot formation and predispose to pulmonary embolism.

1. Alterations or damage to the vascular lining activates the coagulation cascade. This occurs following venipuncture or distention of or trauma to a vein, and in association with inflammatory vascular disease, atherosclerosis, and varicose veins.

2. Venous stasis delays the removal of activated clotting factors from the veins in which clots are formed. Venous stasis is commonly associated with bed rest or sitting for long periods of time, obesity, congestive heart failure, shock states, dehydration, and hypovolemia. Fibrillating atria may also contain clots.

3. Hypercoagulability is linked with pregnancy, carcinoma, fever, the use of oral estrogens, polycythemia vera, and postoperative and trauma states.

Once formed, the clot may experience several fates. It may be lysed by the proteolytic activity of the fibrinolytic system; scar tissue may infiltrate the clot which then becomes a part of vessel wall (organized); or the clot may fragment or become dislodged by sudden changes in venous pressure associated with standing, walking, a Valsalva maneuver, and so on. Once dislodged, the clot then travels up the vena cava, through the right heart, and impacts in the pulmonary circulation.

Pathophysiology

Once the clot becomes dislodged, it reaches the lungs in seconds. A cessation of blood flow to the lung distal to the occlusion causes both pulmonary and hemodynamic abnormalities.

Pulmonary Abnormalities

Since ventilated nonperfused lung cannot participate in gas exchange (increased alveolar dead space volume), any ventilation of the involved lung segment is wasted. In addition, the involved area of lung constricts owing to local abnormalities in alveolar gas tensions and local release of biochemical agents (serotonin, histamine) from the lung itself. A significant local surfactant deficiency and resulting atelectasis occur within 24 hours of embolization, which furthers local lung shrinkage. Fewer than 10% of pulmonary emboli cause pulmonary infarction because of the dual (bronchial and pulmonary arterial) vascular supply to the lung tissue. Pulmonary infarction is characterized by necrosis of alveolar walls and an inflammatory response. On chest radiograph this is seen as a localized infiltrate.

Hemodynamic Abnormalities

Occlusion of a portion of the pulmonary circulation results in a decrease in the cross-sectional area of the pulmonary arterial bed. A greater than 50% reduction in the size of this vascular bed requires an increase in pulmonary artery pressure to maintain blood flow through the pulmonary circulation. This increase in pulmonary artery pressure is termed precapillary hypertension since it is associated with a normal pulmonary capillary hydrostatic pressure (as estimated clinically by PWP). The increase in pulmonary artery pressure increases the work load and oxygen consumption of the right ventricle. The thin-walled right ventricle is not anatomically or physiologically designed to accept heavy pressure loads and is unable to maintain pulmonary blood flow and left ventricular filling when acutely presented with a mean pressure demand greater than 35 to 45 mm Hg. As a consequence of right ventricular failure, cardiac output falls and right atrial and right ventricular end-diastolic pressures increase.

Overall, the hemodynamic derangements and pathophysiologic consequences depend on the degree of obstruction, the rate of obstruction, and the preexisting cardiovascular and pulmonary status of the individual. Given these variables, it is not surprising that pulmonary embolism does not present with a classic constellation of symptoms or signs and consistent laboratory findings. Indeed, the clinical presentation and laboratory values are very inconsistent and often mimic other cardiopulmonary disorders. A high index of suspicion in a patient with risk factors is essential for early recognition and appropriate management.

Hemodynamic Profile

Arterial Pressure. In most cases, there is no change from the patient's normal values (Table 15–1). Hypotension, with a systolic pressure less than 100 mm Hg, occurs in less than 3% of patients and relates to impaired left ventricular filling and decreased cardiac output secondary to a massive pulmonary embolism. When hypotension is present, however, it appears that the decrease in systemic arterial pressure is greater than what would be expected for the level of fall in cardiac output. This exaggerated fall in arterial pressure may be due to impaired baroreceptor reflexes; the cause for this impaired vascular reflex response is not known. With massive pulmonary embolism, the pulse pressure is likely to be narrowed, giving the arterial pressure waveform a damped appearance.

Systemic Vascular Resistance. With submassive pulmonary embolism, this value is likely to be in the normal range. Systemic vascular resistance

TABLE 15–1. General Anticipated Direction of Change in Hemodynamic Parameters in Pulmonary Disorders

Disorder	*Arterial Pressure*	*Pulse Pressure*	*Systemic Vascular Resistance*	*Pulmonary Vascular Resistance*	*Central Venous Pressure*	*Pulmonary Artery Pressure*	*P.A. Wedge Pressure*	*Cardiac Output*	S_vO_2
Chronic obstructive pulmonary disease (COPD)	~	~	~↓	↑	~↑	↑	~	~	↓
Massive pulmonary embolism	~↓	~↓	~↑	↑	↑	↑	~↓	~↓	↓
High-pressure (cardiogenic) pulmonary edema	↑	~↓	↑	↑	~↑	↑	↑	↓	↓
Adult respiratory distress syndrome (ARDS)									
Stage 1—Injury	Specific to type of injury								
Stage 2—Latent period	~	~	~	~	~	~	~	~	~↓
Stage 3—Respiratory failure	~	~	~↓	~↑	~	~↑	~	~	↓
Stage 4—Severe respiratory distress (preterminal)	~	~	~↓	↑	~↑	↑	~	~↓	↓

KEY: ↑, increase; ↓, decrease; ~, no change.
NOTE: The magnitude or direction of change can be modified by coexisting factors or complications (hypovolemia, fluid overload, severity of the primary problem, adequacy of compensatory mechanisms).

will be increased with perfusion failure accompanying massive pulmonary embolism.

Pulmonary Vascular Resistance. The increase in pulmonary vascular resistance is proportional to the amount of obstruction and consequent decrease in the cross-sectional area of the pulmonary arterial bed.

CVP or RA Pressure. There is no change from the patient's normal values with submassive pulmonary embolism. Elevation of the right atrial pressure and CVP is seen in massive pulmonary embolism and reflects right ventricular failure. The right atrial waveform may be altered with increased amplitude of the *a* wave, which reflects increased resistance to filling of the failing right ventricle during atrial systole (Fig. 15–2).

Pulmonary Artery and Wedge Pressure. An increase in pulmonary artery systolic and diastolic pressure occurs with massive pulmonary embolism. The PWP may be in the normal range or decreased due to impaired left ventricular filling; therefore, the pulmonary artery diastolic to wedge pressure (PAd-PWP) gradient increases (Fig. 15–3).

Preexisting cardiopulmonary disease, however, may confuse the hemodynamic diagnosis since preexisting pulmonary disease may have caused abnormalities in pulmonary artery pressure (COPD, pulmonary fibrosis), and coexisting left heart dysfunction will elevate the pulmonary artery as well as

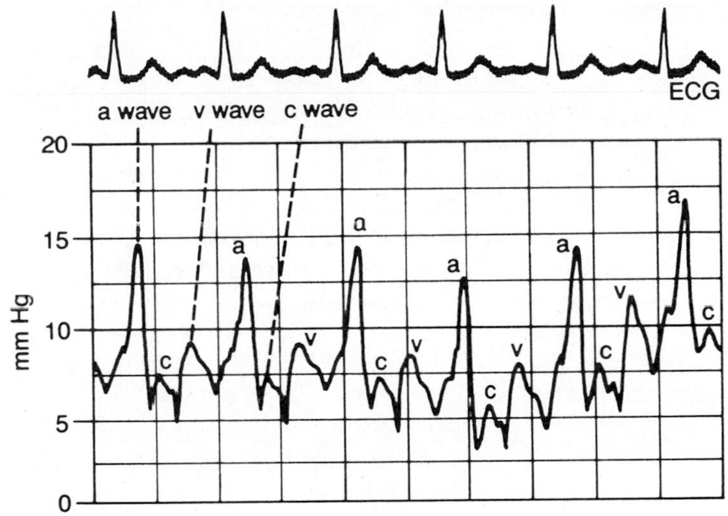

FIGURE 15–2. A right atrial pressure tracing taken from a patient with a massive pulmonary embolism. Note the increased amplitude *a* waves.

wedge pressures. The contour of the waveforms is unchanged, although in severe cases a pulmonary artery pulsus alternans may be noted, which reflects severe right ventricular dysfunction.

Cardiac Output. A decrease in cardiac output accompanies massive occlusion of the pulmonary arterial circulation.

Mixed Venous Oxygen Saturation (SvO_2). This value is decreased if perfusion failure or hypoxemia or both complicates pulmonary embolism.

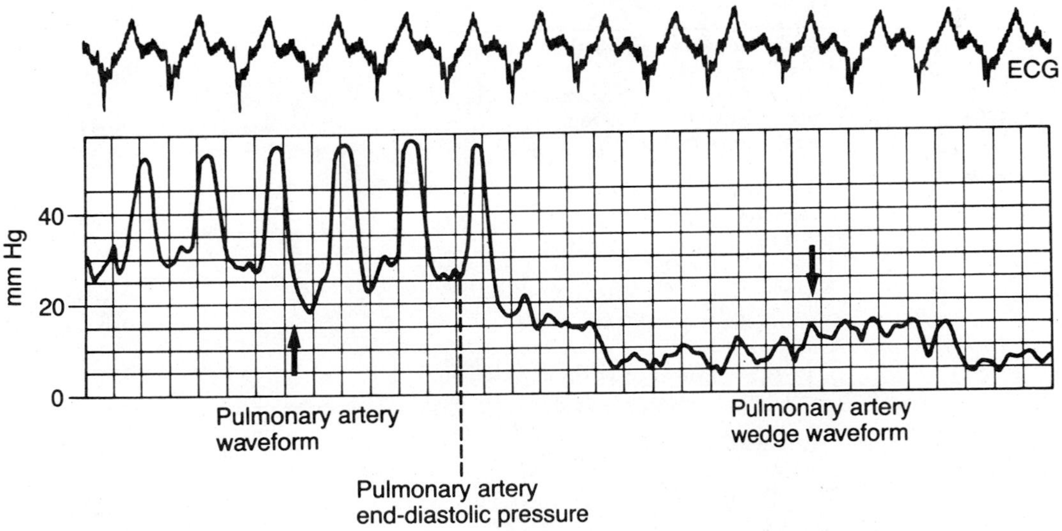

FIGURE 15–3. Pulmonary hypertension secondary to a massive pulmonary embolism. Note the increased pulmonary artery diastolic to wedge pressure (PAd-PWP) gradient.

Clinical Presentation

The findings in Table 15–2 support the statement that no single sign or symptom complex is diagnostic of pulmonary embolism. The signs and symptoms are also commonly associated with other cardiopulmonary diseases; therefore, pulmonary embolism commonly masquerades as and can be mistaken for other disorders.

Palpation of the Precordium. A right ventricular thrust may be present over the left sternal border and suggests massive pulmonary embolism with pulmonary hypertension.

Laboratory Studies

There is no specific diagnostic test for pulmonary embolism. The following tests may be helpful but most are nonspecific. Associated abnormalities may produce positive results not related to pulmonary embolism, and all may be negative in the presence of pulmonary embolism.

ECG. The ECG may be completely normal or there may be only nonspecific ST-T wave abnormalities. The effects of a massive pulmonary embolism on the right heart are manifest as the sudden development of an S-wave in Standard Lead I, a Q-wave in Standard Lead III, and an inverted T-wave in Standard Lead III (SI, Q3, T3) (Fig. 15–4). The sudden onset of complete or

TABLE 15–2. Frequency of Signs and Symptoms in 327 Patients with Documented Pulmonary Embolism

Signs	*Per Cent*
Respiratory rate greater than 16/min	92
Rales (crackles)	58
Increased pulmonic component of the second heart sound (S2)	53
Pulse greater than 100/min	44
Temperature greater than 37.8 C	43
Phlebitis	32
Gallop rhythm	34
Diaphoresis	36
Edema	24
Heart murmur	23
Cyanosis	19
Symptoms	***Per Cent***
Chest pain	88
Pleuritic (typically, sharp and stabbing)	74
Nonpleuritic (substernal, may mimic MI)	14
Dyspnea	84
Apprehension	59
Cough	53
Hemoptysis	30
Sweats	27
Syncope	13

(From Bell WR, Simon TL, Demetes DL: The clinical features of submassive and massive pulmonary emboli. *Am J Med* 1977; 62:358.)

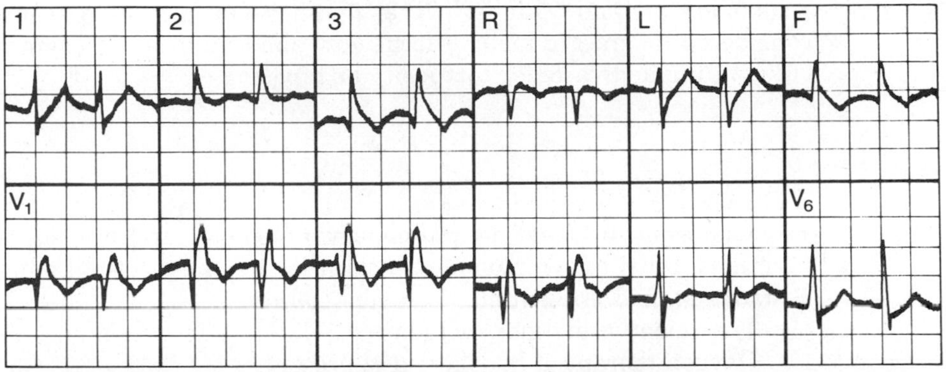

FIGURE 15–4. Acute cor pulmonale from a patient with massive pulmonary embolism. Note the T-wave inversion in the inferior (III, aVF) and anteroseptal leads (V1-4), the S wave in Lead I, the Q wave in Lead III, and right bundle branch block. (From Marriott HJL: *Practical Electrocardiography,* ed 7. Baltimore, Williams & Wilkins Co., 1983, p 459.)

incomplete bundle branch block or supraventricular or ventricular arrhythmias should raise the index of suspicion of pulmonary embolism in patients who are prone.

Chest Radiographs. X-ray abnormalities may vary considerably. The chest film may be completely normal. Important changes to look for include elevation of the hemidiaphragm on the affected side, unexplained densities, pleural effusion, a dilated central pulmonary artery, abrupt cutoff of a pulmonary artery, or locally decreased vascular markings.

Lung Perfusion Scan. False-positive scans may occur if there are other causes for perfusion defects such as blebs, tumors, pneumonia, or redistribution of pulmonary blood flow due to congestive heart failure. A completely normal perfusion scan rules out pulmonary embolism.

Ventilation Scan. The ventilation scan may increase specificity to the perfusion scan. Patients with pulmonary embolism usually have normal ventilation in areas of perfusion defects; however, total occlusion of a pulmonary vessel may, with time, result in destruction of the alveoli. Therefore, ventilation as well as perfusion defects may be present.

Serum Enzymes. Serum lactic dehydrogenase (LDH), serum glutamic-oxaloacetic transaminase (SGOT), and bilirubin values are neither specific nor sensitive. Serum enzymes may all be abnormal, all normal, or variably abnormal.

Blood Gases. Approximately 11% of patients with documented pulmonary embolism have a PaO_2 above 80 mm Hg; none have a PaO_2 greater than 90 mm Hg while breathing room air. The PaO_2 is less than 60 mm Hg in approximately 50% of documented pulmonary embolism cases. Hypocapnia and respiratory alkalosis are present secondary to the hyperventilation that accompanies this disorder.

Pulmonary Angiography. This is the definitive and most reliable study, but it too has pitfalls. It should be performed within 24 to 72 hours of the suspected event; otherwise, resolution of the clot may occur and yield a false-negative study. Positive findings include intraluminal “filling defects” and pulmonary arterial "cutoffs." Other findings that may be present but are not considered diagnostic include focal flow abnormalities or asymmetrical vascular filling and vascular tortuosity or tapering.

Treatment

The goals in treating pulmonary embolism are the support of vital functions, relief of symptoms, reduction in the extent of pulmonary vascular obstruction, and prevention of reembolization.

Treatment guidelines include:

Oxygen therapy if hypoxemia is present.

Prompt anticoagulation with heparin. Heparin does not directly lyse the clot or clots but interferes with coagulation at several steps in the coagulation cascade, thus preventing more clot formation or distal extension of the existing clots. Heparin is given IV to a usual total of 25,000 to 30,000 units per 24 hours by continuous IV infusion or by intermittent bolus for 7 to 10 days. The PTT should be maintained at 1½ to 2½ times the pretreatment value, assuming this value was previously normal.

Bed rest is instituted and the patient is instructed against any activity, such as a Valsalva maneuver, that would produce sudden changes in venous pressure. Bed rest is maintained for approximately 7 to 10 days or until it is felt that any existing deep venous thrombi are dissolved by the fibrinolytic system.

Vasopressor therapy may be used in patients with severe circulatory failure.

Sedative or analgesic agents, such as morphine sulfate or meperidine (Demerol), are administered to relieve pain and apprehension. Sedative agents and narcotic analgesia should be administered very cautiously to patients with preexisting pulmonary disease.

Fluid therapy may be indicated in shock to restore left ventricular filling pressure to a level sufficient to maintain systemic perfusion.

Thrombolytic therapy accelerates lysis of clots, whereas traditional heparin therapy only prevents extension of preexisting clots or more thrombus formation. Therefore, these drugs alleviate the acute, severe hemodynamic derangements associated with involvement of more than 50% of the pulmonary circulation, such as pulmonary hypertension and right heart failure. The risk of bleeding associated with the use of these agents outweighs the benefit in the majority of patients with pulmonary embolism. Most commonly used is streptokinase; a dose of 250,000 units is administered IV over 30 minutes, followed by 100,000 units per hour for the next 24 hours for pulmonary embolism and 72 hours for deep venous thrombosis.

Minimize stress for the patient because stress is associated with increased platelet adhesiveness, which may exacerbate or produce a hypercoagulable state. Stress is also known to predispose to various other physiologic abnormalities (arrhythmias, hypertension) all of which may worsen the clinical and hemodynamic picture.

CHRONIC OBSTRUCTIVE PULMONARY DISEASE (COPD)

Chronic obstructive pulmonary disease is a catchall term used to describe a varying combination of pulmonary diseases in a given patient including:

—Chronic bronchitis, defined as sputum production on most days of the week for at least three months of the year for two or more consecutive years. It is characterized by increased mucus production and inflammatory swelling of the bronchial air passages.

—Emphysema, a condition characterized by destructive changes of the alveolar walls leading to a reduced number and enlarged size of air spaces distal to the terminal bronchioles. These changes result in a reduction in the surface area of the alveolar-capillary membrane and loss of the natural recoil property of the lung.

—Asthma, defined as increased reactivity of the airways to numerous stimuli such as pollens, dust, exercise, strong-smelling perfumes, cigarette smoke, and so on. Hyperreactivity of the airways is manifest as increased mucus production, bronchial mucosal swelling, and bronchial smooth muscle contraction.

Chronic bronchitis and emphysema nearly always coexist in varying degrees. Episodic asthma commonly complicates the clinical picture.

Causes

Both chronic bronchitis and emphysema are closely linked to cigarette smoking or inhaled pollutants or both, although individual susceptibility to these risk factors is variable. In some persons, a genetically acquired deficiency of serum antiproteolytic activity (alpha$_1$-antitrypsin deficiency) is associated with an increased incidence of COPD even in the absence of identifiable risk factors.

Pathophysiology

COPD is characterized by airflow obstruction due to airway narrowing caused by bronchial smooth muscle spasm, airway mucosal edema, and the accumulation of mucus. Poorly ventilated alveoli either fail to be efficient gas-exchanging units or shrink and collapse and do not participate in gas exchange at all. In addition, because of loss of the elastic recoil property of the lung (emphysema), expiration becomes a forced effort that further favors small airway collapse and promotes air trapping and hyperinflation in the distal alveoli. Impaired alveolar ventilation (impaired delivery of oxygen to alveoli and removal of carbon dioxide) is reflected in arterial hypoxemia and hypercapnia. Secondary to pulmonary vasoconstriction induced by hypoxemia, pulmonary artery systolic and diastolic pressures rise. Through hypertrophic adaptation to the increased pressure load, the right ventricle may maintain a compensated cardiovascular status. However, acute respiratory failure in COPD of any cause may suddenly confront the right ventricle with a pressure load beyond its work capacity, and signs and symptoms of right ventricular failure (acute cor pulmonale) ensue.

Causes of Acute Respiratory Failure in COPD

Most instances of acute respiratory failure have an acute precipitating factor. The natural progression of the disease may reach an end point with a clinical presentation identical to that of acute respiratory failure. Acute precipitating events include:

Infection. This accounts for approximately 55% of cases of acute respiratory failure. The patient typically complains of increasing dyspnea and cough with purulent sputum production. Fever may or may not be present.

Left Ventricular Failure. Left ventricular failure worsens pulmonary function by increasing pulmonary vascular blood volume. The subsequent increase in pulmonary capillary hydrostatic pressure (measured by PWP) favors the development of pulmonary edema, which then worsens pulmonary gas exchange. Unfortunately, elderly patients in the COPD age group commonly have hypertensive, valvular, or ischemic heart disease, all of which may produce pulmonary edema. The clinical diagnosis is made difficult because the usual signs of pulmonary edema (tachypnea, dyspnea, crackles, and wheezes) are commonly always present with COPD. In addition, the sound of a gallop rhythm may be completely swamped by noisy breath sounds.

Acute Pulmonary Embolism. This is a very common complication in patients with COPD owing to the chronic presence of risk factors such as immobility, increased blood viscosity, and coexisting heart failure. COPD patients showing sudden worsening of symptoms or hypoxia with a slight fall rather than rise in $PaCO_2$ should be suspected of having acute pulmonary embolism.

With the passage of time, the showers of pulmonary emboli take their toll as more of the pulmonary circulation is lost, thus worsening pulmonary hypertension and its resultant cor pulmonale.

Injudicious Use of Narcotic or Sedative Agents. These agents blunt the ventilatory drive. Because the COPD patient at peak function may barely be able to maintain marginal arterial oxygenation and carbon dioxide elimination, the administration of drugs that blunt the ventilatory drive risks a severely decompensated state.

Surgery or Trauma about the Chest or Abdomen. This causes pain, which limits ventilatory movements and may result in a deterioration in blood gases.

Total Parenteral Nutrition. TPN normally delivers a large carbohydrate load to the patient. The end products of carbohydrate metabolism are water, energy, and carbon dioxide. The COPD patient is unable to increase ventilation commensurate with increased carbon dioxide production, and the normally elevated steady state $PaCO_2$ may rise further to reach intolerable levels.

Injudicious Use of Oxygen in the Spontaneously Breathing Patient. This practice may raise the PaO_2 above a critical level and may eliminate the hypoxic drive to breathe. Ventilation is normally stimulated more efficiently by hypercapnia than by hypoxia in the healthy person. Because of a chronically elevated $PaCO_2$, the chemoreceptors of the COPD patient become insensitive to carbon dioxide, and the primary drive to breathe is hypoxemia. Correction of hypoxemia eliminates the only stimulus to breathe; carbon dioxide levels continue to rise, with consequent central nervous system depression that may end in stupor or coma.

Hemodynamic Profile

Arterial Pressure. Systemic arterial pressure is not significantly affected by COPD (see Table 15–1).

Systemic Vascular Resistance. This value may be slightly decreased relative to the degree of hypoxemic and hypercapnic vasodilation associated with the patient's condition.

Pulmonary Vascular Resistance. This parameter is typically increased to a level proportionate to the degree of hypoxemia, acidemia, and anatomic distortion of the pulmonary circulation, ie, pulmonary emboli.

CVP or Right Atrial Pressure. These parameters remain within the normal range if the hypertrophied right ventricle remains compensated. With the development of right ventricular failure (hypertrophy and dilatation), CVP and right atrial pressures rise. A prominent *a* wave in the right atrial tracing may be present and is produced when the right atrium contracts and encounters resistance to filling within the cavity of the noncompliant or failing right ventricle. The *x* descent, which occurs with right atrial relaxation, becomes brisker and more conspicuous.

Pulmonary Artery and Wedge Pressure. Pulmonary artery systolic and diastolic pressures increase relative to the level of hypoxemia, hypercapnia, and pulmonary vascular changes. If the patient has had multiple pulmonary emboli, pulmonary artery pressures may reach systemic levels. In addition, any factor that increases cardiac output (fever, catecholamines, shivering, seizure activity, or exercise) results in further increases in pulmonary artery pressure because the increased pulmonary blood flow cannot be accommodated by the constricted or damaged pulmonary vascular bed. The left heart pressures, as reflected by PWP, are normal unless there is associated left heart disease. Therefore, the pulmonary artery diastolic pressure no longer reflects the left atrial or left ventricular end-diastolic pressure, but the PWP does. The increased pulmonary artery diastolic to wedge pressure (PAd-PWP) gradient is the result of blood gas or anatomic changes in the pulmonary vessels that increase resistance to run-off of blood through the pulmonary circulation in diastole. In the pulmonary artery wedged position there is no run-off of blood distal to the catheter tip, and the PWP–left atrial pressure relationship remains close. Obtaining an accurate PWP reading, however, may be difficult due to the positive intrathoracic pressures induced by pursed-lip breathing or forced expiration typically seen in patients with COPD. In this context, certainty of the accuracy of the PWP may be impossible; therefore, sequential readings with analysis of trends coupled with observed changes in clinical status are necessary.

Cardiac Output. This value usually is near normal at rest unless there is associated heart disease.

Mixed Venous Oxygen Saturation (SvO_2). This parameter is typically decreased proportionate to the level of arterial hypoxemia, heart failure, or both.

Clinical Presentation

Clinical findings are quite variable and depend on the stage of the disease, the amount of bronchitic and emphysematous involvement, the presence or absence of heart failure, and the presence of complicating factors such as infection.

Mentation. In uncomplicated COPD, the level of mentation is unremarkable. The patient may exhibit personality characteristics such as irritability, manipulative dependent behavior, and so on that not uncommonly accompany chronic, debilitating illness. Acute changes in cerebral function, such as lethargy, slurred speech, confusion, and emotional instability, accompany the sudden deterioration in blood gases associated with acute respiratory failure.

Cutaneous. Hypoxemia, coupled with elevated hemoglobin and hematocrit values, results in a significant amount of desaturated hemoglobin in the capillaries, and central cyanosis is evident.

Heart Rate and Character of Pulse. Tachycardia is frequently present due to hypoxemia and hypercapnia, and the pulse tends to be strong.

Heart Sounds. An early sign of pulmonary hypertension is an accentuation of the pulmonic component of the second heart sound, which may also be palpable. A high-pitched systolic ejection click from accentuated right ventricular ejection vibrations may be heard over the pulmonic area, and a right-sided S_3, best heard near the lower left sternal border or in the epigastrium, relates to right ventricular failure. It may be difficult to hear the heart sounds because of the damping effect of air in the hyperinflated lungs on the sounds or presence of adventitious breath sounds.

Palpation of the Precordium. The apex beat very likely will be difficult to palpate because of the increased anterior-posterior dimensions of the thorax (barrel chest), characteristic of emphysema.

Neck Veins. If right heart failure complicates the clinical picture, venous distention and dependent edema are noted and, if severe, are associated with an enlarged, pulsatile liver.

Respiratory Rate and Character of Breathing. The respiratory rate is typically greater than normal. Labored breathing, commonly through pursed lips, may be present only with exertion but in advanced stages of COPD is present even at rest. The patient much prefers a sitting position, bent forward, and commonly utilizes the accessory muscles of ventilation.

Lung Sounds. Crackles and wheezes are commonly heard diffusely over both lung fields.

Acid/Base. Patients with pure emphysema tend to hyperventilate and maintain near-normal arterial oxygen tensions—hence the name "pink puffers." Pure bronchitic patients have a decreased arterial oxygenation and increased $PaCO_2$ and may also have right heart failure and generalized edema secondary to hypoxemia-induced pulmonary hypertension—hence the name "blue bloaters." The pulmonary hypertension and cor pulmonale in COPD are closely related to the severity of the hypoxemia and become apparent when the resting PaO_2 falls below 45 mm Hg. The great majority of patients with COPD have varying components of emphysema and bronchitis.

Laboratory Studies

ECG. Low QRS voltage is a common finding. In the presence of cor pulmonale, there is commonly evidence of right ventricular hypertrophy, with prominent R-waves in the anterior precordial leads and deep S-waves in the left precordial leads. Atrial arrhythmias are common and ventricular arrhythmias may be observed in severely hypoxic patients.

Chest Radiographs. Changes develop late. Overinflation of the lungs (hyperlucent lungs), with flattening of the hemidiaphragms and widening of the intercostal spaces, is noted in advanced disease. Enlargement of the pulmonary artery trunk and main branches, associated with attenuation of the peripheral branches, relates to the development of pulmonary hypertension. Radiographic enlargement of the right ventricle becomes evident only after considerable dilation has occurred.

Hematology. Chronic hypoxemia is associated with a compensatory increase in the red blood cell count and hemoglobin concentration.

Treatment

Therapy is directed at treatment or prevention of infection, improvement in airflow, control of correctable components of the disease (hypoxemia, hypercapnia, and cardiovascular problems) and avoidance of factors that may worsen the condition, such as cigarette smoking and sedatives. The following directives are specific for care in the acute care setting:

Improvement in Arterial Oxygenation. This serves two important goals: improving tissue oxygenation and reducing pulmonary hypertension. Indeed, the pulmonary artery pressures may become nearly normal by improvement in the blood oxygen content. Right ventricular hypertrophy may be stabilized or actually reversed. In addition, improvement in arterial oxygenation decreases hypoxemia-related bronchoconstriction, which then favors improved alveolar ventilation. Thus, frequent blood gas values should be determined and vigorous therapeutic attempts made to correct abnormalities. Generally, patients do best if their arterial PaO_2 is 55 to 60 mm Hg. Because an improvement in arterial PaO_2 may blunt the patient's hypoxemic ventilatory drive, a rise in $PaCO_2$ may occur with oxygen administration. This is not ground for alarm as long as the patient remains lucid, is easily arousable, and does not develop a pH less than 7.25.

Improvement in Airflow. Measures that promote meticulous bronchial hygiene such as percussion, coughing, and suctioning are indicated. Further improvement in airflow may necessitate the use of corticosteroids to reduce airway inflammation and edema. Inhaled sympathomimetic bronchodilators such as metaproterenol (*Alupent, Metaprel*), isoetharine (*Bronchosol*), and terbutaline (*Brethine, Bricanyl*) are commonly used and have selective action on the bronchial tree, termed beta-2 activity. This is a distinct advantage to the older, nonselective bronchodilators such as epinephrine (*Adrenalin*) and isoproterenol (*Isuprel*), which also have cardiovascular stimulant effects, termed beta-1 activity. These may be particularly harmful when used in patients with ischemic heart disease, often present in this elderly patient population.

Intravenous theophylline (aminophylline) is also a useful drug in COPD. In addition to its effect on the airways, it improves right ventricular performance, increases mucociliary clearance, renders the diaphragm less susceptible to fatigue, and improves the ventilatory response to hypoxemia. However, careful evaluation of serum levels is very important, as toxicity may easily develop despite administration within the recommended dose range. The elderly COPD or critically ill patient has several characteristics which are known to decrease theophylline metabolism and increase blood levels (Table 15–3). As theophyline is a central nervous system and cardiovascular stimulant, signs of toxicity include tachycardia, ectopic activity, restlessness, and seizure activity. Nausea and vomiting may also occur. The therapeutic range of serum theophylline is 10 to 20 mg per liter. Seizures and cardiac arrhythmias occur at levels greater than 25 mg per liter.

Provide Adequate Hydration. Dehydration may thicken bronchopulmonary secretions. However, overhydration may precipitate pulmonary edema.

Mechanical Ventilation. This therapeutic choice is avoided whenever possible because of the difficulties encountered in weaning and the problems

TABLE 15–3. Factors That Decrease Theophylline (Aminophylline) Metabolism

Advanced age
Caffeine
Cimetidine (Tagamet)
Congestive heart failure
Cor pulmonale
Erythromycin
Propranolol

related to barotrauma. The decision to provide ventilatory support is based on the patient's mental and physical status rather than blood gas values alone.

PULMONARY EDEMA

Pulmonary edema is an abnormal accumulation of fluid outside the vascular space of the lung. This fluid may be in the interstitial space, the alveoli, or the cells. All body tissue has continuous two-way movement of fluid from the intravascular and interstitial space across the capillary membrane. This is the means by which nutrients are delivered to the cells and metabolic waste is removed. The factors that determine the intravascular versus extravascular fluid volume are the oppositely directed forces of osmotic and hydrostatic pressures in both spaces and the permeability (porosity) of the capillary membrane. (See Chapter 4, The Circuit—Capillaries). Overall, a greater net force directs fluid *out* of the systemic and pulmonary capillaries. In the lung under normal conditions, this results in an extravasation of approximately 10 to 20 ml of fluid an hour. The pulmonary lymphatics act as a skimming pump returning this watery extract of plasma to the venous circulation. Should greater than normal amounts of fluid enter the lung, the lymphatics can step up their pumping capacity tenfold, thus maintaining the lung in its normal, relatively dry state. When the amount of fluid entering the lung exceeds the maximum lymphatic pumping capacity to remove it, pulmonary edema develops.

Sequence of Formation

The sequence of formation of pulmonary edema appears to be the same regardless of cause. The pathophysiologic, radiologic, and clinical progression will be examined in three phases:

Phase 1. There is an increase in the amount of fluid moving from the pulmonary capillaries into the lung tissue. However, as a result of a compensatory increase in lung lymph flow, there is no measurable increase in lung fluid volume because incoming and outgoing fluid are in balance. Other than a mild tachypnea, which is thought to augment lymphatic drainage by a massaging effect on lymphatic vessels, there are no other associated clinical findings and the chest radiograph is normal. Essentially at this stage, pulmonary edema is undetectable and, in an absolute sense, is not pulmonary edema since there is no abnormal fluid accumulation in the lung. However, it does represent an abnormal or altered state of pulmonary fluid dynamics. The initiating process may spontaneously resolve and the normal state be reestablished, the patient may plateau at this level, or the underlying condition may worsen and progress to Phase 2.

Phase 2. When the pumping capabilities of the lymphatics are exceeded by the additional influx of fluid, the interstitial space becomes progressively engorged with fluid. Fluid first accumulates in pools in the loose interstitial tissue surrounding blood vessels and airways. At this point, the alveoli remain dry and gas exchange remains acceptable. There are no clinical signs, the lungs are clear to auscultation, and there is no subjective complaint of dyspnea. Tachypnea increases because of excitation of sensory nerve endings in the alveolar walls, *J* receptors (see Chapter 2, Control of Ventilation), by the increase in lung fluid. Radiographically, the edema fluid in the tissue surrounding blood vessels produces a clouding and poor definition of the vascular markings. Overall, the lung has a hazy appearance. The interlobar septa that separate the secondary lobules of the lung become edematous and produce linear densities, originally described by Peter Kerley, a British radiologist. Kerley B lines are short, horizontal, linear densities that extend out a few centimeters from the pleural edges and are seen most commonly at the lung bases. Centrally located Kerley A lines are longer than B lines and may course in any direction. With worsening of the patient's condition, pulmonary edema may progress to Phase 3.

Phase 3. A continuous fluid leak not matched by removal saturates the interstitial space, and edema breaks through the alveolar walls and fills the air spaces. In the normal adult, the interstitial space can maximally accommodate 200 to 300 ml of fluid, so substantial fluid collects in the lung before alveolar flooding and its associated clinical signs occur. The early, clinically recognizable signs and symptoms of pulmonary edema do not reflect early pulmonary edema, but rather its end-stage—alveolar flooding.

Initially, fluid accumulates at the corners of some alveoli. This small fluid accumulation alters surface tension and, as the alveolus shrinks, gas is replaced by pulmonary edema fluid. The characteristic of alveolar flooding is such that the alveolus is either completely air or fluid filled. This creates a tissue mosaic of functional (aerated) and nonfunctional (fluid-filled) alveoli. With the advent of alveolar flooding, crackles become apparent. Initially, they are fine (Velcro-like) and are heard near the peak of inspiration. As fluid moves into the larger airways, the auscultated sound takes on a coarse and then a gurgling quality. With progression of the process, gurgling may be inspiratory as well as expiratory.

As the number of fluid-filled alveoli increases, lung compliance decreases, the work of breathing increases, vital capacity and other lung volumes decrease, and the arterial PaO_2 worsens relative to the increasing number of shunt units (perfused but not ventilated alveoli). The point at which the patient complains of dyspnea relates to the patient's sensitivity to body sensations and activity level. Narrowing of bronchi and bronchioles due to edema and reflex bronchospasm increases airway resistance and wheezing may become apparent. Initially the $PaCO_2$ is decreased secondary to hyperventilation. If the patient is overcome with exhaustion, however, ventilatory movements become inadequate and the $PaCO_2$ climbs to normal and then increased levels. Should the fluid reach the level of the trachea, it may be expectorated as pulmonary edema froth. Radiographically, patchy, fluffy opacities in the lungs appear as air is replaced by fluid. The distribution of these opacities varies with the type of pulmonary edema.

Types of Pulmonary Edema

An increased movement of fluid into the lung resulting in pulmonary edema may be due to an imbalance in the protein hydrostatic and osmotic pressures or to increased permeability of the pulmonary capillary membrane. These are discussed below.

High Pressure (Cardiogenic, Hydrostatic) Pulmonary Edema

The most common form of pulmonary edema is due to volume/pressure overload of the pulmonary circulation, most commonly from left heart dysfunction and failure—hence, the names high pressure, cardiogenic, or hydrostatic pulmonary edema. The increase in pulmonary capillary hydrostatic pressure, as estimated clinically by measured pulmonary artery wedge pressure (PWP) or left atrial pressure, increases the amount of fluid movement from the pulmonary vascular to tissue space. When the amount of fluid entering the lung is greater than the lymphatics' capacity to remove it, x-ray and/or physical signs of pulmonary edema develop. This is typically associated with a PWP greater than 18 to 20 mm Hg.

Causes. In most instances, high pressure pulmonary edema is caused by a passive increase in pulmonary intravascular volume and pressure due to elevated left heart pressures, secondary to heart disease, although in some cases there is no cardiac disease or dysfunction. Causes include:

Intravascular Volume Overload. In this circumstance, there is volume overload of the entire cardiovascular system. This will produce a general increase in pressures throughout the cardiac and vascular structures. Intravascular volume overload may be due to: overtransfusion, fluid retention as in inappropriate antidiuretic hormone (ADH) secretion, or oliguric renal failure.

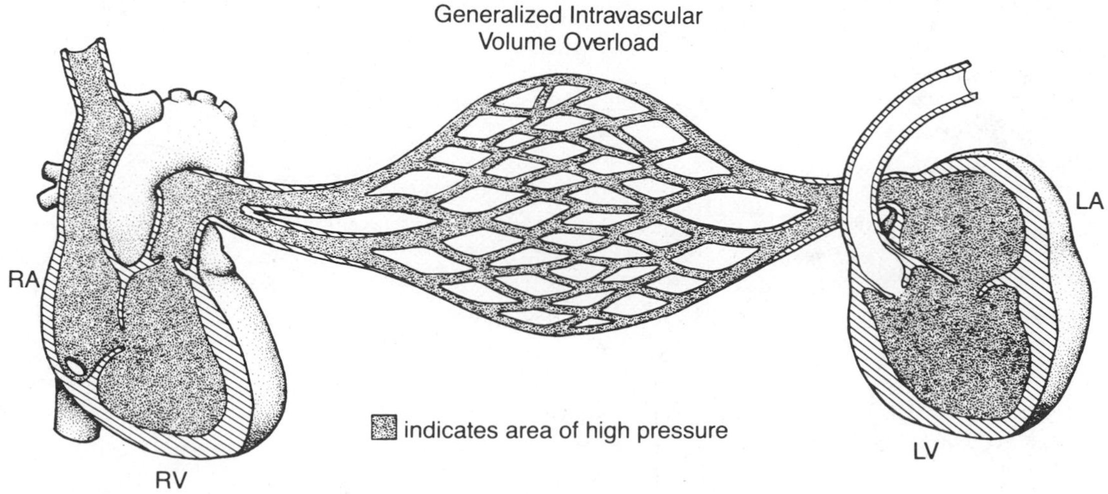

INCREASED PULMONARY VENOUS PRESSURE. Obstructive diseases involving the pulmonary veins are rare but may cause generalized or localized pulmonary edema. The elevated pulmonary venous pressure is passively transmitted back to the pulmonary capillaries. Pulmonary venous hypertension may be due to mediastinitis with scarring, mediastinal tumor, or pulmonary venous occlusive disease.

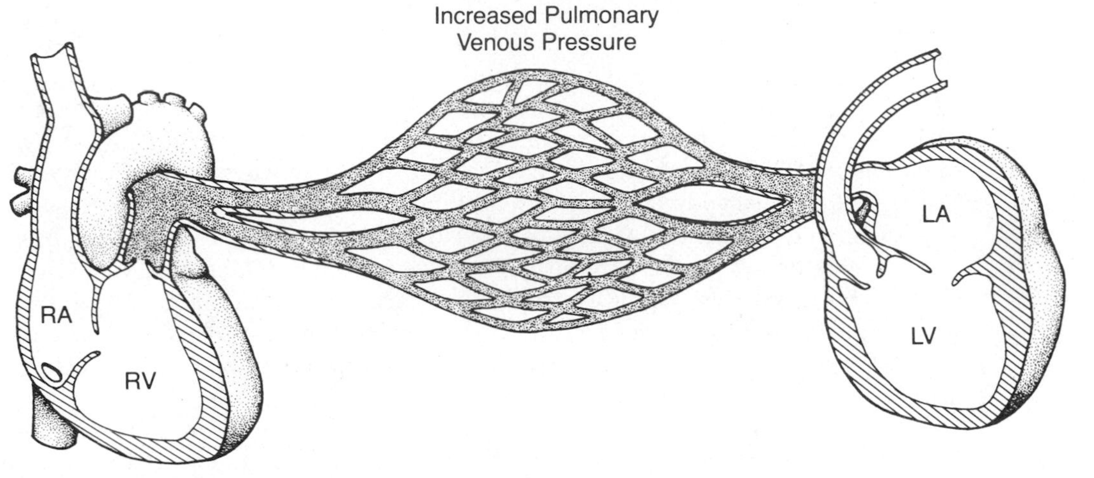

INCREASED LEFT ATRIAL PRESSURE. In this circumstance, left ventricular function may be normal but blood is dammed upstream of the high-pressure left atrium because of left ventricular inflow obstruction. Mean left atrial pressure may also be elevated because of regurgitant flow across an incompetent mitral valve. Left atrial pressure may be increased in mitral valve disease, including mitral stenosis, mitral regurgitation, and prosthetic mitral valve dysfunction; or left atrial myxoma.

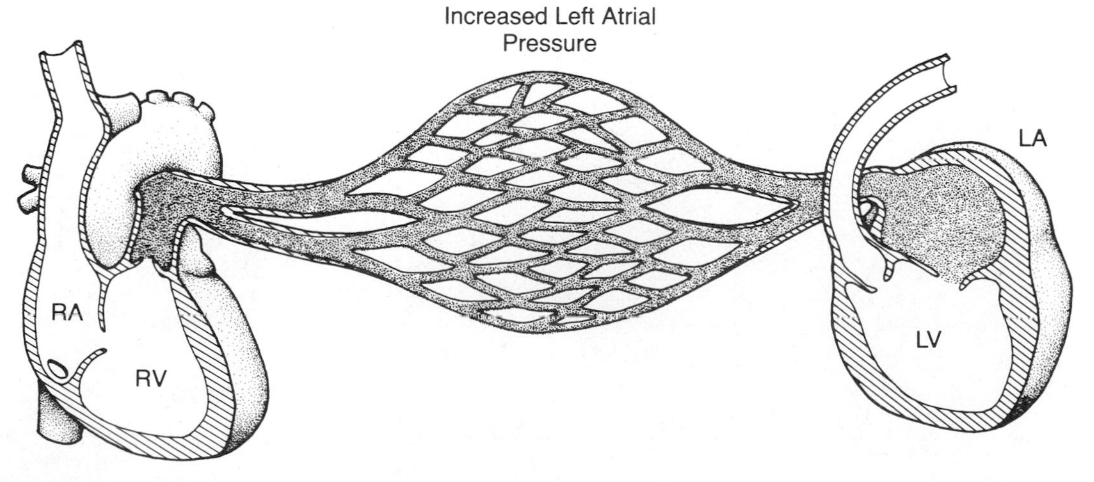

INCREASED LEFT VENTRICULAR END-DIASTOLIC PRESSURE. In circumstances of left ventricular dysfunction, the elevated LVEDP is reflected back to the left atrium, pulmonary veins, and pulmonary capillaries with transudation of fluid into the lung.

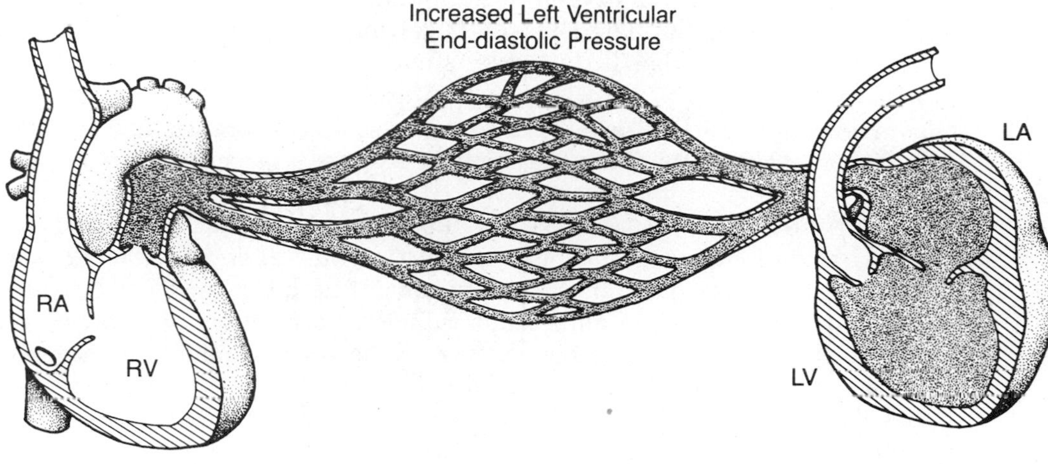

Increased LVEDP may be due to: ischemic heart disease, including angina, acute myocardial infarction, and left ventricular aneurysm; cardiomyopathy; pericardial disease, including constrictive pericarditis; aortic valvular disease, including aortic stenosis and aortic regurgitation; hypertensive crisis, including pheochromocytoma and malignant hypertension; arrhythmias; and high cardiac output states, including severe anemia, thyrotoxicosis, A-V fistula, and extreme fever.

Factors Precipitating Acute Pulmonary Edema. The most common cause of acute high pressure pulmonary edema is an exacerbation of preexisting heart failure or sudden-onset disease or dysfunction within the left heart. The cause of the sudden deterioration in cardiovascular status or altered physiologic state that allowed elevation in left atrial pressure must be identified and corrected in order to allow return to the patient's previous steady state. Factors known to precipitate acute pulmonary edema include ischemic events that may be silent; pulmonary or systemic infection; excessive or rapid IV transfusion; anemia; thyrotoxicosis; sodium excess; physical exertion; or emotional stress such as anger, fear, or intense anxiety.

Pathophysiology. Fluid accumulation in the lung interferes with gas exchange and results in hypoxemia and also causes increased stiffness of the lungs. Noncompliant lungs require a greater inspiratory pressure and work of breathing to maintain a physiologically acceptable tidal volume. Airway narrowing also increases the effort associated with exhalation; the respiratory rate also progressively increases. The feeling of breathlessness and accumulation of pulmonary edema froth create a sensation of suffocation and drowning. The associated intense fear and anxiety coupled with systemic underperfusion increase sympathetic nervous system stimulation that, together with the increased work of breathing, increase the work of the heart and produce a generalized increase in oxygen consumption. The patient requires progressively more oxygen but paradoxically is getting less, and the failing heart is required to work harder. If this cycle is not interrupted, it will quickly lead to death (Fig. 15–5).

Hemodynamic Effects. A sudden worsening of preexisting left heart failure or sudden onset of left heart failure results in two circulatory derangements:

THE FORWARD COMPONENT OF LEFT HEART FAILURE. Due to a loss of power (acute ischemic event), flow obstruction (mitral stenosis, aortic stenosis), or regurgitant flow (mitral insufficiency) the heart may not be able to maintain forward flow in an amount sufficient to meet the metabolic needs of the body. Compensatory sympathetic nervous system–induced vasoconstriction helps maintain mean arterial pressure despite the reduction in stroke volume; however, increased systemic vascular resistance increases left ventricular afterload and may worsen failure.

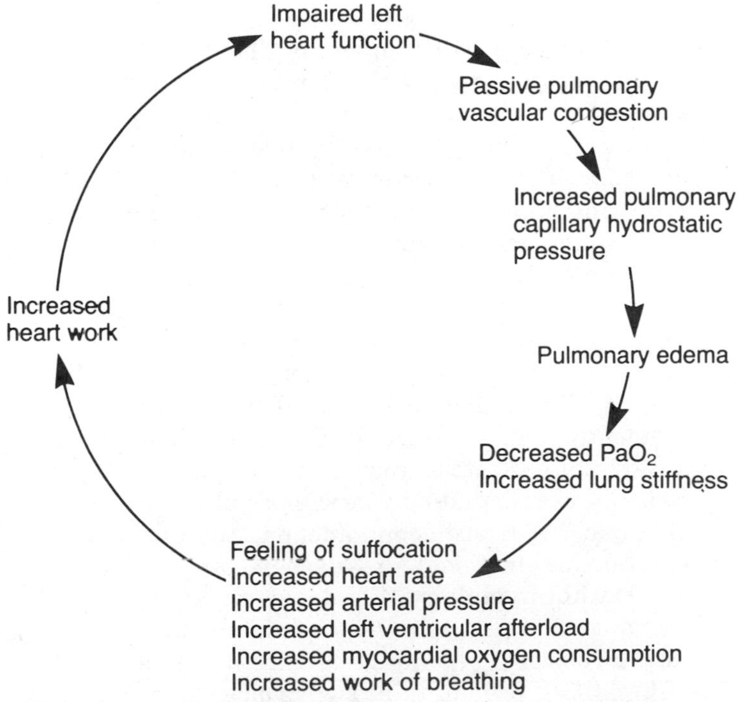

FIGURE 15–5. The vicious cycle of cardiogenic pulmonary edema.

THE BACKWARD (CONGESTIVE) COMPONENT OF LEFT HEART FAILURE. Because the left heart is unable to pump out all the blood brought to it, blood will passively accumulate in the pulmonary circulation, thus elevating pulmonary intravascular volume and pressure. Regardless of the initiating mechanism, an increase in PWP (a close correlate of pulmonary capillary hydrostatic pressure) of greater than 18 to 20 mm Hg is met with increased movement of a watery extract of plasma into the lung. As PWP increases, progressively greater extravascular fluid shifts occur. Generally, a PWP of 30 to 35 mm Hg is associated with massive transudation of fluid into the lung and is incompatible with life beyond a few hours.

There are two exceptions to this numerical yardstick for the development of pulmonary edema:

1. Patients with slow-onset, long-standing elevations in left atrial pressure, such as mitral stenosis or mitral insufficiency, may tolerate a very high PWP rather well. Three mechanisms develop over a period of time that tend to protect the patient from pulmonary edema even with left atrial pressures as high as 35 mm Hg: supernormal pulmonary lymph flow, diminished permeability of the pulmonary capillary membrane, and reactive constriction of the pulmonary arterioles that reduces pulmonary blood flow (see Chapter 16, Mitral Stenosis—Hemodynamic Effect).

2. Patients with low plasma protein concentration may develop clinical pulmonary edema at relatively low left atrial pressures. Low plasma protein levels decrease the threshold pulmonary capillary hydrostatic pressure at which fluid begins to accumulate in the lung (Fig. 15–6). In a classic study,[2] Guyton demonstrated that when the plasma protein concentration was re-

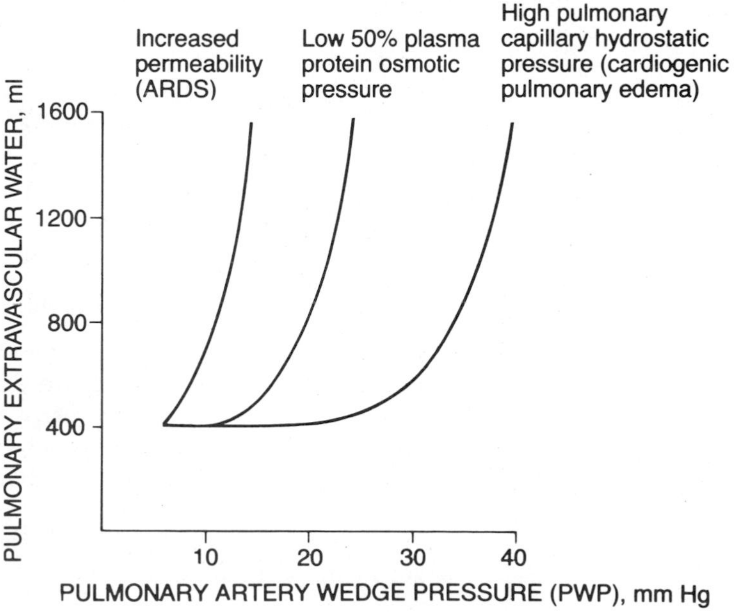

FIGURE 15–6. Threshold pulmonary capillary hydrostatic pressure levels at which fluid accumulates in the lung with various physiologic and/or hemodynamic abnormalities.

duced to approximately 50% of normal value by plasmapheresis, pulmonary edema developed at a PWP of 11 mm Hg. Some authorities,[3, 4] therefore, suggest that monitoring the colloid osmotic–pulmonary artery wedge pressure (COP-PWP) gradient may be helpful in predicting the predisposition to pulmonary edema in critically ill patients, many of whom are known to be hypoproteinemic.

Hemodynamic Profile. ARTERIAL PRESSURE. (See Table 15–1.) The blood pressure is typically elevated unless the patient is in cardiogenic shock. The waveform may appear damped if there are significant reductions in stroke volume and pulse pressure.

SYSTEMIC VASCULAR RESISTANCE. This value is typically elevated secondary to generalized vasoconstriction due to high endogenous catecholamine blood levels.

PULMONARY VASCULAR RESISTANCE. Increases in left atrial pressure result in the opening of pulmonary vascular channels in the least dependent areas of the lung by back pressure. Although this would ordinarily decrease pulmonary vascular resistance, with the onset of pulmonary edema this effect is overridden by hypoxemia-induced pulmonary vasoconstriction as well as by the reduction in pulmonary vascular luminal size created by the cuffs of pulmonary edema fluid that form around blood vessels. Therefore, the overall effect is an increase in pulmonary vascular resistance that will be worsened by complicating respiratory or metabolic acidosis.

CVP OR RA PRESSURE. These values may be normal if the right ventricle is able to increase performance commensurate with increases in afterload. However, when mean pulmonary artery pressure exceeds 35 to 45 mm Hg, the right ventricle typically fails. CVP values greater than 20 cm H_2O are not uncommon in cardiogenic pulmonary edema. In the presence of right ventricular failure, a dominant *a* wave may be noted in the right atrial tracing reflecting increased resistance to right ventricular filling during atrial systole.

PULMONARY ARTERY AND WEDGE PRESSURE. These values are increased owing to passive congestion of the pulmonary circulation with blood. The PWP is greater than 18 mm Hg in a person with a previously normal left atrial pressure or is significantly higher than previous values in patients with chronically elevated values, ie, mitral stenosis. The waveform may appear damped but the overall contour is unchanged unless the primary disturbance produces an altered waveform such as giant *v* waves in mitral regurgitation.

CARDIAC OUTPUT. A decrease in cardiac output accompanies pulmonary edema because of left heart dysfunction. Cardiac output may be normal or increased if pulmonary edema is due to intravascular volume overload or a high cardiac output state such as arteriovenous fistulas.

MIXED VENOUS OXYGEN SATURATION (SvO_2). This value is decreased because of decreasing peripheral blood flow, hypoxemia or both.

Clinical Presentation. The clinical presentation of pulmonary edema represents a spectrum of signs and symptoms that relate to the stage or severity of the process. In the earlier stages, it may be manifest only as exertional dyspnea, tachypnea, and orthopnea. The clinical presentation discussed below relates to advanced, severe pulmonary edema.

MENTATION. The patient with acute pulmonary edema is almost always terrified and may be very restless and thrash about. Cerebral hypoxia may produce changes in mentation such as confusion, irritability, and obtundation.

CUTANEOUS. In low cardiac output states, the patient is typically diaphoretic and the skin is usually cool, particularly at the extremities. The complexion is pale, and peripheral cyanosis may be noted. In pulmonary edema accompanying high cardiac output states (volume overload, arteriovenous fistulas, extreme fever) the skin may be warm and pink.

HEART RATE AND CHARACTER OF PULSE. Weak peripheral pulses and tachycardia accompany pulmonary edema caused by cardiac failure. The rapid pulse may be bounding in high cardiac output states such as fever.

AUSCULTATION OF THE CHEST. Marked adventitious lung sounds, which begin in the dependent portions of the lungs and extend upward to varying heights such as the level of the scapula, may obscure the S_3 and S_4 gallops characteristic of a failing, noncompliant ventricle. In the end stage, gurgling may be heard across the room—the ominous death rattle.

PALPATION OF THE PRECORDIUM. If pulmonary edema is due to heart failure, the apex beat is displaced downward and to the left, covers a large area, and may be more sustained.

NECK VEINS. The external jugular veins are visibly distended, reflecting elevated venous pressure secondary to right heart failure, if present.

RESPIRATORY RATE AND CHARACTER OF BREATHING. Respirations are markedly labored, shallow, and rapid. The nares are flared; intercostal, suprasternal, supraclavicular, and substernal retractions reflect the increased negative intrathoracic pressure required for inspiration.

PULMONARY EDEMA FLUID. The expectorated or suctioned froth may be clear and colorless, apricot-colored, or blood-tinged.

ACID/BASE. Hypoxemia is characteristic of pulmonary edema. Tachypnea initially produces respiratory alkalosis; however, when the patient cannot keep up with the work of breathing, respiratory acidosis prevails. With severe perfusion failure, metabolic acidosis will worsen the acidemic state.

Laboratory Studies. ECG. Changes will be noted specific to the cause of the pulmonary edema, such as ischemia or infarct patterns.

CHEST RADIOGRAPH. The fluffy-appearing densities in the lung form a "butterfly wing" distribution to the edema pattern. Increased density at the hilum radiates out to the periphery. Heart size is enlarged if the primary defect is ventricular failure. There are limitations of the chest radiograph in diagnosing pulmonary edema secondary to left heart dysfunction. A known diagnostic lag period exists in which pulmonary artery pressures may be elevated but edema may not be apparent on chest film. On the other hand, it may take 12 to 48 hours for radiographic evidence of pulmonary edema to clear after therapy has normalized hemodynamic parameters.

MANAGEMENT. Acute pulmonary edema is the most dramatic and terrifying consequence of left heart failure. While the prognosis is good if it is not due to overwhelming heart disease, it may rapidly lead to death if not quickly diagnosed and aggressively treated. The following measures are directed at resolving the acute process.

- *Maintain adequate arterial oxygenation.* Supplemental oxygen is given to maintain a PaO_2 of at least 65 mm Hg. A mask may be used or, if ventilatory movements weaken, intubation with mechanical support with or without PEEP is generally required.
- *Place the patient in a sitting position with feet down.* The patient will spontaneously assume the sitting postion when able. When upright, three fourths of the blood displaced to the dependent parts of the body comes from the pulmonary circulation, and one fourth from the heart and great vessels. Overall, this results in an approximate 25% reduction in pulmonary blood volume.[5] On the other hand, laying the upright patient down to obtain an ECG or PWP reading may produce intolerable overload of the central circulation and risks cardiac arrest. It is common to find patients in acute pulmonary edema in the emergency department, ICU, or CCU being managed in a high Fowler position while on a cart or bed. This has two disadvantages: 1) With the legs held horizontally, the forces of gravity are not maximized to unload the cardiopulmonary unit. 2) Patients typically slip down and don't remain in the high Fowler position longer than about five minutes. If the patient is too weak to sit upright at the side of the bed or in a chair, the patient may be placed in a semiupright position by placing shock blocks at the head portion of the bed while a foot board prevents downward slippage out of the bed. A pillow placed vertically between the scapulae additionally brings the shoulders back and facilitates effective ventilatory movements in the bedridden patient.
- *Morphine sulfate* carefully given in 3 to 5 mg increments IV to a possible total of 15 mg has several very beneficial effects in the treatment of pulmonary edema. The narcotic promotes a sense of well-being and the sympathetically induced arteriolar and venous constriction is diminished. Thus, preload, afterload, and heart work are reduced while stroke volume increases. Nevertheless, the patient should be observed carefully for respiratory depression, the main adverse effect of the drug. Morphine may have to be avoided if the patient has a decreased level of consciousness, hypotension, or chronic pulmonary disease. Nausea and vomiting may also occur with the use of the drug.
- *Preload reduction.* Although morphine sulfate is a venodilator, additional preload reduction may require the use of a diuretic such as furosemide, which additionally increases venous capacitance. Venodilation may also be accomplished with the use of nitroglycerin given sublingually, topically, or intravenously.
- *Afterload reduction.* Nitroprusside (Nipride) has a venous dilator action, thereby reducing preload, and the arterial dilator action reduces systemic vascular resistance. The latter effect is very useful for patients in whom arterial pressure remains elevated.

- *Theophylline (aminophylline)*, by its bronchodilator effect, is useful when bronchospasm complicates pulmonary edema. It additionally has a mild positive inotropic and diuretic effect in patients not on aminophylline therapy. The 5 mg/kg IV dose is infused slowly over a period of 10 to 15 minutes.
- *Positive inotropic agents.* By increasing cardiac output, these agents improve perfusion of the systemic circulation and may reduce the PWP by increasing stroke volume.

Permeability Pulmonary Edema (Adult Respiratory Distress Syndrome)

The adult respiratory distress syndrome (ARDS) is a severe form of acute respiratory failure that may occur in people with or without preexisting pulmonary disease. Increased permeability of the pulmonary capillary membrane allows a transudation of proteinaceous fluid into the interstitial and alveolar spaces. Thus, the patient presents with a clinical and pathophysiologic picture of pulmonary edema. There is no specific laboratory test for ARDS; rather, the diagnosis is strongly considered if the following criteria are fulfilled:

- a pulmonary artery wedge pressure of less than 18 mm Hg;
- hypoxemia that responds with less than a 10 mm Hg increase in PaO_2 to a 20% increase in FIO_2;
- the appearance of bilateral, diffuse infiltrates on chest x-ray film; and
- no other reason for hypoxemia and radiographic changes.

The use of these diagnostic criteria may be complicated because pneumonia and/or left ventricular failure frequently complicate ARDS.

Clinically, ARDS is characterized by dyspnea; tachypnea; a progressive decrease in lung compliance; and, terminally, hypercapnia. ARDS is known by many names, some descriptive of the clinical setting and some descriptive of the pathophysiologic process (Table 15–4).

Incidence and Mortality. There are an estimated 150,000 cases of ARDS annually in the United States, with a mortality rate of approximately 50 to 70%.

TABLE 15–4. Alternative Names for Permeability Pulmonary Edema (ARDS)

Descriptive of Pathophysiologic Features	*Descriptive of Clinical Setting*
Adult respiratory distress syndrome (ARDS)	Shock lung
Adult hyaline membrane disease	Transplant lung
Congestive atelectasis	Posttransfusion lung
Noncardiogenic pulmonary edema	Da Nang lung
Progressive respiratory distress	Septic lung
Respiratory insufficiency syndrome	
Stiff lung	
Wet lung	
White lung	
Liver lung	

TABLE 15–5. Causes of Permeability Pulmonary Edema (ARDS)

Shock	***Hematologic Disorders***
All types	Massive blood transfusion
Trauma	Disseminated intravascular coagulation
Direct lung injury	Prolonged cardiopulmonary bypass
Nonthoracic trauma	Thrombotic thrombocytopenic purpura
Fracture of the long bones	Leukemia
Inhalation of Noxious Substances	***Metabolic Disorders***
Aspiration of gastric contents	Diabetic ketoacidosis
Near drowning (fresh or salt water)	Uremia
Irritant gases	Pancreatitis
Smoke inhalation	***Miscellaneous***
Sustained high FIO_2 (50 to 60% or greater)	Eclampsia
Infectious Causes	Air or amniotic fluid emboli
Viral or bacterial pneumonia	Radiation
Septicemia	Heat stroke
Drug Overdose	
Heroin	
Methadone	
Acetylsalicylic acid (aspirin)	
Barbiturates	
Colchicine	
Propoxyphene (Darvon)	
Chlordiazepoxide (Librium)	

Causes. ARDS may be precipitated by a widely diverse group of physical insults (Table 15–5).

Pathophysiology. The common denominator in ARDS is a serious insult to the body that directly or indirectly targets the lung. When not due to direct lung injury, such as aspiration of gastric contents or smoke inhalation, the mechanisms that provoke lung damage appear to be biochemical and immunologic, secondarily affecting the lung through blood-borne mediators. These substances lead to damage and disruption of the pulmonary capillary membrane. The development of "pores" in the capillary wall allows a fluid leak from the vascular to the interstitial spaces despite normal-to-low pulmonary intravascular pressures. Hence, the names "permeability pulmonary edema" or "noncardiogenic pulmonary edema." The vascular pores may be of sufficient size to allow formed elements of blood, such as red blood cells, to escape into the extravascular space. In addition, the damaged capillary endothelium is no longer able to retain plasma proteins, such as albumin and fibrinogen, in the vascular space. Thus, the protein content of the edema fluid and interstitial protein osmotic pressure are nearly identical to those of plasma. For this reason, the pulmonary capillary hydrostatic pressure, as estimated by PWP, becomes a critical factor in determining lung water, and pulmonary edema can be rapid in onset and catastrophic with even relatively small increases in PWP (Figs. 15–6 and 15–7).

Other pathophysiologic features of this unfortunate syndrome are small airway disease and diffuse atelectasis. There also appears to be disruption of the structure of the interstitium as well as plugging of the pulmonary

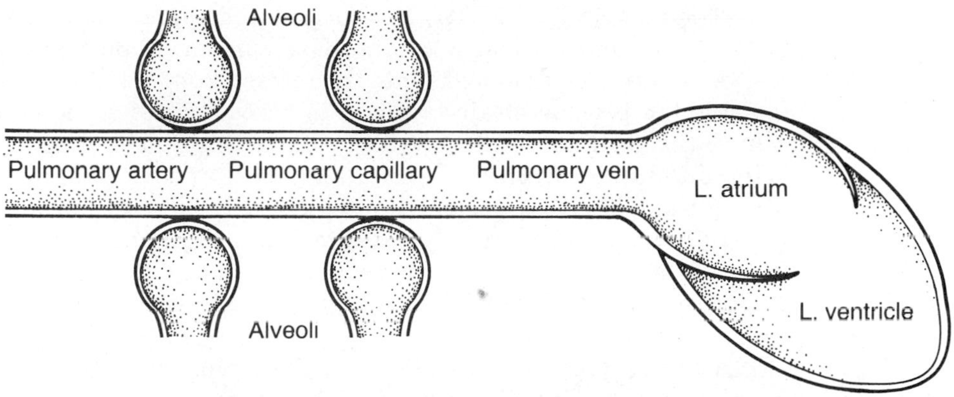

FIGURE 15–7. In diastole, there is a continuous open passage from the left ventricle to the pulmonary arteries. Therefore, pulmonary artery diastolic and wedge pressures approximate pulmonary capillary hydrostatic pressure, pulmonary venous pressure, left atrial pressure, and left ventricular end-diastolic pressure. Because pulmonary capillary hydrostatic pressure is an important determinant of fluid movement into the lung, reducing PWP reduces fluid flux into the lung in ARDS.

microcirculation by intravascular aggregates of fibrin and blood cells (microthrombi).

Four clinical stages characterize the course of ARDS.

1. INJURY. This stage is associated with metabolic and perfusion abnormalities as the body attempts to "adapt and survive" in response to the insult. The resulting biochemical and/or perfusion abnormalities may initiate and set the stage for subsequent pulmonary damage.

Hemodynamic Profile. This will be specific to the type of injury (hypovolemia secondary to hemorrhage, septicemia, drug overdose, and so on (see Table 15–1).

Clinical Presentation. PHYSICAL EXAMINATION. Unless associated thoracic or upper airway trauma are present, there is no evidence of respiratory distress and the lungs are clear to auscultation.

CHEST RADIOGRAPH. The chest film is typically normal in the absence of other complicating problems such as hemothorax and pneumothorax.

PAO_2. The arterial oxygen tension is slightly decreased below the patient's normal values. Given previously normal arterial oxygenation, one may anticipate a PaO_2 of 70 to 80 mm Hg while the patient is breathing room air (FIO_2, 0.21).

$PACO_2$. There is respiratory alkalosis due to the hyperventilation that typically accompanies physiologic or psychologic stress. In a previously healthy person, one may anticipate a $PaCO_2$ of 30 to 40 mm Hg.

MIXED VENOUS OXYGEN SATURATION (SvO_2). This value falls secondary to decreased arterial oxygenation and/or perfusion deficit accompanying the insult.

2. THE LATENT PERIOD. This period of apparent stability may last from 12 to 48 hours. Because of the development of pulmonary vascular "pores," a protein-rich fluid leaks into the interstitium of the lung. The edema compresses the peripheral airways and is associated with increased airway resistance that will not be perceived by the patient at this time.

Hemodynamic Profile. PULMONARY ARTERY AND WEDGE PRESSURE. These values are within normal limits, given cardiovascular stability and normal intravascular volume. A possible increase in the pulmonary artery systolic and diastolic pressures, with a widening of the pulmonary artery diastolic-to-wedge pressure (PAd-PWP) gradient, reflects an increase in pulmonary vascular resistance.

PULMONARY VASCULAR RESISTANCE. This value may be within normal limits or increased. The reason for the increase is poorly understood.

Clinical Presentation. PHYSICAL EXAMINATION. The chest is clear to auscultation. There is no cough or declared or apparent respiratory distress. Hyperventilation continues and may be slightly increased.

CHEST X-RAY FILM. There are minimal or no infiltrates. The appearance of the lung fields may be consistent with interstitial pulmonary edema.

PAO_2. This value decreases and may approximate 60 to 80 mm Hg while the patient is breathing environmental air. Although this value is considered physiologically acceptable, it is not normal for a previously healthy adult.

$PACO_2$. This value decreases to approximately 25 to 35 mm Hg secondary to hyperventilation.

MIXED VENOUS OXYGEN SATURATION (SvO_2). This value continues to fall proportionate to decreases in arterial saturation.

3. ACUTE RESPIRATORY FAILURE. Proteinaceous edema fluid and formed elements of blood now enter the lung tissue and alveoli. The first physical signs of pulmonary edema now appear and relate to the alveolar flooding.

Hemodynamic Profile. The "numbers" may yet be essentially within normal limits unless cardiovascular disease coexists or heart failure compounds the problem. Elevation of pulmonary artery pressures with widening of the PAd-PWP gradient is likely becoming more pronounced (see Table 15–1).

Clinical Presentation. PHYSICAL EXAMINATION. The patient now complains of dyspnea and may be restless. Crackles and wheezes may be noted on auscultation, and the patient may occasionally cough.

CHEST X-RAY FILM. Scattered infiltrates begin to coalesce diffusely throughout the lungs. The diffuse infiltrates are due to the accumulation of lung fluid as well as diffuse atelectasis.

PaO_2. This value continues to decrease and may approximate 50 to 60 mm Hg. This is physiologically unacceptable. Unfortunately, it is common to take first serious notice of blood gases when the "numbers" are outside the physiologically acceptable limits; earlier careful evaluation of laboratory data would reveal the developing defect (decreasing PaO_2) before values are at levels that threaten adequate tissue oxygenation. At this time the disease is well established and mortality is approximately 50%.

$PaCO_2$. This value decreases to approximately 20 to 35 mm Hg owing to continuing hyperventilation, which may now be further increased.

MIXED VENOUS OXYGEN SATURATION (SvO_2). This value continues to fall relative to worsening hypoxemia.

4. SEVERE RESPIRATORY FAILURE (Preterminal). There is gross distortion of the lung tissue. The number of functional, perfusing pulmonary capillaries is markedly reduced owing to microthrombolytic obstruction. The protein-rich fluid in the alveoli may become organized and transformed into fibrous tissue. Lung compliance is greatly decreased, and the work of breathing is tremendously increased because of increasing lung stiffness secondary to pulmonary edema, fibrosis, and massive, diffuse atelectasis.

Hemodynamic Profile. PULMONARY ARTERY AND WEDGE PRESSURE. Pulmonary artery pressures are now commonly markedly elevated, reflecting increased pulmonary vascular resistance secondary to acute lung injury (see Table 15–1). This increases right ventricular afterload and may result in right ventricular failure. In the absence of left ventricular dysfunction, the PWP will be normal to low. An example of hemodynamic measurements in Stage 4 is right atrial pressure (CVP), 10 mg Hg; PA systolic pressure, 60 mm Hg; PA diastolic pressure, 30 mm Hg; PWP, 5 mm Hg; and PAd-PWP gradient, 25 mm Hg (normal, 1 to 3 mm Hg).

CARDIAC OUTPUT. Cardiac function and output are usually normal in patients with ARDS, although in Stages 3 and 4 cardiac output may be low secondary to a decreased left ventricular filling volume that occurs as a consequence of increased pulmonary vascular resistance and right heart failure.

Clinical Presentation. PHYSICAL EXAMINATION. The patient is in obvious respiratory distress and may be using accessory muscles to generate wider swings in intrathoracic pressure to move air in and out of increasingly stiff lungs. These exaggerated alterations in intrathoracic pressure reflect the vasculature of the thorax and produce a roller coaster appearance to the movement of the pulmonary artery and wedge waveforms (see Chapter 9, Ventilatory Effects, Pulmonary Artery Pressure Measurements). Intercostal, suprasternal, substernal, and supraclavicular retractions are usually evident. Diaphoresis, mental obtundation, and nasal flaring may be noted as diffuse wheezes and crackles continue, although crackles tend to be less pronounced in ARDS pulmonary edema than in high-pressure (cardiogenic) pulmonary edema. Breath sounds diminish, reflecting decreasing movement of air through diffusely atelectatic lungs. Tachypnea continues with grunting respirations. If the patient is being supported with mechanical ventilation, peak inspiratory pressures required to deliver a given tidal volume progressively increase. While they may be in the range of 20 to 30 cm H_2O early in the course of ARDS, they may progress to levels as high as 70 to 80 cm H_2O or greater terminally.

PaO_2. Arterial oxygen tensions progressively decrease, with very poor response to increased levels of FIO_2. Indeed, the PaO_2 may be as low as 40 mm Hg while the patient is receiving 100% oxygen.

$PaCO_2$. Terminally, the $PaCO_2$ increases beyond 45 mm Hg despite adequate ventilatory movements. Because carbon dioxide normally is easily diffused across the alveolar-capillary membrane, the increase in $PaCO_2$ levels is a grave prognostic sign as it suggests severe damage to lung tissue. If the patient is spontaneously breathing, hypercapnia may be compounded by respiratory muscle fatigue.

MIXED VENOUS OXYGEN SATURATION (SvO_2). This value is typically very low relative to the severity of hypoxemia.

Treatment. To date, there is no generally agreed-upon therapy that prevents the development or progression of lung injury or promotes lung healing once injury is established. Given these dismal facts, it is not surprising that the mortality rate remains above 50 per cent. Current management is directed toward patient support in the hope that the process will spontaneously resolve and the lung will heal and recover normal function. Management guidelines include:

1. Correction of the primary problem and any associated abnormalities such as acid-base or electrolyte disorders.

2. Correction of arterial hypoxemia. Typically this entails the use of supplemental oxygen. However, pulmonary oxygen toxicity is predicted to occur when an FIO_2 of greater than .50 to .60 is administered for an extended period of time. Ironically, the clinical, pathophysiologic, and laboratory picture of pulmonary oxygen toxicity is identical to that of ARDS. The length of time that it takes for toxicity to occur is variable and cannot be predicted individually. Depending on the dose of oxygen (FIO_2) and individual susceptibility, this may be clinically significant within a few days. Therefore, the lowest FIO_2 that provides an acceptable PaO_2 (approximately 60 mm Hg) should be used. Lower levels of FIO_2 may be achieved with the use of positive end-expiratory pressure (PEEP). PEEP, compared with ventilatory support using atmospheric end-expiratory pressure, prevents small airway and alveolar collapse and also recruits previously collapsed alveoli. These effects maintain or increase the surface area of the lung available for the diffusion of gases and may also reduce lung stiffness. Nevertheless, at levels higher than 10 to 15 cm H_2O PEEP frequently makes determination of accurate pulmonary artery and wedge pressures difficult (see Chapter 9, Ventilatory Effects, Pulmonary Artery Pressure Measurements). It also has the potential to depress cardiac output by: 1) decreasing the venous return to the heart by compression of the compliant venae cavae; 2) compression of the pulmonary capillaries by PEEP-distended alveoli. Because this might impair right ventricular emptying, high levels of PEEP have the potential to decrease blood flow to the left heart and left ventricular filling volume; and 3) producing a tamponade effect on the ventricles in diastole that may interfere with ventricular filling.

At levels of PEEP greater than 15 cm H_2O, equalization of right and left ventricular filling pressures (as measured clinically by right atrial pressure and PWP) may occur secondary to impaired right ventricular emptying. The resulting increase in right ventricular diastolic pressure may shift the ventricular septum toward the left ventricle, thereby reducing its internal dimensions. Thus, for a given ventricular filling volume, ventricular filling pressures increase, although these effects of PEEP on hemodynamics and pressure measurements cannot be accurately predicted. The stiff, noncompliant lungs of ARDS tend to prevent transmission of airway pressure to the cardiovascular structures and, therefore, have a protective effect on cardiac output. The degree of lung stiffness is quite variable from person to person, within the same individual during the course of the disease, and regionally within the same lung.

The goal in management of ARDS is to use a level of PEEP that provides the maximum increase in PaO_2 with the minimum decrease in cardiac output.

3. Frequent position changes. Repositioning the patient every 30 minutes to 1 hour can significantly reduce the tendency toward pooling of secretions, hypostatic pneumonia, and atelectasis.

4. Good tracheal-bronchial hygiene. This involves suctioning the intubated patient or encouraging coughing and deep breathing frequently in the spontanously breathing patient.

5. Elevation of the head and thorax. The upright position produces the best overall ventilation/perfusion ratios throughout the lung, increases vital capacity, eases the work of breathing, and lowers pulmonary capillary hydrostatic pressure.

6. Maintenance of adequate cardiac output. As increasing left ventricular filling pressures may increase fluid movement into the lung in ARDS, an inotropic agent such as dopamine may be required to increase or maintain dequate cardiac output in lieu of volume loading. Attempts are usually made to keep left ventricular filling pressures (PWP) in the low range of normal (see Figs. 15–6 and 15–7).

REFERENCES

1. Dalen JE, Alper JS: Natural history of pulmonary embolism. *Prog Cardiovasc Dis* 1975; 17:259.
2. Guyton AC, Lindsey AW: Effect of elevated left atrial pressure and decreased plasma protein concentration on the development of pulmonary edema. *Cir Res* 1959; 7:649–657.
3. Rackow EC, Fein IA, Siegel J: The relationship of the colloid osmotic–pulmonary artery wedge pressure gradient to pulmonary edema and mortality in critically ill patients. *Chest* 1982; 82:433–437.
4. Weil, MH, Hennig RJ, Morassette M, et al: Relationship between colloid osmotic pressure and pulmonary artery wedge pressure in patients with acute cardiorespiratory failure. *Am J Med* 1978; 64:643–650.
5. Gunttopalli KK: Acute pulmonary edema. *Cardiol Clin* 1984; 2:183–200.

SUGGESTED READING

General

Groves BM, Reeves JT: Pulmonary hypertension. In Horwitz LD, Groves BM (eds): *Signs and Symptoms in Cardiology*. Philadelphia, JB Lippincott, 1985.

Pulmonary Edema

Balk R, Bone RC: The adult respiratory distress syndrome. *Med Clin North Am* 1983; 67:685–700.

Bone RC (ed) The Adult Respiratory Distress Syndrome. *Clin Chest Med* 1982; 3:1–212.

Boyson PG, Modell JH: Pulmonary edema. *In* Shoemaker W, Thompson WL, Holbrook PR (eds): Philadelphia, WB Saunders, 1984.

Depman ST, Wendel CH: Congestive heart failure and pulmonary edema. *Primary Care* 1986; 13:71–75.

Donat WE, Weiner BH: Syndromes of left ventricular failure. *In* Rippe JM, Irwin RS, Alpert JS (eds): *Intensive Care Medicine.* Boston, Little, Brown, 1985.

Fishman DP, Renkin EM: *Pulmonary Edema.* Bethesda, MD, American Psychological Society, 1979.

Ingram RH, Braunwald E: Pulmonary edema, cardiogenic and noncardiogenic. *In* Braunwald E (ed): *Heart Disease, A Textbook of Cardiovascular Medicine.* Philadelphia, WB Saunders, 1984.

Lake KB: Adult respiratory distress syndrome (high permeability pulmonary edema). *In* Burton GC, Hodgkin JE (eds): *Respiratory Care, A Guide to Clinical Practice,* ed 2. Philadelphia, JB Lippincott, 1984.

Matthay MA: Pathophysiology of pulmonary edema. *Clin Chest Med* 1985; 6:301–314.

Prewitt RM, Matthay MA, Ghignone M: Hemodynamic management in the adult respiratory distress syndrome. *Clin Chest Med* 1983; 4:251–268.

Shapiro BA: Noncardiogenic edema, adult respiratory distress syndrome, and PEEP therapy. *In* Cane RD, Shapiro BA (eds): *Case Studies in Critical Care Medicine.* Chicago, Year Book Medical Publications, 1985.

Sibbald WJ: Pulmonary edema. *In* Sibbald WJ (ed): *Synopsis of Critical Care,* ed 2. Baltimore, Williams & Wilkins, 1984.

Spano JF, Hurst JW: The recognition and management of heart failure. *In* Hurst JW (ed): *The Heart.* New York, McGraw-Hill, 1982.

Wilson RF: Acute respiratory failure. *In Principles and Techniques of Critical Care.* Kalamazoo, MI, The Upjohn Company, 1976.

Pulmonary Embolism

Bell WR, Simon TL, DeMets DL: The clinical features of submassive and massive pulmonary emboli. *Am J Med* 1977; 62:355–360.

Benotti JR, Dalen JE: Pulmonary embolism. *In* Horwitz LD, Groves BM (eds): *Signs and Symptoms of Cardiology.* Philadelphia, JB Lippincott, 1985.

Hayes SP, Bone RC: Pulmonary emboli with respiratory failure. *Med Clin North Am* 1983; 67:1179–1191.

Hinshaw HC, Marray JF: Pulmonary Thromboembolism. *In Diseases of the Chest,* ed 4. Philadelphia, WB Saunders, 1980.

Matthay MA, Matthay RA: Pulmonary thromboembolism and other pulmonary vascular diseases. *In* George RB, Light RW, Matthay RA (eds): *Chest Medicine.* New York, Churchill Livingstone, 1983.

Chronic Obstructive Pulmonary Disease (COPD)

Burrow B: Chronic Airways Disease. *In* Wyngaarden JB, Smith LH (eds): *Cecil Textbook of Medicine,* ed 17. Philadelphia, WB Saunders, 1985.

Francis PB: Acute respiratory failure in obstructive lung disease. *Med Clin North Am* 1983; 67:657–668.

Hinshaw HC, Marray JF: Chronic bronchitis and emphysema. *In Diseases of the Chest,* ed 4. Philadelphia, WB Saunders, 1980.

Matthay RA, Berger HJ: Cardiovascular function in cor pulmonale. *Clin Chest Med* 1983; 4:269–295.

Sherter CB, Polnitsky CA, Matthay RA: Chronic obstructive pulmonary diseases (asthma, bronchitis, emphysema, bronchiectasis and cystic fibrosis). *In* George RB, Light RW, Matthay RA (eds): *Chest Medicine.* New York, Churchill Livingstone, 1983.

Wilson RF: Chronic Respiratory Failure. *In Principles and Techniques of Critical Care.* Kalamazoo, MI, The Upjohn Company, 1976.

Monitoring the Patient with Cardiovascular Disease

16

MELISSA TOBIN, MSN, RN
GLORIA DAROVIC, RN, CCRN, CEN

Cardiovascular disease is the leading cause of death in the industrialized world. Despite major advances in diagnostic and therapeutic modalities, millions of people succumb to disorders of the cardiovascular system each year. Many are left with major disabilities and impaired lifestyles. The physical, emotional, and financial toll that cardiovascular disease takes on our society is of enormous proportions.

Over the past few decades, dramatic improvement has been made in the ability to diagnose and treat various forms of cardiovascular disease in the acute care setting. For example, through the utilization of bedside hemodynamic monitoring devices, the clinician is able to assess cardiac function quickly and accurately, and then guide therapy accordingly.

PRINCIPLES THAT PLAY A ROLE IN CARDIOVASCULAR FUNCTION

Several of the major cardiovascular disorders are presented in this chapter. Although each disorder may not be directly related to the others, the following principles play a critical role in cardiovascular function in both normal and disease states.

- *Myocardial oxygen supply must equal demand to maintain normal myocardial function.* In response to hypoxia secondary to hypoperfusion or decreased arterial oxygen content, the myocardium becomes electrophysiologically unstable and/or poorly contractile. Many patients with cardiovascular disease (valvular, cardiomyopathy, hypertensive, coronary artery) may be asymptomatic without functional disability for a long period of time. Then some mechanism unfavorably tips the balanced scale of myocardial oxygen supply and demand and renders the patient symptomatic with some degree of cardiac decompensation. The precipitating factor may be tachycardia, anemia, infection, exercise, pregnancy, or trauma. Most of the therapeutic interventions in caring for the patient with cardiovascular disease manipulate the myocardial oxygen supply/demand equation in some way. Depending on the primary disorder, the patient will generally be stabilized if the balance is restored.

- *Within physiologic limits, an increase in the volume of the ventricle at the end of diastole (preload) results in an increase in the force of the subsequent contraction and stroke volume (Starling's law).* Clinically, this filling volume correlates well with the measured filling pressure (PWP, PAd, LA pressure) if the ventricle has normal compliance. This relationship is illustrated in the ventricular function curve, which plots stroke volume against end-diastolic volume and sarcomere length. However, as a result of changes in ventricular compliance (distensibility) and contractility imposed by myocardial disease, each patient has an optimal point on the ventricular function curve at which stroke volume is maximized at a particular level of end-diastolic pressure. This value may also suddenly change in the same patient in response to acute physiologic changes in the myocardium (see Fig. 16–1). The Starling effect is therefore a very important consideration in managing the acutely ill patient with cardiovascular disease. By assessing preload and its relationship to stroke volume, the optimum level of cardiac output can be achieved while guarding against the development of pulmonary edema in the individual patient. This is accomplished by manipulation of preload with volume challenges, diuretics, and/or venodilators.
- *Sudden changes in afterload may produce sudden changes in ventricular performance.* It is well known that increases in afterload decrease the ventricle's ability to eject its contents, particularly in a diseased state. Through evaluation and manipulation of pulmonary artery and aortic diastolic pressures, as well as pulmonary and systemic vascular resistance by vasodilators, right and left ventricular performance may be optimized.
- *The contractile or inotropic state of the myocardium exerts a potent influence on ventricular performance, stroke volume, and myocardial oxygen consumption.* Myocardial disease or negative inotropic agents such as beta or calcium channel blockers reduce myocardial contractility, stroke volume, and myocardial oxygen consumption for any given level of preload or afterload. Positive inotropic agents such as digitalis increase contractility, myocardial oxygen consumption, and stroke volume. Thus, stroke volume and myocardial oxygen consumption may be influenced by administering agents that either increase or decrease contractility.
- *Ventricular wall motion abnormalities, such as those that occur with ischemic disease, or poorly coordinated ventricular contractile dynamics, such as occurs with ventricular ectopy, have the potential to decrease stroke volume and cardiac output.*
- *There is a predictable relationship between ventricular radius, intramyocardial wall tension, and myocardial oxygen consumption (law of Laplace).*

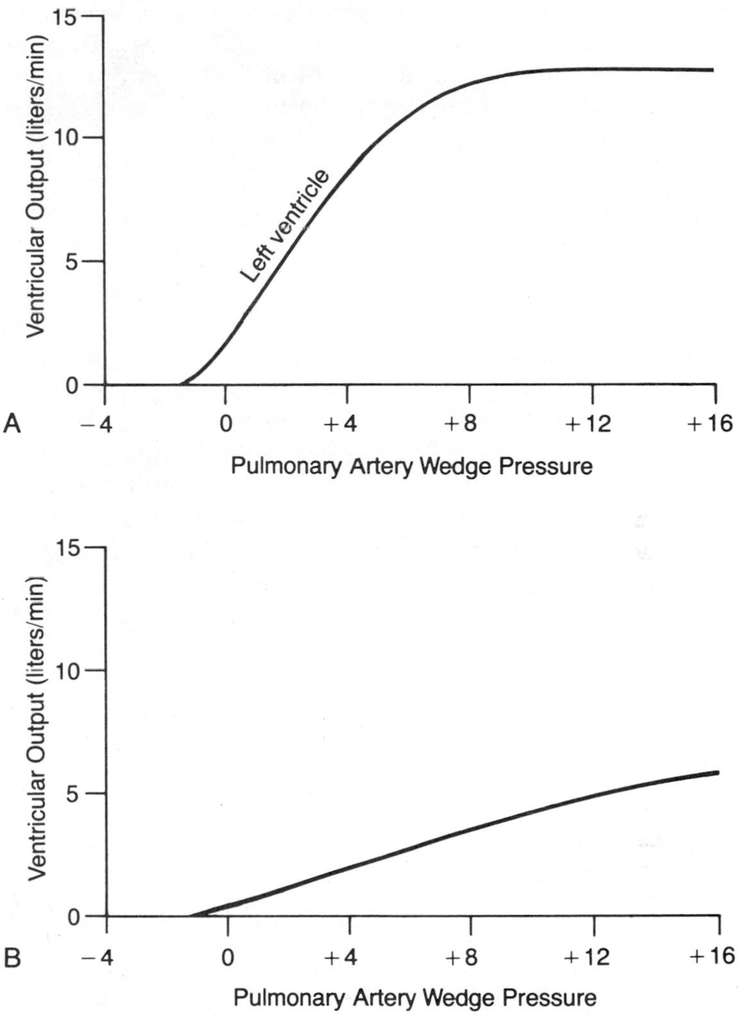

FIGURE 16–1. *A.* In a patient with known coronary artery disease with no acute ischemic episode and normal ventricular function, peak left ventricular performance is attained with a level of preload, as measured by pulmonary artery wedge pressure, of 8 to 10 mm Hg. A PWP of 4 mm Hg still produces a cardiac output that is quite acceptable under a varied range of activities. *B.* In the same patient during an acute ischemic attack, the sudden-onset left ventricular dysfunction and decreased compliance acutely alter the ventricular function curve so that a PWP of 15 mm Hg is required to optimize left ventricular performance. Note that even at that increased level of preload, maximum cardiac output is far less than under normal circumstances and may be inadequate for many activities.

Because myocardial oxygen consumption increases in direct proportion to peak intramyocardial systolic pressure, an increase in ventricular end-diastolic volume will increase the radius of the ventricle, its intramyocardial systolic pressure, and oxygen consumption. Thus, ventricular dilatation, secondary to heart failure, can significantly increase myocardial work and oxygen consumption in the patient with cardiovascular disease. An unfavorable shift in the Laplace relationship may be a factor in rendering the clinically stable patient unstable or the unstable patient more unstable as a result of increasing myocardial oxygen demand in a circumstance where a compensatory increase in oxygen supply is not possible (coronary artery disease).

Often, a change in one or more of the above variables renders the patient unstable. In the clinical setting, this may be due to hypovolemia, acute ischemic attacks, ventricular ectopy, systemic or pulmonary hypertension, and/or emotional or physiologic stress. Only by removing or correcting the inciting event and instituting therapy to optimize ventricular performance can improved cardiac performance and tissue perfusion be attained.

HEART FAILURE

Any form of cardiovascular disease or dysfunction can ultimately result in heart failure. Heart failure may be defined as a pathologic state in which an abnormality in cardiovascular function renders the heart unable to pump out blood at a rate equal to body requirements, provided that there is normal venous return to the heart.

Although anatomically one organ, functionally the heart is two distinct pumps serving two distinct circulations. The *right heart* (right atrium and right ventricle) receives systemic venous deoxygenated blood and pumps it through the pulmonary circulation. The *left heart* (left atrium and left ventricle) receives pulmonary venous oxygenated blood and pumps it into the systemic circulation. Even though both ventricles share the intraventricular septum, one ventricle typically fails before the other. The terms *left heart* or *left sided* and *right heart* or *right sided* failure are used to designate the side of the heart that is primarily impaired or that produces the predominance of physical signs and symptoms.

Left Heart Failure

Heart failure most commonly begins with the left heart because valvular and ischemic disease, as well as hypertension, most frequently affect the left heart and arterial circulation.

Forward failure refers to the decrease in the left ventricular output, which results in systemic underperfusion. This can be related to specific organ systems. In the gastrointestinal tract, this is manifest clinically and pathophysiologically as anorexia, indigestion, and poor absorption of nutrients; in the kidneys as salt and water retention; and in skin and skeletal muscle as pallor, weakness, tiredness, cool extremities, and exercise intolerance. In response to the decrease in cardiac output, the peripheral arterioles constrict to maintain mean arterial pressure and adequate cerebral and coronary perfusion pressure. In extreme cases, however, systemic perfusion may be impaired so severely that the patient goes into shock.

Backward failure, the congestive component of left heart failure, relates to the damming up of blood in the pulmonary circulation. This results in increased pulmonary vascular pressures, pulmonary vascular congestion, and interstitial and alveolar edema. Clinically, backward failure manifests as dyspnea, tachypnea, breathlessness, hypoxemia, cough, and crackles and wheezes on auscultation. Ultimately, the right ventricle will have to develop a higher systolic pressure to empty into the higher-pressure pulmonary circulation. It may adequately meet this pressure demand until right ventricular afterload exceeds its physiologic capacity and right ventricular failure ensues.

Right Heart Failure

When referring to the right heart, the term *forward failure* relates to decreased forward blood flow, which results in decreased pulmonary blood flow and decreased left ventricular filling. This, in turn, may reduce the output of the left ventricle. Left heart failure is the most common cause of right heart failure, and the dyspnea of pulmonary edema may be somewhat relieved as the right ventricular output falls and pulmonary vascular congestion diminishes. The sign and symptom complex relating to *backward* or congestive failure of the right heart relates to physical changes that occur secondary to elevated volume and pressure in the systemic veins and capillaries. The visible veins, especially the external jugular veins, become distended. The liver becomes enlarged and tender, and extravasation of fluid from the systemic capillaries, which are now under back pressure, causes ascites and systemic edema.

When either ventricle fails, its diastolic volume increases because it cannot pump out all the blood it receives. Stroke volume, therefore, may increase somewhat by the Starling effect.

Since both ventricles are part of a continuous and closed circuit and share a common septum, it is obvious that in the absence of anatomic abnormalities, the right or left ventricle cannot pump more or less blood than the other ventricle for any significant amount of time. Because of this ventricular functional and anatomic interdependence, pure failure of one side of the heart will ultimately produce hemodynamic and anatomic abnormalities in the contralateral ventricle, resulting in bilateral ventricular dysfunction.

Effects of Heart Failure on Hemodynamic Parameters

In the circulation distal to the failing ventricle, the pulse pressure is generally narrowed (reflecting a decreased stroke volume). The levels of systolic and diastolic pressure are variable depending on vascular resistance in the receiving circulation and the severity of cardiac dysfunction. Typically, venous pressure is elevated (congestive component of failure) proximal to the failing chamber.

The anticipated hemodynamic profile specific to each form of heart disease is outlined in the individual sections on each defect

The Ejection Fraction

The ventricles do not empty completely with each heart beat. In a normal person in the recumbent position, the ratio of stroke volume to ventricular end-diastolic volume is approximately 65 ± 8%. This value is termed the *ejection fraction*. For example, a patient with a ventricular end-diastolic volume of 110 ml and a stroke volume of 70 ml will have an ejection fraction of 64%. This angiographically calculated value is considered to be the most useful index of ventricular function. Increased contractility typically increases the stroke volume and ejection fraction, whereas heart disease usually reduces stroke volume and ejection fraction.

ISCHEMIC HEART DISEASE

Ischemic heart disease is characterized by physiologic changes in the myocardium caused by a deficiency in arterial blood supply. This entity encompasses a wide pathophysiologic spectrum ranging from transient, reversible myocardial ischemia to permanent, irreversible myocardial damage and necrosis.

Causes. Ischemic heart disease usually results from atherosclerotic lesions that obstruct normal coronary artery blood flow. The major causes of myocardial ischemia are listed in Table 16–1. The primary defect in each is a deficiency in myocardial oxygen supply.

Ischemic heart disease resulting from coronary atherosclerosis is the most common cause of heart disease in the industrialized world. It most often becomes clinically significant during middle age, and men are more vulnerable than women. The major risk factors for ischemic heart disease include family history, hypertension, diabetes mellitus, smoking, defects in lipid metabolism, and emotional factors. Obesity, a sedentary lifestyle and a diet high in cholesterol and saturated fats have also been implicated.

Pathophysiology. The normally functioning myocardium requires an adequate oxygen supply to meet its metabolic demands. These demands vary considerably depending on the workload imposed upon the myocardium by

TABLE 16–1. Major Causes of Myocardial Ischemia

Obstructive coronary atherosclerosis
Aortic valvular disease
Hypertrophic cardiomyopathy
Coronary embolism
Inflammatory disease of the coronary arteries
Congenital anomalies of the coronary circulation
Coronary vasoconstriction or spasm
Severe hypotension
Rapid ventricular rate

exercise, emotional disturbances, fever, infection, or any physiologic or psychologic stress. Since the myocardium extracts 70 to 80% of the oxygen from its arterial blood at rest, increased myocardial oxygen needs can be met only by increased coronary blood flow mediated by coronary vasodilation. Coronary artery disease may impose severe limits to increasing coronary blood flow in times of stress and additionally may produce critical reductions in flow at rest (coronary artery spasm, thrombosis, atheromatous obstruction). Should the myocardial oxygen supply/demand equation become imbalanced, compensatory mechanisms—including local autoregulatory changes (dilatation of the vasculature distal to the lesion), the development of a collateral circulation, and anaerobic metabolism—attempt to maintain the viability of the myocardium. Nevertheless these mechanisms may not contribute significantly to maintaining myocardial function and tissue viability. For example, autoregulatory mechanisms may not be of further benefit in the setting of an acute ischemic attack since the vasculature of the ischemic bed may have been already maximally dilated as a result of chronic obstruction of a coronary artery. The development of a collateral circulation may provide increased myocardial blood flow, but the extent of development varies among individuals and is known to be a long-range (not acute) adaptation to chronic coronary artery disease. Anaerobic metabolism is not only inefficient but ineffective in maintaining tissue viability because the myocardium can metabolize anaerobically for only a few minutes before severe functional deficits and profound metabolic changes occur.

The force of myocardial contraction relates directly to myocardial oxygen availability. For example, with a 10% reduction in coronary blood flow, the myocardium continues to contract but with slightly less force. With a 50% reduction in coronary blood flow, the force of contraction is markedly weaker, and the myocardium begins to produce lactic acid. With an 80% reduction in coronary blood flow, the myocardium essentially ceases to contract—a condition appropriately termed *the ischemic freeze* or *ischemic paralysis*. The metabolic changes in myocardial cells that produce these functional derangements occur within 10 to 30 seconds of the reduction in oxygenated blood flow.

Hemodynamic Effects. Systolic as well as diastolic abnormalities leading to severe hemodynamic derangements may occur if the ischemic area is sufficiently large or the ischemic episode is sufficiently profound.

Systolic Abnormalities. In the ischemic involved area, some muscle fibers are not contracting at all (akinesis) while others at the periphery of the ischemic zone are contracting with reduced force (hypokinesis). Weakness or paralytic loss of a functional portion of the myocardium results in an overall diminution in the heart's pumping capabilities and predisposes to heart failure. The remaining adequately perfused ventricle continues to contract, although some of that contractile force is dissipated into pushing blood into the nonfunctional ventricular wall segment, which then bulges outward in systole. This abnormal wall motion (dyskinesis) further impairs pump function and predisposes to heart failure (Fig. 16–2).

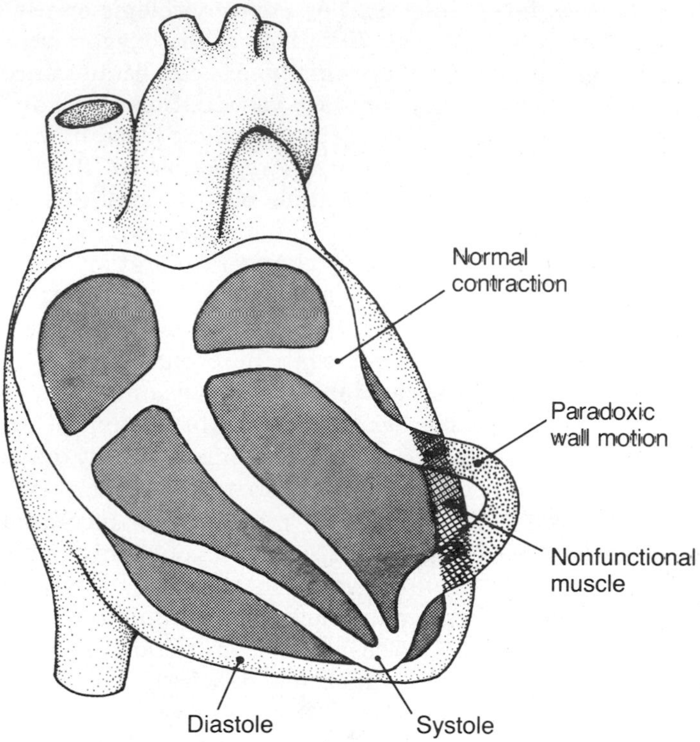

FIGURE 16–2. Abnormal wall motion in acute myocardial infarction. Note the systolic paradoxical outward bulging of the ischemic involved area of myocardium.

Diastolic Abnormalities. The ischemic myocardial fibers become swollen, stiff, and nonyielding. This results in reduced compliance of the ventricle, which interferes with normal diastolic filling. The end-diastolic volume/end-diastolic pressure relationship is thus distorted; for any ventricular filling volume, the ventricular filling pressure will be increased. Whereas the measured PWP may be in the normal range (4 to 12 mm Hg), the intraventricular volume at end-diastole may be inadequate to stretch the normal muscle fibers sufficiently to maintain adequate stroke volume. For this reason, most patients with acute myocardial ischemia require a PWP of 15 to 18 mm Hg to maintain a normal cardiac output.

Compensatory mechanisms attempt to maintain cardiac function and mean arterial blood pressure. The sympathetic nervous system becomes strongly excited and stimulates the remaining normal ventricular muscle mass to increase its work. Unfortunately, this also increases its oxygen consumption in proportion to its increased work load and threatens ischemic injury to this tissue. Mean arterial pressure is maintained by vasoconstriction induced by the sympathetic nervous system, at the price of increasing left ventricular afterload and oxygen consumption. This may worsen the ischemic process. An ischemic myocardium is electrically unstable and prone to arrhythmia. The increased circulating catecholamine levels further increase the arrhythmogenic potential. Indeed, many patients with coronary artery disease die of ventricular fibrillation without having suffered any permanent damage to the myocardium.

If the acutely ischemic myocardium is reperfused within 20 minutes and the oxygen debt is paid, there is no permanent damage to the myocardial cells.

Angina Pectoris

Angina pectoris is pain due to transient myocardial ischemia. It is typically, but not always, brought on by physical stress or strong emotional stimuli and is relieved by rest.

HEMODYNAMIC PROFILE

Arterial Pressure (Table 16–2). This value may fall if there is a significant drop in cardiac output but is more likely to be normal or elevated due to sympathetic nervous system stimulation.

TABLE 16–2. General Anticipated Direction of Change in Hemodynamic Parameters

Disorder	*Arterial Pressure*	*Pulse Pressure*	*Systemic Vascular Resistance*	*Pulmonary Vascular Resistance*	*Central Venous Pressure*	*Pulmonary Artery Pressure*	*Pulmonary Wedge Pressure*	*Cardiac Output*	SvO_2
Angina pectoris	~↑	~↓	↑	~	~	↑	↑	~↓	~↓
Acute myocardial infarction	↓~↑	~↓	↑	~	↓~↑	↓~↑	↓~↑	~↓	~↓
Ventricular septal defect	~↓	~↓	↑	↑	↑	↑	↑	↓	↓
Right ventricle infarction	~↓	~↓	↑	~	↑	~↓	~↓	↓	↓
Mitral stenosis	~	↓	~↑	↑	~↑	↑	↑	~↓	↓
Mitral regurgitation									
Chronic	~	~	~	~	~	↑	↑	~	~
Acute	~↓	↓	↑	↑	↑	↑	↑	↓	↓
Aortic stenosis	~	~↓	~↑	~↑	~↑	~↑	~↑	~↓	~↓
Aortic regurgitation									
Compensated, chronic	↑	↑	~↓	~	~	~	~↑	~	~
Decompensated, chronic	↑	↓↑	~↑	↑	↑	↑	↑	↓	↓
Acute	~	↓↑	↑	↑	~↑	↑	↑	↓	↓
Cardiac tamponade	~↓	↓	↑	~↑	↑	↑	↑	~↓	↓
Dilated cardiomyopathy	~	↓	↑	~↑	↑	↑	↑	~↓	↓

KEY: ↑, Increase; ↓, decrease; ~, no change.

NOTE: The magnitude or direction of change can be modified by coexisting factors or complications (hypovolemia, fluid overload, severity of the primary problem, adequacy of compensatory mechanisms).

Systemic Vascular Resistance. This parameter is likely to be elevated and reflects the vasoconstriction mediated by sympathetic nervous system stimulation.

Pulmonary Vascular Resistance. There is typically no significant change.

CVP or Right Atrial Pressure. These values may be expected to be in the normal range.

Pulmonary Artery and Wedge Pressures. These values tend to increase, reflecting the increased left ventricular end-diastolic pressure associated with the decreased ventricular compliance and stroke volume that occur in conjunction with an acute ischemic attack.

PWP Waveform. Because atrial contraction makes a large contribution to the filling of the stiff, failing ventricle, the atrial *a* wave may be of increased amplitude. In this circumstance, the mean PWP will be lower than left ventricular end-diastolic pressure. Therefore, the PWP *a* wave pressure correlates more closely with pressure in the left ventricle at end-diastole.

Cardiac Output. This measurement may be reduced or may be maintained in the normal range by compensatory tachycardia.

Mixed Venous Oxygen Saturation (SvO_2). This value will be reduced if perfusion failure complicates the anginal attack.

Clinical Presentation

The patient with typical angina pectoris complains of chest pain or discomfort usually brought on by physical stress or emotion. In some cases, however, the discomfort may be brought on by relatively nonstrenuous activities or may even occur at rest. The intensity of the discomfort is variable and can range from a vague sensation of pressure to intolerable pain; the character may be described as a heaviness, pressure, choking, or a tight sensation in the retrosternal region. The discomfort may also radiate to or be limited to the shoulder, arm, throat, jaws, teeth, back, or abdomen. The pain or discomfort usually lasts from 3 to 5 minutes, rarely lasts longer than 20 minutes, and is usually relieved by nitroglycerin or rest. The patient usually remains immobile as any activity increases the discomfort; however, some patients merely slow their activity to obtain relief whereas others become restless.

Mentation. There is usually no change in mentation but the patient may appear anxious. The painful episode may be associated with periods of weakness or dizziness.

Cutaneous. The skin color may be unchanged. If the anginal attack is associated with significant perfusion failure, the skin may be pale, cyanotic, cool, and diaphoretic.

Heart Rate and Character of Pulse. The heart rate is usually elevated above the patient's norm. The pulse may also be irregular due to ectopic beats.

Heart Sounds. When left ventricular compliance is decreased and left ventricular diastolic volume and pressure are increased, the active and rapid filling phases of the ventricle result in increased distending forces. Therefore, atrial systole and the rapid ventricular filling phase may result in an audible and palpable S_4 and S_3 respectively. It must be remembered that an atrial contraction (sinus rhythms, some atrial rhythms) is required for the production of a fourth heart sound. There may also be a transient mitral regurgitant systolic murmur.

Palpation of the Precordium. The third and fourth heart sounds may be palpable. This feature helps distinguish them from the S_3 and S_4 sounds sometimes heard in normal people that are not associated with precordial movements. There may also be a palpable abnormality in left ventricular wall motion, which the examiner perceives as a distinct double impulse separated by a few centimeters.

Neck Veins. Examination of the jugular veins is typically unremarkable.

Respiratory Rate and Character of Breathing. The anginal patient is usually tachypneic and may also be dyspneic.

Lung Sounds. The lungs are typically clear to auscultation.

Acid/Base. Values are usually maintained within normal limits unless persistent perfusion failure produces metabolic acidosis.

Laboratory Exam

ECG. In ischemic disease, the ECG taken at rest with the patient free of pain is often normal. With acute ischemia, the ECG may remain normal or reveal peaked or inverted T waves as well as ST segment depression or elevation. With ischemic relief, the ST segment and T waves return to their normal position. Ventricular ectopy commonly accompanies an acute ischemic episode.

Echocardiogram. Transient wall motion abnormalities are noted.

Thallium Scan. Because thallium is taken up preferentially by nonischemic myocardial cells, areas of ischemia appear as *cold spots* on thallium scintigraphy.

Cardiac Catheterization. This is a useful diagnostic test since 15% of patients with chest pain have no significant coronary artery disease. This procedure helps to localize the site and extent of the lesion or lesions and additionally may help distinguish a fixed lesion from coronary artery spasm.

Treatment

The goals of therapy during an anginal attack are to optimize the balance of myocardial oxygen supply and demand, to prevent myocardial infarction, and to promote patient comfort. If it is deemed that the patient requires CCU admission (unstable angina), the patient is placed on bed rest with continuous ECG monitoring and frequent vital sign checks. Invasive hemodynamic monitoring is not usually required. The patient is kept NPO till stabilized

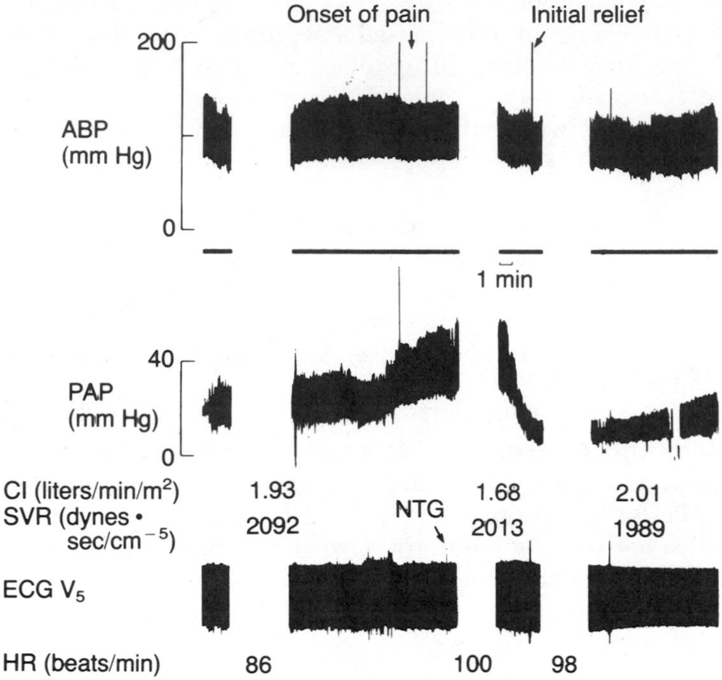

FIGURE 16–3. These simultaneous systemic and pulmonary arterial pressure tracings were obtained during an acute ischemic episode from a patient with resting angina. The level of arterial systolic and diastolic pressure remained unremarkable throughout the ischemic episode. The first evidence of a change from the norm is the abrupt increase in pulmonary artery diastolic pressure (a close correlate of LVEDP) from approximately 15 mm Hg to greater than 25 mm Hg. This pressure increase relates to sudden-onset ventricular dysfunction or decreased compliance or both. The increase in pressure is then followed by the patient's complaint of chest pain; the pain was a relatively late symptom of the ischemic attack.

Owing to nitroglycerine-induced venodilation and decreased venous return to the heart (arrow), ventricular filling pressure, heart size, and myocardial oxygen consumption were reduced, and the patient obtained relief from pain. (Courtesy of H. J. C. Swan, M.D., Cedars-Sinai Medical Center, Los Angeles.)

since emergent cardiac catheterization and/or surgery may be indicated if the pain is not relieved by standard therapy or the patient's condition deteriorates.

Oxygen Therapy. Supplemental oxygen is advocated as a method of supplying more oxygen to the ischemic areas of myocardium.

Medications. Many pharmacologic agents are variably used in the management of angina pectoris.

NITRATES. Nitroglycerin is a mainstay of therapy for myocardial ischemia. The primary mode of action is as a venodilator, which promotes venous pooling. This produces an immediate reduction in preload and myocardial oxygen consumption (Fig. 16–3). The slight arterial dilator properties of the drug reduce systemic vascular resistance, thus facilitating left ventricular unloading. Coronary vasodilator properties may improve global as well as regional ventricular function.

BETA BLOCKING AGENTS. This group of drugs decreases myocardial oxygen consumption by decreasing heart rate, contractility, and arterial blood pressure. Because stroke volume may fall secondary to decreased contractility, the patient should be closely observed for the indications of congestive heart failure (weight gain, orthopnea, etc.).

CALCIUM CHANNEL BLOCKING AGENTS. These agents increase myocardial oxygen supply by decreasing coronary vasomotor tone and are particularly helpful in patients who are prone to coronary artery spasm. They also decrease myocardial oxygen consumption by reducing contractility and arterial blood pressure.

NARCOTICS. If the anginal pain is not relieved by nitrates, morphine sulfate is used for its analgesic, calming, and preload reducing effects.

ANTICOAGULANTS. Mini-dose heparin may be used to prevent thromboembolic events if the patient is being maintained on bed rest.

STOOL SOFTENERS. Stool softeners are prescribed because straining at stool is prohibited. The patient commonly is permitted to use the bedside commode as this is less taxing and stressful than the bedpan.

ANTIARRHYTHMIC AGENTS. Xylocaine (lidocaine) may be used to prevent or reduce the severity of ventricular arrhythmias.

Acute Myocardial Infarction

Acute myocardial infarction relates to acute myocardial necrosis due to ischemia. If adequate oxygenated blood flow is reestablished within 20 minutes of an ischemic event, normal myocardial cell metabolism and function return. However, if ischemia persists for the next 30 minutes to 2 hours, scattered cells begin to die within the blighted, ischemic zone and the infarct formation begins. By four to six hours following the onset of the ischemic attack, there is usually massive cellular necrosis with swelling and functional impairment of the tissue immediately surrounding the infarcted area. The actual rate of progression and extent of necrotic damage are related to the degree of coronary artery occlusion, the size of the involved vascular bed, the adequacy of existing collateral circulation, and the interplay of myocardial oxygen supply and demand. For example, if the patient is allowed to remain in pain, the arterial pressure remains elevated; if the patient is stressed psychologically or physiologically, myocardial oxygen demand further increases in excess of the fixed, reduced supply, and infarct formation will occur more rapidly and extensively.

The actual mechanism producing the reduction in coronary blood flow varies among individuals. A thrombus may occlude the artery at the site of the atheromatous lesion or hemorrhage may occur beneath the plaque. Coronary vasospasm or less severe increases in coronary vasomotor tone have also been implicated in acute myocardial infarction.

The ischemic process begins and is commonly most severe at the inner one third of the myocardium (subendocardium), because oxygen consumption is greatest in this area. In addition, systolic compression of the penetrating coronary artery branches is greatest in the subendocardium, thus preventing systolic blood flow. In addition, intramyocardial diastolic pressure (influenced by ventricular diastolic pressure) is greater than in any other area of myocardium. In other words, even under normal conditions the vulnerable subendocardium consumes the most oxygen but gets the least oxygenated blood flow in systole or diastole. The infarct may be limited to just the subendocardium or may move, like a wave front, toward the epicardium until the ischemic damage involves the entire thickness of the muscle (transmural infarction).

It is theorized that in the fully developed acute myocardial infarction, three zones of functional and electrophysiologic abnormalities relate to the regional severity of oxygen deprivation. These are not sharply defined anatomic or functional areas but, rather, blend imperceptibly (Fig. 16–4).

The center area of *necrosis* receives no blood supply or so little blood supply that it is unable to sustain life. It is noncontractile, painless, and electrically inert. This is seen on the ECG leads oriented to this area as a deep or wide Q wave (Fig. 16–5). The area of *injury* immediately adjacent to the necrotic area is undergoing severe metabolic alterations, is noncontractile, and is potentially painful. The electrophysiologic instability of this area predisposes to ectopic arrhythmias. ECG leads oriented toward this area record S–T segment elevation. The area of *ischemia* surrounding the area of injury is undergoing less severe metabolic change and is likely poorly contractile, electrically unstable, and potentially painful. ECG leads oriented to the area of ischemia demonstrate T wave inversion.

The hemodynamic status of the individual patient relates to the size of the ischemic bed as well as the functional status of the noninvolved myocardium and heart valves. In the patient with preexisting heart disease or dysfunction, a relatively small infarct may precipitate a hemodynamic disaster.

The full spectrum of cardiac function in acute myocardial infarction, therefore, may range from essentially normal hemodynamic parameters and systemic perfusion to profound pump failure and cardiogenic shock.

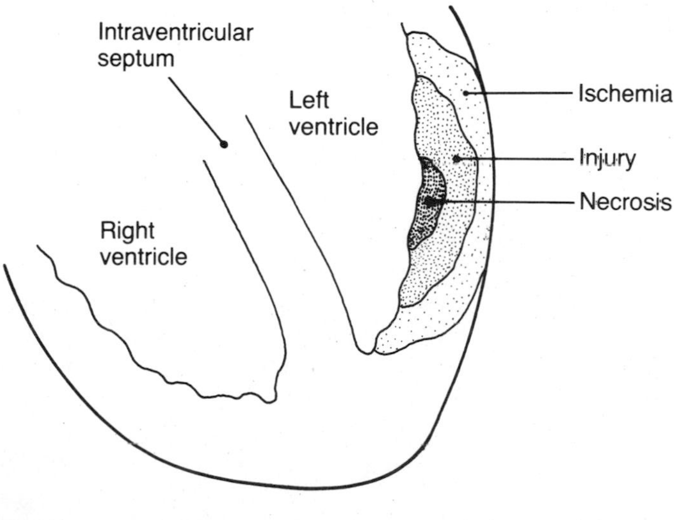

FIGURE 16–4. Zones of functional and electrophysiologic abnormalities in acute myocardial infarction.

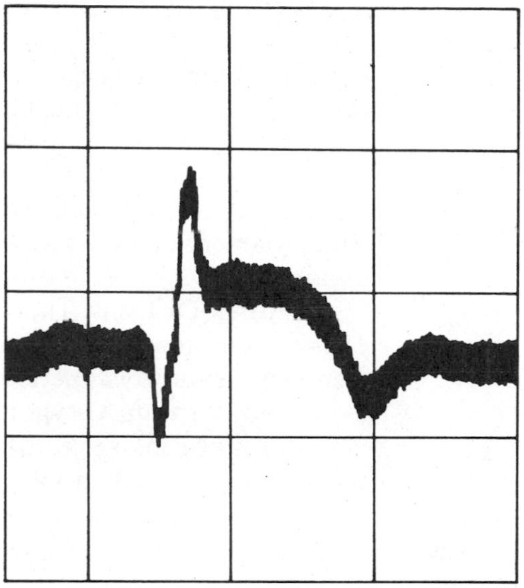

FIGURE 16–5. Electrocardiographic evidence of acute myocardial infarction. The Q wave reflects the area of necrosis, the ST segment elevation reflects the area of injury, and T wave inversion reflects the most peripheral area of ischemia. (With permission of Marriott HJL: *Practical Electrocardiography*, ed 7. Baltimore, Williams & Wilkins, 1983.)

HEMODYNAMIC PROFILE

Arterial Pressure (see Table 16–2). This value is variable. If blood catecholamine levels are very high secondary to sympathetic nervous system overdrive, the patient may be hypertensive. Values may also be relatively normal. If ventricular function and cardiac output are severely depressed, the patient will experience a significant drop in blood pressure. A small percentage of patients are hypovolemic due to nausea, vomiting, diaphoresis, diuretic overresponse, and/or hyperventilation. In this circumstance, a careful physical assessment and patient history or other hemodynamic parameters may disclose that the narrowed pulse pressure and perhaps hypotension are due to volume depletion.

If the force of left ventricular ejection and stroke volume fall, the rate of rise of the upstroke of the arterial pressure waveform is delayed and the pulse pressure is narrowed. This gives a damped appearance to the waveform. Pulsus alternans implies severe left ventricular dysfunction.

Systemic Vascular Resistance. This value is commonly elevated owing to sympathetic nervous system stimulation and/or reflex response to low cardiac output. A small percentage of patients with cardiogenic shock (see Chapter 14) exhibit an inappropriate vascular response to a drop in cardiac output. These people may not constrict sufficiently to maintain arterial blood pressure. Systemic vascular resistance may actually decrease.

Pulmonary Vascular Resistance. This value is usually normal unless hypoxemia or pulmonary edema complicates the clinical picture. In these circumstances, pulmonary vascular resistance will be elevated.

CVP or RA Pressure. Volume depletion will lower this value. In the presence of right ventricular failure, this value will be elevated.

Pulmonary Artery and Wedge Pressure. These values will be below normal if the patient is hypovolemic. Values will be normal in patients who maintain relatively normal ventricular function. In those with a significant reduction in ventricular compliance and ventricular failure, values will be elevated. In general, patients with elevated PWP tend to have more severe coronary artery disease and wall motion abnormalities than those with normal pulmonary artery wedge pressure.

Cardiac Output. This parameter will be maintained within normal limits in uncomplicated acute myocardial infarction but will be decreased when ventricular dysfunction or other abnormalities complicate the picture.

Mixed Venous Oxygen Saturation (SvO_2). This value is maintained in the normal range if cardiac output is maintained. Values fall relative to decreases in cardiac output.

Clinical Presentation

The character of acute myocardial infarction pain is the same as that of anginal pain, but the duration is more prolonged and may last for several hours until it spontaneously resolves or analgesics are given. The intensity of the pain may also be more severe, and it does not respond to two or more nitroglycerin tablets. The pain may also be associated with nausea, vomiting, or epigastric distress. However, 15 to 30% of myocardial infarction patients have no pain. They are most often blacks, diabetics, and patients with chronic atrial fibrillation and hypertension; why these particular groups of individuals tend to be pain-free is not known. Nevertheless, in these persons myocardial infarction may only be indicated with syncope, gastrointestinal upset, arrhythmias, extreme weakness or fatigue, or sudden onset of pulmonary edema.

Mentation. The level of mentation is typically normal, but patients are anxious during periods of pain and may also complain of lightheadedness. Changes in mentation occur relative to the severity of perfusion failure when present.

Cutaneous. Pallor and diaphoresis may be associated with the period of pain at the onset of myocardial infarction, although some patients maintain a normal complexion. Overall, the skin color and temperature are variable, depending on the absence or presence and severity of perfusion failure.

Heart Rate and Character of Pulse. Sinus tachycardia may be produced by fever, anxiety, heart failure, or hypovolemia. Sinus bradycardia may be present in patients with lesions of the right coronary artery. Arrhythmias or conduction disturbances commonly cause abnormalities in heart rate and rhythm. With significant heart failure, the pulses are of low volume.

Heart Sounds. An atrial gallop (S_4) is very frequently audible and, if failure is present, will be accompanied by a ventricular gallop (S_3). With weakened ventricular contractions, the heart sounds are muffled with dimin-

TABLE 16–3. The Killip Scale

Class	Description	Incidence (%)	Mortality (%)
I	No pulmonary rales or S_3	33	6
II	Bibasilar rales which persist after cough, and/or an S_3	38	17
III	Rales over one half of the lung fields, with pulmonary edema on chest radiography	10	38
IV	Pulmonary edema with cardiogenic shock	19	81

ished intensity of the first heart sound. A transient systolic regurgitant murmur may result from ischemic dysfunction of a papillary muscle.

Palpation of the Precordium. Rarely is the apical impulse completely normal in acute ischemic disease. The atrial gallop may be palpable. Failure and dilatation of the ventricle tend to displace the apex beat downward and to the left. A decreased force of the apex beat with an increased duration is also characteristic of left ventricular failure due to ischemic disease; the ventricular gallop may also be palpable. The examiner may also perceive regional abnormalities in wall motion (dyskinesis) as an extra impulse at a site a few centimeters away from the apex beat.

Neck Veins. If hypovolemia complicates acute myocardial infarction, the external jugular veins will be collapsed while the patient is in the supine position. In patients with severe left ventricular failure and secondary right ventricular involvement, the external jugular veins will be visibly distended. Ordinarily, the neck veins are unremarkable.

Respiratory Rate and Character of Breathing. Hyperventilation commonly accompanies pain. Otherwise, the rate and character of breathing are normal in the absence of pulmonary edema.

Lung Sounds. Breath sounds are normal unless left ventricular failure produces pulmonary edema. The severity of cardiac dysfunction in acute myocardial infarction may be classified according to the Killip scale, which relates auscultatory and radiographic findings to the severity of heart failure (Table 16–3).

Urine Output. Urine volume is typically well maintained unless the patient is in cardiogenic shock.

Acid/Base. If the patient is hyperventilating from anxiety, pain, or pulmonary edema, a mild-to-moderate respiratory alkalosis will be present. Severe perfusion failure results in metabolic acidosis.

Laboratory Examination

The diagnosis of acute myocardial infarction should be based on the clinical presentation and history, diagnostic enzyme levels, and ECG changes. These may be additionally supplemented by various other laboratory tests.

ECG. Although the ECG is fundamental in the diagnosis of acute myocardial infarction, certain pitfalls in its use must be emphasized. For example, T wave abnormalities may be delayed for over a week after the infarction; sometimes none of the typical changes develop. In addition, the papillary muscles, septum, atria and right ventricle may have significant damage but manifest no ECG changes. In addition, ST and T wave changes relate not only to acute infarction but to electrolyte abnormalities, medications, anxiety, hyperventilation, recent meal ingestion, and so on. Figure 16–5 illustrates the total constellation of typical ECG changes in a fully evolved acute myocardial infarction viewed by leads oriented to the infarcted area.

Chest Radiograph. In the absence of heart failure, the lung fields and heart size are normal. Cardiac enlargement and signs of pulmonary congestion secondary to left ventricular dysfunction may be present even when other clinical signs and symptoms of heart failure are absent. Diffuse pulmonary infiltrates are present with clinically overt pulmonary edema, although there is a known lag time from the appearance of monitored hemodynamic alterations (elevated PAP and PWP) to the appearance of radiographic evidence of pulmonary edema. Likewise, it may take from 12 to 48 hours for radiographic evidence of pulmonary edema to clear following normalization of hemodynamic parameters.

Echocardiogram. Paradoxic systolic expansion of the severely ischemic or necrotic area (dyskinesis) or reduced excursions (hypokinesis) of the less severely involved areas may be evident. In addition, any complications of acute myocardial infarction (papillary muscle rupture, ventricular septal defect) may be visualized on the echocardiogram.

Radionuclide Studies. Technetium scans are useful in confirming the diagnosis of acute myocardial infarction. The isotope is taken up by acutely damaged myocardial cells and results in a *hot spot*. The scan becomes positive within 12 to 36 hours after the infarct and remains positive for six to ten days. Radionuclide ventriculograms define cardiac function by assessing wall motion. Gated cardiac blood pool imaging makes possible the noninvasive assessment of ventricular ejection fraction and the evaluation of ventricular wall motion.

Cardiac Catheterization. In selected cases, visualization of the coronary anatomy helps guide therapy by localizing the site and extent of the coronary lesion or lesions. Depending on the facilities available at a given institution or nearby hospital, the use of percutaneous transluminal coronary angioplasty (PTCA) or thrombolytic agents may be considered. The need for emergency surgery, as in the case of left main coronary artery disease, may be more carefully defined. In addition, coronary vasospasm may be ruled out.

Serum Enzymes and Other Laboratory Studies. Serum enzymes—including creatine phosphokinase (CPK), serum glutamic oxaloacetic transaminase (SGOT), and lactic dehydrogenase (LDH)—are elevated in 90% of patients with acute myocardial infarction. The isoenzyme of CPK (CPK-MB) is considered to be the best laboratory parameter for the diagnosis of acute myocardial infarction. For values and time references of these enzymes, refer

TABLE 16–4. Serum Enzymes in Myocardial Infarction

Enzyme	Onset of Elevation (Hrs)	Peak Elevation	Return to Normal (Days)
CPK	6–12	24 hours	3–4
SGOT	8–12	36 hours	3–4
LDH	24–48	3–6 days	8–14

to Table 16–4 and Figure 16–6. These levels should be obtained on admission, every eight hours for 24 hours, and then daily.

The white blood cell count and sedimentation rate will be elevated in acute myocardial infarction by the second day. The degree of elevation is related to the extent of myocardial damage and to the degree of inflammation present. The hematocrit often rises slightly. The blood sugar should initially be elevated as part of the normal sympathoadrenal (stress) response.

TREATMENT

The goals of therapy in acute myocardial infarction are to limit infarct size, promote electrical stability, promote patient comfort, and prevent complications. As in angina pectoris, some of these goals are accomplished with bed rest, morphine analgesia, anticoagulation, and supplemental oxygen. In a few cases, additional pharmacologic or mechanical interventions are required to optimize cardiac function and prevent complications. These interventions relate to the manipulation of preload, afterload, and contractility

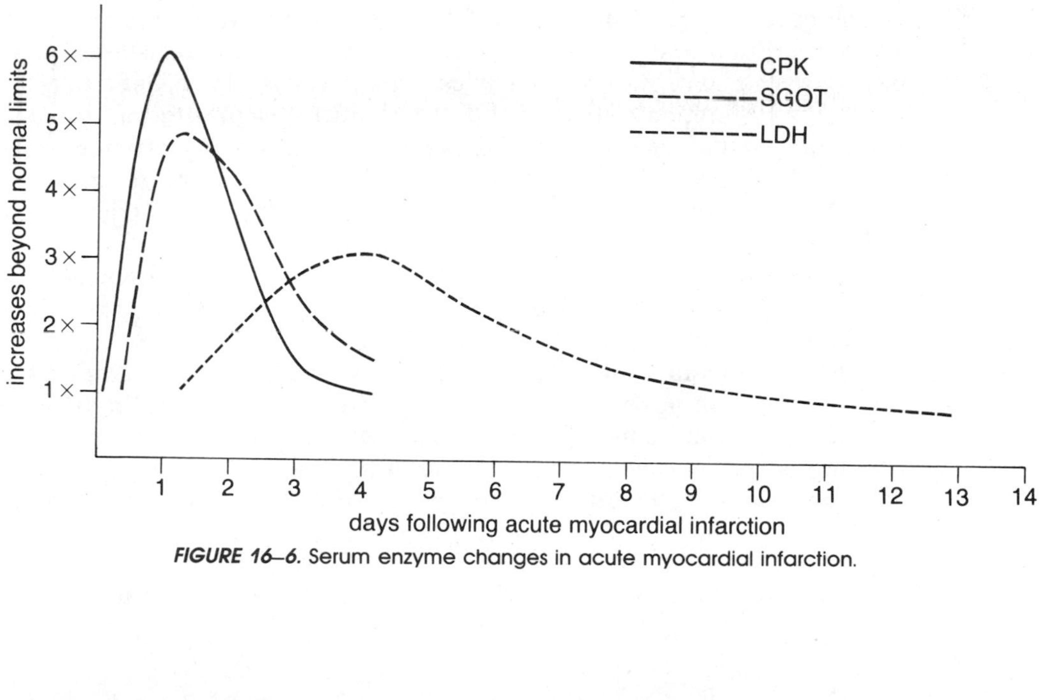

FIGURE 16–6. Serum enzyme changes in acute myocardial infarction.

(the primary determinants of heart work and oxygen consumption). In most cases, the safe and efficacious use of these pharmacologic and mechanical interventions mandates the use of invasive hemodynamic monitoring.

Antiarrhythmic Therapy. Some physicians prefer to prescribe a lidocaine infusion routinely on all CCU admission as prophylaxis against ventricular arrhythmias and sudden cardiac death. If the patient is not receiving lidocaine, a syringe filled with 100 mg of lidocaine should be at the patient's bedside for at least the first two to three days after the acute infarction.

Preload Reduction. By decreasing the volume of blood brought to the left ventricle, ventricular size and oxygen consumption are reduced. In addition, if the PWP is greater than 20 mm Hg, aggressive preload reduction is necessary to prevent or treat pulmonary edema. The primary effect of furosemide (Lasix) on preload reduction is by venodilation. This effect is achieved within the first five minutes of administration and results in the pooling of significant amounts of blood in the systemic veins. Secondarily, its diuretic effect reduces preload by reducing the circulating blood volume. Additional preload-reducing agents are nitroglycerin (sublingual, topical, intravenous drip) given to maintain a level of preload (as measured by PWP) that provides the maximum reduction of pain with the least reduction in cardiac output. When stroke volume and cardiac output are low due to inadequate ventricular filling, preload may have to be increased by volume infusion—for example, 50 to 100 ml of normal saline infused over a 15-minute period with close clinical and hemodynamic evaluation.

Afterload Reduction. A reduction in systemic vascular resistance, accomplished by the administration of arterial dilator agents, reduces the impedance to left ventricular ejection. Consequent to the vasodilator effect, stroke volume is increased and myocardial oxygen consumption is reduced. An increase in cardiac output up to 25% (relative to the functional state of the myocardium and original level of systemic vascular resistance) may be anticipated in some patients. Afterload reduction is also beneficial in acute myocardial infarction complicated by acute mitral regurgitation or an acute ventricular septal defect. In these cases, a reduction in systemic vascular resistance improves forward systemic blood flow and decreases regurgitant flow (acute mitral regurgitation) or left-to-right shunt (ventricular septal defect).

Inotropic Agents. Agents that improve contractility, thereby enhancing ventricular emptying and systemic blood flow, may be required. These include dopamine, dobutamine, and amrinone.

Other Pharmacologic Agents. It has been suggested that administering infusions containing potassium chloride, glucose, and insulin (polarizing solutions) may reduce infarct size and the incidence of arrhythmias. However, evidence is not yet conclusive that this therapeutic intervention is beneficial.

The Intra-Aortic Balloon Pump (IABP). (See Chapter 14, Treatment of Cardiogenic Shock.) If other measures do not *quickly* stabilize the patient and relieve pain, the IABP should be strongly considered. Balloon counterpulsation augments arterial pressure during diastole, thereby increasing coronary perfusion pressure and coronary blood flow. In ventricular systole, afterload reduction eases ventricular ejection and improves systemic perfusion. Cardiac function may improve 30 to 50%. Therefore, the patient is hemodynamically stabilized and pain is either completely or greatly relieved. The IABP is additionally helpful in stabilizing the patient during cardiac catheterization and induction to anesthesia, and during and following any required surgical interventions (aortocoronary bypass surgery, repair of a ventricular septal defect, and so on).

Surgical Intervention. Although controversy exists regarding indications for aortocoronary bypass grafting, there is general agreement that it is indicated for left main coronary artery disease, triple vessel disease, refractoriness to medical therapy, and IABP dependence in a patient with an operable coronary anatomy. In the emergency setting, if bypass surgery is performed within the first four hours of the onset of pain of myocardial infarction, there may be substantial salvage of functional myocardium.

COMPLICATIONS OF ACUTE MYOCARDIAL INFARCTION

Complications may occur at any time in the peri- and postinfarction period but are most common in the initial seven to ten days after the acute event. Arrhythmias (supraventricular, ventricular, and conduction defects) are very common and may be controlled by measures directed at restoring physiologic stability. These include the correction of electrolyte imbalances, provision of adequate systemic and myocardial oxygenation, reduction of sympathetic nervous system stimulation, and reduction in myocardial and total body oxygen requirements. Antiarrhythmic agents and/or pacing may be additionally required. Heart failure generally portends a poor prognosis and correlates with the proportion of ventricular muscle mass that has become nonfunctional. Less than 25% death or dysfunction of the left ventricular muscle mass generally does not produce signs or symptoms of heart failure during hospitalization. If heart failure is present, diuretic and unloading agents as well as inotropic support of the heart may provide symptomatic relief.

Mechanical complications of acute myocardial infarction may range from those that produce minor hemodynamic dysfunction to those that are immediately fatal. Four types of mechanical complications can occur.

Papillary Muscle Dysfunction or Rupture. Normal papillary muscle function is essential for proper coaptation (meeting and closure) of the mitral valve leaflets: therefore, ischemic dysfunction or rupture of the papillary muscle results in failure of normal systolic mitral valve closure and regurgitant flow (see Acute Mitral Regurgitation).

This complication more commonly affects the posterior papillary muscle because its only blood supply is from the posterior descending branch of the right coronary artery. The anterior papillary muscle has a dual circulation from the left anterior descending and circumflex arteries. Abnormalities in papillary muscle function, therefore, are more commonly associated with posterior or inferior wall infarctions.

Ischemic dysfunction may be transient and may only present during episodes of angina pectoris. Depending on the volume of regurgitant flow into the left atrium relative to forward flow into the aorta, symptoms may be mild or profound. Consequently, the patient may have baseline periods of hemodynamic stability punctuated by episodes of varying degrees of acute-onset hemodynamic deterioration with an accompanying sudden-onset systolic murmur.

Complete rupture should be suspected when acute pulmonary edema, shock, an apical thrill, and a high-pitched, holosystolic decrescendo murmur develop in a patient with a recent myocardial infarction. A large regurgitant orifice and poorly contractile ventricle may make the murmur inaudible and thus prevent its detection. Complete rupture is an absolute surgical emergency as rapid clinical deterioration and death (mortality greater than 50% by 24 hours) can be anticipated. Rapid diagnosis therefore is essential and lifesaving if followed by valve replacement or repair.

Medical management is directed at reducing or eliminating the regurgitant stream and increasing systemic perfusion. Reduction in left ventricular volume (preload) reduces the regurgitant orifice size. Reduction in resistance to left ventricular outflow (afterload) enhances forward blood flow and systemic perfusion. A balanced venous and arterial dilator such as nitroprusside, administered by careful hemodynamic monitoring, may help stabilize the patient prior to surgery or during a period of severe, transient mitral valve dysfunction. The IABP may be used additionally to reduce left ventricular outflow resistance while augmenting aortic diastolic pressure and coronary blood flow. Dobutamine, the inotrope of choice, may be used to further improve left ventricular performance without increasing systemic vascular resistance.

Acute Ventricular Septal Defect. Rupture of the intraventricular septum is a potentially lethal event that may complicate anterior or inferior wall infarctions within two to ten days of the acute event.

During systole, left ventricular blood that is 97 to 99% saturated with oxygen is shunted through the ventricular septal defect into the right ventricle (Fig. 16–7). There it is added to and mixes with systemic venous deoxygenated blood. Thus an increased volume of blood with an increased oxygen saturation flows into the pulmonary circulation. Flow overload of the pulmonary circulation and left heart predisposes to pulmonary edema. At the same time, however, systemic perfusion failure occurs because a decreased volume of blood is ejected by the left ventricle into the general circulation. The volume of the shunted blood and the severity of the hemodynamic abnormality depend on the size of the defect and the systolic pressure difference between the two ventricles.

Hemodynamic deterioration is sudden in onset and often relentless. Initially, the arterial pressure is normal but progressively falls relative to decreasing left ventricular outflow. Right atrial pressure is typically markedly elevated as are right ventricular and pulmonary artery pressures. The PWP

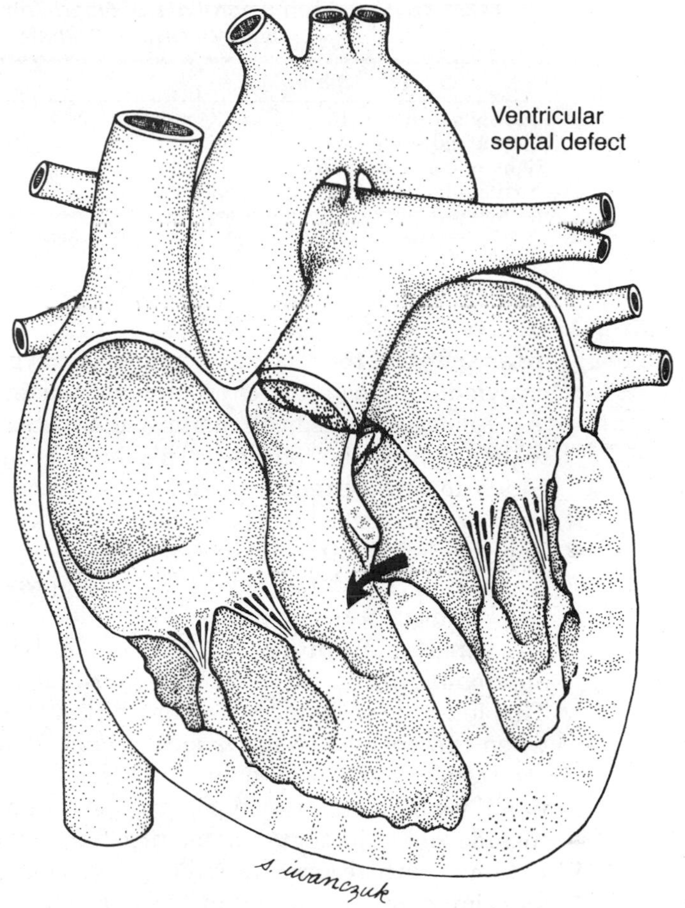

FIGURE 16–7. Flow abnormality in ventricular septal defect.

is additionally elevated and, although the PWP waveform usually appears normal, in a small number of patients it may be distorted by large *v* waves. These are produced by the increased systolic volume of blood entering the normal left atrium via the pulmonary circulation from the acute left-to-right shunt.

The clinical picture may be indistinguishable from that of acute, severe mitral regurgitation. Acute pulmonary edema, low cardiac output progressing to shock, and a pansystolic decrescendo murmur are common to both. In acute ventricular septal defect, however, the murmur is most audible at the lower sternal border and may be accompanied by a palpable thrill over the same area. The pulmonary artery catheter is a very helpful tool in differentiating acute mitral regurgitation from acute ventricular septal defect. Patients with the latter have an oxygen saturation step up in excess of 5% from blood gas samples obtained from the right atrium to the right ventricle or pulmonary

TABLE 16–5. Oxygen Saturations of Blood Samples Drawn During Flotation of a Pulmonary Artery Catheter in Acute U.S.D.

Sample	%
Arterial saturation drawn from the radial artery	96
Right atrial sample	71
Right ventricular sample	87
Proximal pulmonary artery sample	89

artery. Table 16–5 is an example of oxygen saturations of blood samples drawn during flotation of a pulmonary artery catheter.

Emergency medical therapy is directed toward reducing the impedance to left ventricular outflow. This may be accomplished with nitroprusside, which lowers systemic vascular resistance, thus improving left ventricular outflow and reducing the severity of the shunt. Dobutamine may further improve left ventricular performance without increasing systemic vascular resistance. Additional hemodynamic improvement may be achieved with the IABP. Surgical repair of the defect affords an excellent long-term survival.

Cardiac Rupture. Rupture of the left ventricular free wall occurs in approximately 3% of acute transmural acute myocardial infarction patients. This lethal event typically occurs within the first ten days of the acute infarct when the necrotic tissue is most friable. The rupture occurs at the border of the transmural infarction because the area between the normal and dysfunctional myocardium is the point of maximum stress. Patients at greatest risk include older patients; women; patients with sustained hypertension; and patients with recurrent, severe chest pain. This catastrophic event may be associated with straining at stool or by other sudden physical stress such as coughing or sneezing.

The rate of progression and severity of symptoms are determined by the rate and volume of blood flow into the pericardial sac. The hemodynamic profile and clinical presentation are nearly identical to those of cardiac tamponade. The patient is hypotensive and has elevated venous pressures, distended neck veins, dyspnea, distant heart sounds, equalization of right and left heart pressures in diastole, and pulsus paradoxus. Sudden-onset sinus bradycardia followed by a junctional or idioventricular rhythm and decreased amplitude QRS complexes may precede electromechanical dissociation and death. Emergency surgery may save the patient's life if blood loss into the pericardium is slow and myocardial performance has not been severely compromised.

Right Ventricular Infarction. The right coronary artery supplies vessels to both the inferior wall of the left ventricle and the right ventricular wall. Total occlusion of the right coronary artery, therefore, produces right ventricular infarction in most patients, and estimates suggest occurrence rates of between 19 and 43% in all patients with inferior wall myocardial infarction. The area of damage is generally the posterior right ventricular wall, but in a small number of cases the damage also involves the anterolateral wall. Isolated ischemic damage to the right ventricle is rare. There is almost always a variable amount of damage to the inferior wall of the left ventricle as well.

The ischemia-damaged right ventricle is unable to generate sufficient power to drive adequate amounts of blood through the pulmonary circulation and fill the left ventricle. As a result, left ventricular stroke volume falls by the Starling effect. If left ventricular filling and performance are sufficiently depressed, the arterial pressure falls.

The rigid parietal pericardium limits outward expansion of the often massively dilated failing right ventricle, which then encroaches on the limited pericardial space and increases intrapericardial pressure. This may produce a hemodynamic profile similar to that of constrictive pericardial disease in which diastolic pressures of the right and left ventricle are equal. In less severe cases, right atrial and right ventricular end-diastolic pressures increase to levels greater than the left ventricular end-diastolic pressure, which may be low, normal, or elevated depending on the functional state of the left ventricle and adequacy of left ventricular filling. In addition, the intraventricular septum may shift toward the left ventricle reducing its internal size and altering the left ventricular diastolic volume/pressure relationship. Therefore, for any left ventricular filling volume (the determinant of end-diastolic fiber length and stroke volume), the left ventricular filling pressure, as measured by PWP, may be deceptively high.

The clinical spectrum of right ventricular infarction ranges from normal findings in patients with minimal right ventricular dysfunction to systemic hypotension, clear lungs, and marked jugular venous distention and venous hypertension in patients with a severely impaired right ventricle. The 12-lead ECG reflects damage to the inferior wall of the left ventricle. More specific information relating to the right ventricle may be obtained from right precordial leads such as V_{4R} whose lead position is identical to that of V_4, but which is recorded on the right chest.

Since the left ventricle is the prime mover of blood, treatment is directed toward increasing left ventricular filling so that cardiac output and arterial pressure are restored to acceptable levels. Intravascular volume is expanded until the PWP reaches 15 mm Hg or the arterial pressure and cardiac output normalize. This may require up to 6 liters of fluid over 24 hours. Inotropic agents—such as dobutamine, dopamine, amrinone—may be required when hypoperfusion persists after adequate volume loading. Some patients may respond favorably to agents that reduce right ventricular afterload, such as nitroprusside or nitroglycerin. By decreasing pulmonary vascular resistance, these agents favor passive filling from the right ventricle to the left side of the heart; however, they must be used very cautiously in patients whose systemic arterial pressure is marginal or low.

VALVULAR HEART DISEASE

The cardiac valves are responsible for maintaining unidirectional flow of blood through the cardiac circuit. Valvular heart disease describes cardiac dysfunction that results from structural and/or functional abnormalities of one or several cardiac valves. The valvular abnormality may result in regurgitation or stenosis. *Regurgitation* is the backflow or reflux of blood through an incompetent valve because it fails to close sufficiently. *Stenosis* is impairment to normal opening of a valve that results in obstruction to blood flow across the valve orifice.

Valve dysfunction may be pure (stenosis *or* regurgitation) or mixed (stenosis *and* regurgitation). Only one valve may be functionally abnormal, such as congenital aortic stenosis, or multiple valves may be involved, such as mitral and aortic dysfunction due to rheumatic fever. The more complex the value dysfunction and the more valves involved in any patient, the greater potential for hemodynamic compromise. In this chapter only pure valve lesions are discussed. Stenotic lesions are more common than regurgitant lesions, and aortic valvular disease is more common than mitral valvular disease. Tricuspid and pulmonic valvular disease is not common and will not be discussed.

Mitral Stenosis

Mitral stenosis is a valvular disorder in which there is obstruction to forward blood flow from the left atrium into the left ventricle owing to functional impairment of the valve and narrowing of the valve orifice. This results in an inability of the left atrium to empty and fill the left ventricle adequately.

CAUSES AND PATHOPHYSIOLOGY

The most common cause of mitral stenosis is rheumatic fever. Progressive inflammatory changes eventually cause scarring as well as fibrosis, fusion, and shortening of the chordae tendineae and distortion of the valve leaflets. Calcium, which may also be deposited on the valve leaflets, further impairs valve mobility. Altogether, these physical changes result in obstruction to blood flow across the mitral valve. Valve scarring and deformity occur slowly, so functional valve impairment sufficient to produce symptoms typically does not develop until 3 to 25 years after the episode of rheumatic fever. Less common causes of mitral stenosis include congenital abnormalities (seen commonly in infants and children), active infective endocarditis, carcinoid disease, and calcium accumulation in the mitral valve annulus (ring).

Hemodynamic Effects

In the normal heart, blood flows freely through the mitral valve through a principal orifice or several secondary orifices that lie between the chordae. Chordal fusion, calcium deposits, adhesions, or vegetations narrow or obliterate the secondary orifices and reduce the principal orifice size in mitral stenosis. As the valve orifice becomes significantly narrowed, obstruction to blood flow and a pressure gradient between the left atrium and left ventricle develop in diastole.

The severity of this pressure gradient can be demonstrated by simultaneous pressure measurements from the left atrium and ventricle obtained in a cardiac catheterization laboratory (Fig. 16–8). This pressure gradient may suddenly increase further if blood flow through the heart increases (exercise, emotional stress) and/or diastole is shortened (tachycardia, irregular heart rhythms). As the size of the pressure gradient increases, left atrial pressure

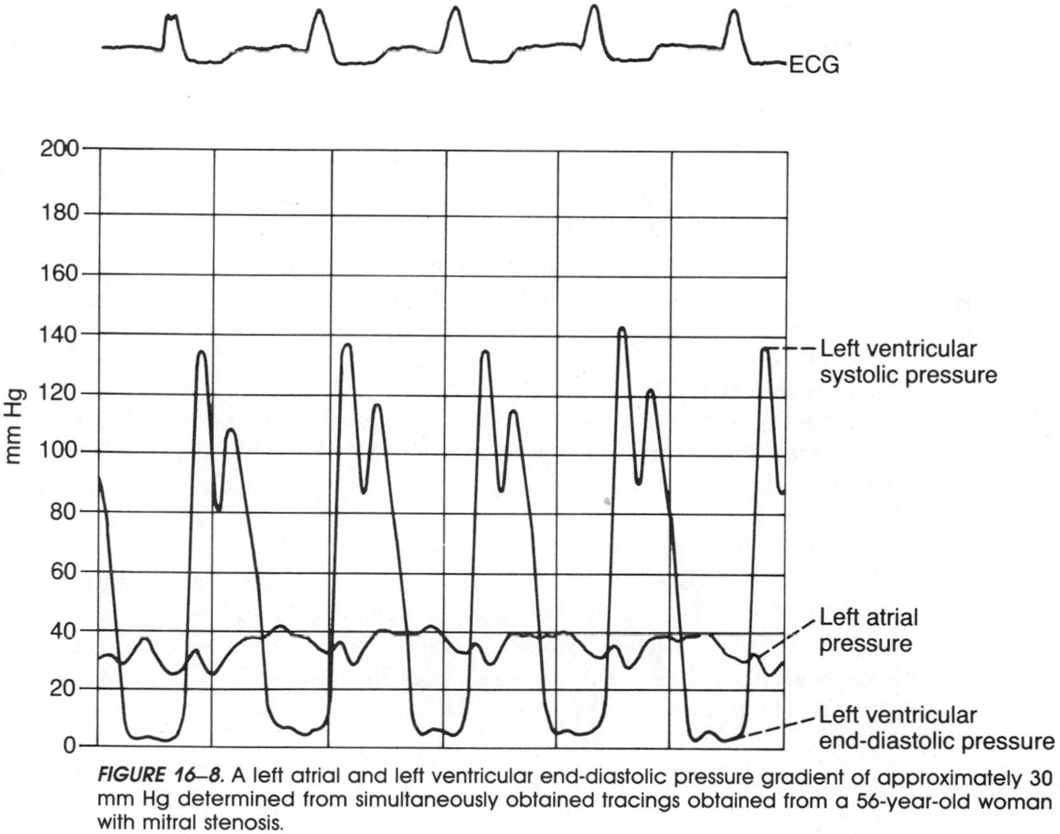

FIGURE 16–8. A left atrial and left ventricular end-diastolic pressure gradient of approximately 30 mm Hg determined from simultaneously obtained tracings obtained from a 56-year-old woman with mitral stenosis.

rises and left ventricular filling is reduced. The consequences of both are discussed below.

ELEVATED LEFT ATRIAL PRESSURE. Chronic elevation of left atrial pressure results in chronically increased pressures in the entire pulmonary circulation. A reduction in the mitral orifice size from the normal 4 to 5 cm^2 to less than 1 cm^2 (critical mitral stenosis) requires a left atrial pressure of approximately 25 mm Hg to maintain a normal cardiac output. Exercise or tachycardia results in greater sudden increases in left atrial pressure. The patient, therefore, is very predisposed to pulmonary edema, particularly upon exertion. However, with the progression of time and the severity of the stenosis, compensatory changes occur in the lung that elevate the threshold level necessary to produce pulmonary edema. These occur variably among individuals and include:

(1) The development of supernormal pulmonary lymph flow, which drains off the excess fluid entering the lung; (2) diminished permeability of the alveolar capillary membrane; and (3) hyperplasia and hypertrophy of the pulmonary arterioles, which then become capable of considerable amounts of spasm. Pulmonary capillary hydrostatic pressure (the prime determinant of fluid movement into the lung) is determined by the resistance to blood flow from the lung, as determined by pulmonary venous or left atrial pressure, and the amount of blood flowing into the pulmonary capillary bed. Therefore, pulmonary arteriolar constriction may reduce pulmonary blood flow to a level sufficient to protect against pulmonary edema. Pulmonary arteriolar constriction results in increased pulmonary vascular resistance and a widening of the pulmonary artery diastolic to pulmonary artery wedge pressure gradient.

Secondary to the increase in pulmonary artery pressures due to reactive constriction of the pulmonary arterioles and elevated left atrial pressure, the right ventricle hypertrophies and eventually fails. The patient then develops peripheral edema, fatigue, distention of the visible veins, and abdominal tenderness and swelling.

As the high-pressure left atrium progressively dilates, atrial fibrillation develops transiently and then permanently. Stasis of blood in the enlarged, fibrillating atrial chambers predisposes to clot formation along the atrial walls (mural thrombi). These may detach or fragment and produce pulmonary or systemic embolic problems.

REDUCTION IN LEFT VENTRICULAR FILLING. Cardiac output falls as left ventricular filling is impaired across the stenotic mitral valve. With time, the left ventricular cavity may become smaller and the muscular wall thinner. The decreased cardiac output causes a reduced tolerance to exercise and progressive weakness and fatigue.

HEMODYNAMIC PROFILE

The hemodynamic features of mitral stenosis at any given severity are largely determined by the cardiac output, heart rate, and pulmonary vascular resistance (see Table 16–2).

Arterial Pressure. This value remains normal until cardiac output falls significantly such as during tachycardia. The pulse pressure is narrowed proportionate to reductions in stroke volume.

Systemic Vascular Resistance. As cardiac output falls, systemic vasoconstriction increases resistance to peripheral run-off of blood.

Pulmonary Vascular Resistance. This value may be normal with mild mitral stenosis or may be tremendously high with severe disease (2000 dynes/sec/cm^{-5}).

CVP or Right Atrial Pressure. These values may be normal in the early stages of the disease but will increase as prolonged, severe increases in pulmonary vascular resistance result in right ventricular failure. The right atrial waveform in patients with sinus rhythm shows a prominent *a* wave (reflecting increased resistance to filling the hypertrophied, failing right ventricle). In atrial fibrillation, due to loss of the atrial kick, there is only one crest, the *v* or *c-v* wave.

Pulmonary Artery Pressure. In mild disease, this value is normal. With progression of the disease, pulmonary artery systolic and diastolic pressures become elevated and, in the presence of extreme elevations of pulmonary vascular resistance, may exceed systemic arterial pressure (Fig. 16–9).

Pulmonary Artery Wedge Pressure. The measured PWP correlates well with mean left atrial pressure, which is typically elevated in other than mild disease. However, because valvular obstruction prevents equilibration between the left atrium and left ventricle in diastole, the PWP does not reflect the usually low left ventricular end-diastolic pressure. In mitral stenosis with sinus rhythm, the PWP waveform shows a prominent *a* wave and a gradual pressure decline following mitral valve opening (*y* descent). In addition, a widening of the pulmonary artery diastolic-to-pulmonary artery wedge pressure gradient will occur when pulmonary vascular changes increase pulmonary vascular resistance. The size of the gradient relates to the severity of the vascular change.

Cardiac Output. In mild cases of mitral stenosis where obstruction to flow across the valve has not yet occurred, cardiac output is normal. Cardiac output tends to decrease in relation to the flow obstruction across the valve. The output of the heart is additionally fixed and, although it may be adequate if the patient is at rest, the heart cannot increase output in response to increased tissue needs (fever, exercise, sepsis, shivering).

Mixed Venous Oxygen Saturation (SvO_2). This value falls relative to the severity of systemic underperfusion and/or hypoxemia.

Clinical Presentation

Symptoms do not usually appear until the mitral valve orifice is reduced to 2.5 cm^2 or less. The onset of symptoms is gradual and is usually related to exertion or exercise. Other factors that precipitate symptoms are pregnancy, atrial fibrillation, emotional stress, and respiratory infection. The severity of

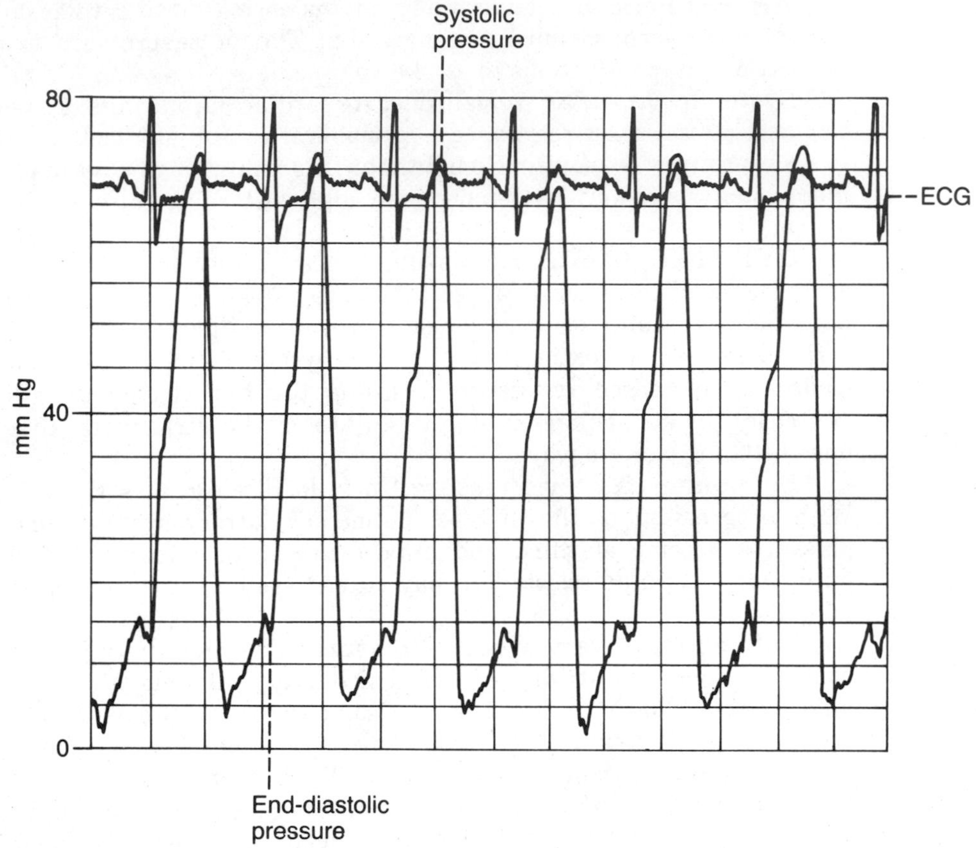

FIGURE 16–9. In the presence of pulmonary hypertension from any cause, an abnormally high afterload is imposed on the right ventricle. With gradually increasing pulmonary artery pressures, the right ventricle hypertrophies and is able to meet the abnormally high pressure demand. In this tracing, right ventricular systolic pressure approaches 80 mm Hg.

symptoms is related to the degree of valvular dysfunction and the disturbances in heart rate and rhythm. The principal symptoms of mitral stenosis and their causes are shown in Table 16–6.

Mentation. This is usually normal unless embolization from a left atrial thrombus has resulted in cerebral infarction.

Cutaneous. A pinkish-purple discoloration of the cheeks is common. Generally, the complexion is pale, the skin is warm, and peripheral cyanosis may be noted. Peripheral edema will be present with right ventricular failure.

Heart Rate and Character of Pulse. This value is usually normal or slightly tachycardic unless the patient is in uncontrolled atrial fibrillation (rate greater than 100 beats per minute). In more advanced disease, the pulse is small and, in the presence of atrial fibrillation, irregular. A pulse deficit is typical of atrial fibrillation (the apical pulse is greater than the simultaneously counted radial pulse).

TABLE 16–6. Major Symptoms of Mitral Stenosis and Their Causes

Symptom	*Cause*
Dyspnea	Pulmonary venous hypertension
Fatigue	Low cardiac output state
Paroxysmal nocturnal dyspnea; orthopnea; night cough	Redistribution of fluid from the lower extremities and trunk to the lungs with recumbency
Hemoptysis	Pulmonary venous hypertension causing rupture of some vessels
Palpitations	Atrial fibrillation with a rapid ventricular response
Hoarseness	Enlargement of the left atrium and compression of the laryngeal nerve
Hepatic congestion, ascites, dependent edema, and jugular venous distention	Right ventricular failure
Chest pain	Right ventricular hypertension, concomitant coronary artery disease, or coronary embolization
Cerebral findings (stroke or seizures)	Systemic embolization of mural thrombus from the left atrium

Heart Sounds. The typical auscultatory findings occur in the following sequence with progression of severity of the disease. Initially, the first heart sound (S_1) is accentuated because the thickening mitral valve leaflets are maximally open at the onset of systole and must swing through a wide arc to close. The second heart sound (S_2) is normal. Following the second heart sound there is a characteristic opening snap, which is attributed to the abrupt cessation of the outward motion of the mitral valve early in diastole. The opening snap is best heard at the apex with the diaphragm of the stethoscope. With the onset of symptomatic mitral stenosis, a diastolic rumble is audible. It is a low-pitched sound heard best with the bell of the stethoscope held over the apical impulse and with the patient lying in the left lateral position. The loudness of the murmur does not accurately correlate with the severity of the stenosis.

Palpation of the Precordium. The apical impulse is of short duration and lightly tapping. A left parasternal lift may be perceived by the examiner's hand and is indicative of right ventricular hypertrophy secondary to pulmonary hypertension.

Neck Veins. The external jugular veins become distended when right ventricular function deteriorates.

Respiratory Rate and Character of Breathing. This increases with the onset of pulmonary congestion and edema and additionally appears labored. Dyspnea may be the first symptom of the disease noted by the patient.

Lung Sounds. The lung sounds are normal. With the onset of pulmonary edema and alveolar flooding, crackles and wheezes are audible.

Acid/Base. These values are normal unless pulmonary edema or profound perfusion failure is present.

LABORATORY STUDIES

ECG. The ECG may be normal in the early stages of the disease. With the onset of obstruction to blood flow across the valve, left atrial enlargement will be manifest by P wave abnormalities (P mitrale). If the pulmonary artery pressure is greater than 35 mm Hg, signs of right ventricular hypertrophy may be noted; a right axis deviation is also common. Atrial fibrillation with coarse fibrillation waves is very commonly observed in patients with disease severe enough to warrant hospitalization.

Chest Radiograph. The appearance of the chest film relates to the severity of anatomic distortion of the cardiac and vascular structures and the degree of pulmonary congestion and edema. In mild mitral stenosis the chest film is usually normal. In more severe cases, there may be increased prominence of the pulmonary arteries and the vascular markings of the upper lobe vasculature relating to redistribution of blood flow toward the apex of the lung. Enlargement of the left atrial appendage produces a straightening of the left heart border. The enlarged left atrium may extend farther to the right than does the right atrium, giving the right atrial shadow the appearance of a "double density." Left atrial enlargement also causes a widening of the angle of the tracheal bifurcation. All signs of pulmonary edema may be present in more advanced disease.

Echocardiogram. Motion of the mitral valve leaflets is diminished. Calcium deposits or vegetations may be visualized. The left atrium is enlarged and left atrial thrombi may be visualized. Echocardiography is additionally useful in evaluating the patient's response to therapy.

Radionuclide Studies. These techniques are used with the patient at rest or during exercise to determine left ventricular end-diastolic volume, left ventricular ejection fraction, and cardiac output. They may also be used to follow the patient's response to therapy.

Cardiac Catheterization. This diagnostic technique is used to measure the gradient across the valve and various chamber pressures, assess ventricular function and cardiac output, and detect concomitant valvular or coronary artery disease.

TREATMENT

The asymptomatic patient with only auscultatory or laboratory signs of mitral stenosis requires no treatment except for endocarditis prophylaxis.

Endocarditis Prophylaxis. Antibiotic therapy is indicated in any patient with anatomic distortion of an endocardial structure who requires a surgical procedure, dental manipulation, or instrumentation that may produce bacteremia (tooth extraction, cystoscopy, gastroendoscopy). With progression of the disease and appearance of symptoms, the following therapeutic interventions are added:

Digitalis. Once atrial fibrillation has developed, cardiac glycosides are used to control the ventricular response. Some patients, however, are very dependent on a sinus mechanism to maintain hemodynamic stability. In these cases, cardioversion may restore sinus rhythm.

Quinidine. This agent is used to maintain sinus rhythm once restored by cardioversion.

Diuretics and Salt Restriction. Since most symptoms relate to the congestive components of left- and right-sided failure, diuretics and salt restriction may be used to reduce blood volume and pulmonary and systemic venous pressures.

Patient Instruction. Strenuous activity or anything that would induce tachycardia should be avoided because the resulting increase in left atrial pressure may predispose to pulmonary edema.

Surgical Therapy. Surgery should be considered once the patient becomes symptomatic despite optimal medical therapy. Surgical options include:

MITRAL COMMISSUROTOMY. For this procedure, either the surgeon's finger or a knife is used to create a larger opening between the mitral valve commissures (sites of junction between the valve cusps). This is the procedure of choice for patients with pure mitral stenosis and relatively pliable, noncalcific valves and may be performed in an open or closed heart. This procedure is merely palliative and not curative; patients usually require reoperation at 5 to 20 years.

MITRAL VALVE REPLACEMENT. For this procedure, the diseased valve is resected and the prosthetic valve inserted in its place. This is the procedure of choice in the setting of combined mitral regurgitation and stenosis and for patients with extensive valvular calcification. Long-term anticoagulation is required.

Mitral Regurgitation

Mitral regurgitation, also called mitral insufficiency, is a valvular disorder in which inadequate closure or incompetence of the mitral valve results in retrograde blood flow from the left ventricle into the left atrium during systole.

Causes and Pathophysiology. Competence of the mitral valve apparatus depends on normal anatomy of the valve leaflets; integrity and proper length of the chordae tendineae; integrity and normal contractile dynamics of the papillary muscle; proper function of the myocardium from which the papillary muscles arise; and proper size of the left ventricle and mitral valve annulus (ring). An abnormality involving any of these structures may prevent the two valve leaflets from making complete contact in systole.

The major causes of mitral regurgitation are:

MITRAL VALVE PROLAPSE. Prolapse of the mitral valve leaflets into the left atrium during left ventricular systole may be due to floppy structure of the valve leaflets secondary to degenerative disease, excessive length of the chordae tendineae, or an enlarged valve annulus. Mitral valve prolapse is a very common cause of mitral regurgitation in adults.

Rheumatic Fever. The associated valvulitis may lead to progressive fibrotic shortening of the mitral valve leaflets and calcification of the valve commissures in a fixed, open position. Secondary further distortion of the valve may be produced by left atrial enlargement, which commonly occurs in mitral disease. An enlarged left atrium pulls the posterior mitral valve leaflet away from the anterior leaflet, thereby accentuating the incompetence of the valve; therefore, mitral insufficiency leads to more mitral insufficiency.

Bacterial Endocarditis. In the septic patient, blood-borne bacteria may become implanted on the valve leaflet and "eat away" the leaflets and/or chordae. Bacterial attack on a valve is more likely to occur in an anatomically altered (rheumatic or congenital) valve leaflet.

Ischemic Heart Disease. Ischemic dysfunction or rupture of the papillary muscle (see Complications of Acute Myocardial Infarction) may cause transient or permanent, mild or severe mitral regurgitation.

Left Ventricular Dilatation; Dilatation of the Mitral Valve Annulus. Dilatation of a failing left ventricle, from any cause, may distort the alignment of the chordae and papillary muscles to the valve leaflets and also increase the size of the valve annulus. The valve leaflets are thus prevented from coapting in systole. This can be expected to occur when the ventricle is significantly dilated.

Trauma. Cardiac injury, secondary to thoracic trauma, on rare occasion may result in traumatic rupture of the papillary muscle or chordae.

Hemodynamic Effects. In left ventricular systole, the total left ventricular stroke volume is distributed between the forward (systemic) stroke volume and the regurgitant volume into the low pressure left atrium. This results in a reduction in forward systemic blood flow and volume overload of the left atrium. The consequent increase in left atrial pressure will then be reflected back to the pulmonary veins, capillaries, and arteries. This predisposes to pulmonary edema and right ventricular failure.

In diastole, the blood, which flowed retrogradely through the mitral valve during ventricular systole, flows back to the left ventricle while the normal blood flow comes in from the pulmonary circulation. This results in flow/volume overload of the left ventricle.

The following factors determine the volume of regurgitant flow.

The Size of the Regurgitant Orifice. Ventricular dilatation, which accompanies failure, enlarges the size of the mitral regurgitant orifice and increases regurgitant flow. On the other hand, reduction in left ventricular size and volume through the use of inotropic or vasodilating agents or diuretics may diminish the size or entirely eliminate the regurgitant orifice and regurgitant flow.

The Pressure Difference Between the Left Atrium and Left Ventricle. Left ventricular systolic pressure, an important and therapeutically alterable factor in the left ventricular–left atrial pressure difference, is dependent on systemic vascular resistance and stroke volume. Any increase in systemic vascular resistance will increase the level of the left ventricular systolic pressure and the severity of the regurgitant flow because more blood will preferentially flow to the area of lesser pressure (the left atrium). Conversely, decreases in systemic vascular resistance, achieved by the use of vasodilator agents, reduce regurgitant volume.

In severe mitral regurgitation, as much as 80% of the total left ventricular stroke volume may flow back into the left atrium.

Chronic, slowly progressing mitral regurgitation is rather well tolerated because compensatory cardioadaptive changes maintain stroke volume and near-normal left atrial pressure. On the other hand, the hemodynamic consequences of acute mitral regurgitation are clinically far more dramatic and poorly tolerated.

Chronic Mitral Regurgitation

The slowly evolving cardiac changes involve both the left ventricular and left atrial chambers.

Over the long term, the *left ventricle* hypertrophies and is able to maintain cardiac output by emptying more completely. In addition, the left ventricle dilates and becomes more distensible (compliant). This permits rapid diastolic filling and accommodation of the large incoming volume with a minimum increase in left ventricular end-diastolic pressure.

Increased compliance and enlargement of the *left atrium* also occur and damp the pressure effect of the regurgitant flow so that significant regurgitation may be present with only mild elevations of mean left atrial and pulmonary vascular pressures. This protects against pulmonary edema and right ventricular failure.

As a result of these compensatory changes, the patient with mild or even moderate regurgitation may be quite stable and relatively symptom-free for years. However, if regurgitation worsens, or another cardiac disorder complicates the picture (myocardial infarction), left ventricular function deteriorates and left ventricular end-diastolic volume and pressure increase progressively. With further ventricular dilatation, the regurgitant orifice may enlarge and cause more regurgitation, and the patient's condition spirals downward. In this setting, the rising left atrial pressure predisposes to pulmonary edema and right ventricular failure. Decreases in forward blood flow predispose to systemic underperfusion.

Hemodynamic Profile. ARTERIAL PRESSURE. (See Table 16–2.) The arterial pressure is normal if the patient maintains a compensated steady state.

SYSTEMIC VASCULAR RESISTANCE. This value generally remains normal. However, any increase in systemic vascular resistance mediated by stress, heart failure, and so on will increase left ventricular outflow resistance and worsen the regurgitant flow.

PULMONARY VASCULAR RESISTANCE. This value may be normal or slightly decreased if the patient has a large, compliant left atrium and relatively mild left atrial pressure elevations. Mild elevations in left atrial pressure result in the opening of pulmonary vascular channels at the uppermost portions of the lung and increase the functional cross-sectional area of the pulmonary circulation. This effect results in a slight decrease in pulmonary vascular resistance. With greater increases in left atrial pressure (above 18 mm Hg) the development of cuffs of fluid around blood vessels and hypoxemia is met with increases in pulmonary vascular resistance.

CVP or Right Atrial Pressure. These values may be normal if the right ventricle maintains normal function.

Pulmonary Artery and Wedge Pressure. The pulmonary artery systolic and diastolic pressures increase in proportion to the increase in left atrial pressure. This value tends to be greater than normal. The level of elevation relates to the volume of regurgitant flow, the compliance and size of the left atrium, and the functional state of the left ventricle. The amplitude of the PWP *v* waves may be deceptively low relative to a large regurgitant volume if an enlarged, compliant left atrium absorbs and accommodates the large regurgitant flow. However, the left ventricular end-diastolic pressure is lower than the mean left atrial pressure if *v* waves are significantly large. If the patient is in sinus rhythm, the *a* wave correlates best with left ventricular end-diastolic pressure. If the patient is in atrial fibrillation, the pre-*v* area of the trace more closely reflects ventricular end-diastolic pressure.

Cardiac Output. This value is normal if the left ventricle remains compensated and the volume of the regurgitant flow is not large.

Mixed Venous Oxygen Saturation (SvO_2). In a compensated state, this value is normal.

Acute Mitral Regurgitation

Acute mitral regurgitation is a potentially lethal event that is characterized by sudden-onset pulmonary edema and severe perfusion failure. It is often due to acute bacterial endocarditis, transient ischemic dysfunction of a papillary muscle, rupture of the head of a papillary muscle, or chordae tendineae. Hemodynamic disturbances are profound because the regurgitant flow is suddenly imposed on a previously normal left atrium and ventricle. The inability of the left atrium and left ventricle to suddenly dilate and increase compliance results in a marked increase in left ventricular end-diastolic pressure and left atrial and pulmonary vascular pressures. Since the regurgitant flow into the left atrium occurs only in ventricular systole, the amplitude of the left atrial *v* wave is increased and may reach levels of 50 to 70 mm Hg. Because the *a* wave is not significantly affected, the mean left atrial pressure rises to levels of approximately 15 to 20 mm Hg above left ventricular end-diastolic pressure. The pressure in the pulmonary vessels and right ventricle rises proportionately; pressure overload on the right ventricle ultimately produces right ventricular failure. Forward systemic blood flow may be sufficiently low to produce shock.

Hemodynamic Profile. ARTERIAL PRESSURE. (See Table 16–2.) Blood pressure may be maintained but the pulse pressure is likely to be narrowed. If the regurgitant leak is sufficiently large, critical reductions in forward flow produce hypotension.

SYSTEMIC VASCULAR RESISTANCE. This value increases relative to the fall in cardiac output. However, the compensatory rise in systemic vascular resistance increases left ventricular outflow resistance and worsens the regurgitant leak.

PULMONARY VASCULAR RESISTANCE. This value increases with the onset of pulmonary edema.

CVP OR RIGHT ATRIAL PRESSURE. With the onset of right ventricular failure, these values increase and the amplitude of the right atrial *a* wave increases.

PULMONARY ARTERY PRESSURE. Pulmonary artery systolic and diastolic pressures increase in proportion to the increase in left atrial pressure. If the regurgitation is severe, the regurgitant waves may be transmitted back to the pulmonary artery and may distort the pulmonary artery waveform.

PULMONARY ARTERY WEDGE PRESSURE. This parameter is elevated, and prominent regurgitant *v* waves are noted. The *a* waves may additionally be of greater amplitude than normal due to resistance to filling of the failing left ventricle at the end of diastole (Fig. 16–10).

CARDIAC OUTPUT. This value can be expected to fall relative to the size of the regurgitant leak as well as the presence of underlying myocardial disease such as acute myocardial infarction.

MIXED VENOUS OXYGEN SATURATION (SvO_2). This value decreases relative to the perfusion status of the patient and pulmonary edema–induced hypoxemia.

Clinical Presentation. People with minimal-to-mild, chronic, well-compensated mitral regurgitation appear healthy and may lead normal lives with no restrictions on activities. On physical examination, the only abnormality noted may be the systolic murmur at the apex. This is sometimes accompanied by a third heart sound that relates to rapid diastolic filling of the ventricle and does not necessarily indicate failure. Because of the low pressure against which the left ventricle ejects (into the left atrium), the valve defect is well tolerated and the asymptomatic clinical course may extend over many years.

If symptoms do arise, they are a function of the severity of the regurgitation, the rate of progression, the level of pulmonary artery pressure, and the presence of associated valvular or coronary artery disease. The clinical picture of moderate-to-severe mitral regurgitation is presented in the following discussion.

MENTATION. The patient may be alert but complains of weakness and fatigue. In acute, severe mitral regurgitation the patient may be obtunded and restless.

CUTANEOUS. The patient appears pale, but the skin is likely to be warm except for the hands and feet, which may be cool. In severe, acute mitral

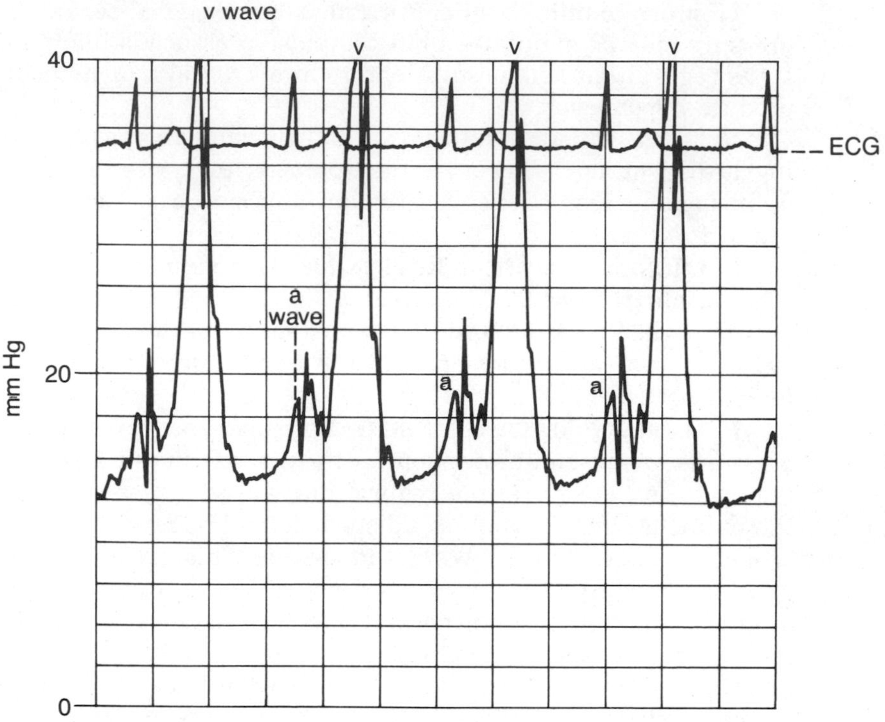

FIGURE 16–10. Pulmonary artery wedge tracing from a patient with acute mitral regurgitation. Note the increased amplitude *a* waves as well as the giant *v* waves that result from regurgitation of blood into a normally small, noncompliant left atrium.

regurgitation, the patient is typically ashen with peripheral cyanosis. The skin is additionally cool and clammy.

HEART RATE AND CHARACTER OF PULSE. The heart rate is increased and the amplitude of the pulse is reduced. With severe left ventricular dysfunction, pulsus alternans may be detected. Rhythm disturbances include sinus arrhythmia, premature ventricular beats, and, commonly, atrial fibrillation,

HEART SOUNDS. The classic auscultatory finding is a holosystolic, blowing, high-pitched murmur, which is maximally heard at the apex and may radiate to the left axilla and left back. In acute-onset, severe mitral regurgitation, the murmur may last only through the first half of systole. An atrial gallop may be heard and a ventricular gallop is common. Usually only a summation gallop is heard because the patient is almost always tachycardic.

PALPATION OF THE PRECORDIUM. In acute, severe mitral regurgitation, the apex beat is in the normal position and is usually hyperactive. A systolic thrill may be palpated over the apex. With chronic, severe regurgitation, the apex beat is laterally displaced, sustained, and covers a large area.

NECK VEINS. The external jugular veins become distended with the advent of right ventricular failure.

RESPIRATORY RATE AND CHARACTER OF BREATHING. The patient will be tachypneic due to pulmonary congestion and edema and prefers to sit upright. Breathing is labored relative to the severity of the pulmonary edema.

LUNG SOUNDS. Pulmonary crackles and wheezing occur in the setting of overt pulmonary edema.

ACID/BASE. If pulmonary edema is present, hypoxemia and respiratory alkalosis are typically present. With severe perfusion failure, the accumulation of lactic acid produces a metabolic acidosis.

Laboratory Studies. ECG. In acute mitral regurgitation, the ECG is usually normal, although there may be frequent ectopy. In chronic mitral regurgitation, the ECG shows evidence of left atrial enlargement with P wave abnormalities. The incidence of left ventricular hypertrophy is 50%; right ventricular hypertrophy, 15%; and atrial fibrillation, 75%. Coarse fibrillatory waves are common.

CHEST RADIOGRAPH. In acute mitral regurgitation, the heart size is normal with only mild left atrial enlargement; however, there is marked evidence of pulmonary edema. Patients with chronic mitral regurgitation commonly manifest cardiomegaly with left ventricular and left atrial enlargement. Right ventricular and pulmonary artery enlargement may be seen in the setting of pulmonary hypertension. The lung fields will be clear if pulmonary vascular pressures are not sufficiently high to produce pulmonary edema.

ECHOCARDIOGRAM. This reveals left atrial and ventricular enlargement and increased wall motion, particularly in systole. The etiology of the regurgitation may be diagnosed, such as rupture of the chordae tendineae, mitral valve prolapse, flail leaflets, and so on. The severity of the regurgitation, however, cannot be adequately quantified.

CARDIAC CATHETERIZATION. This procedure is performed to confirm the diagnosis and to assess ventricular function. The regurgitant fraction and the ejection fraction are measured, as are pressures in the various heart chambers. Concomitant coronary artery or valvular disease can also be assessed.

Treatment. Medical therapy for the asymptomatic patient with mild or moderate mitral regurgitation and good ventricular function is unnecessary, but periodic medical evaluation is mandatory. Prophylactic antibiotics are required prior to dental or invasive medical or surgical procedures. No restriction of activity is required.

With more severe regurgitation, the patient should be instructed to avoid strenuous physical exercise. The following therapeutic interventions help relieve symptoms and maintain hemodynamic stability.

Vasodilators. Arterial and venous dilators reduce the filling volume of the ventricle and decrease systemic vascular resistance. Both interventions help reduce the size of the regurgitant orifice, which, in turn, reduces the regurgitant volume. Afterload reduction additionally increases forward flow.

Digitalis and Anticoagulants. If atrial fibrillation develops, these pharmacologic agents are used to control the ventricular rate and decrease embolic complications.

Salt Restriction and Diuretics. This therapeutic approach helps relieve the congestive components of heart failure.

Surgical Replacement of the Mitral Valve. Surgery should be considered when symptoms of pulmonary congestion or signs of inadequate cardiac output persist despite optimum medical therapy. Following valve replacement, the patient should be carefully observed for the development of left ventricular failure. If the left ventricle is compromised prior to surgery, valve replacement can result in frank failure because the left ventricle is suddenly required to eject its entire contents into the high resistance systemic circulation. The abrupt change in afterload can produce deterioration in left ventricular function.

Aortic Stenosis

Aortic stenosis is a valvular disorder in which there is an impairment to aortic valve opening which then obstructs left ventricular outflow. Aortic stenosis is the most common valve lesion and affects approximately 25% of all patients with chronic valve disease. Obstruction to left ventricular outflow can occur at valvular, subvalvular, or supravalvular locations. This discussion focuses on valvular aortic stenosis since it is the predominant lesion of the three and the most commonly fatal valve lesion.

Causes and Pathophysiology

Aortic stenosis has three primary etiologies: congenital, rheumatic, and degenerative.

Congenital. Congenital aortic valve stenosis may result from a congenital unicuspid or bicuspid valve (instead of the normally tricuspid valve). The congenital bicuspid valve is the most commonly encountered malformation of the aortic valve. With the passage of time, progressive sclerosis and thickening and calcification of the anomalous valve may occur so that the orifice is ultimately reduced to a narrow, slitlike opening.

Rheumatic. Rheumatic aortic stenosis results in progressive cusp fibrosis, valve calcification, and fusion of one to three of the aortic commissures. A history of rheumatic fever is present in 30 to 50% of patients with aortic stenosis.

Degenerative. Degenerative aortic stenosis occurs in patients aged 65 or older as a result of chronic, normal, mechanical, stress "wear and tear" of the valve. In degenerative aortic stenosis, the valve is tricuspid and commissures are not fused, but calcium deposits impair the mobility of the valve cusps. This type of aortic stenosis is more commonly encountered in women and is typically not severe.

Less common etiologies of aortic stenosis include hyperlipidemia, infective endocarditis, metabolic abnormalities, and systemic lupus erythematosus.

Hemodynamic Effects

The spectrum of hemodynamic alterations in aortic stenosis includes primary systolic as well as secondary diastolic abnormalities.

Systolic Abnormalities. The primary hemodynamic abnormality of aortic stenosis occurs during systole when blood is ejected from the left ventricle through a narrowed aortic valve orifice. Obstruction to left ventricular outflow requires the development of an excessively high left ventricular systolic pressure just to maintain a normal or near-normal cardiac output. Left ventricular systolic pressure may reach levels as high as 260 to 300 mm Hg. The generation of these extraordinary systolic pressures results in a proportionate increase in myocardial oxygen consumption. However, the systolic pressure in the aorta is less than that of the left ventricle. The difference between the left ventricular and aortic systolic pressure is termed the aortic valve gradient. A systolic aortic gradient of greater than 50 mm Hg is considered to be representative of critical stenosis.

If, for any reason, significant depression in contractility develops, the drop in cardiac output is compensated by increased systemic vascular resistance. This generalized vasoconstriction attempts to maintain mean arterial pressure and coronary and cerebral perfusion, but this further increases left ventricular afterload and oxygen consumption.

Diastolic Abnormalities. In any type of aortic stenosis, the obstruction develops and increases gradually over a prolonged period of time. The gradually increasing systolic pressure overload of the left ventricle is compensated by an increase in ventricular wall thickness and mass. This concentric hypertrophy without dilatation develops to maintain the functional demands of the left ventricle, that is, to increase systolic pressure sufficient to maintain a normal ejection fraction and cardiac output.

The increase in ventricular mass and concomitant decrease in compliance (increased stiffness) result in a significant increase in left ventricular diastolic pressure, which is further elevated by forceful atrial contraction. In aortic stenosis, atrial systole is especially important to fill the thick, stiff ventricle and may contribute as much as 40% to stroke volume. The required increase in left atrial systolic pressure results in progressive enlargement of the left atrium but does not result in elevation in mean left atrial pressure sufficient to produce pulmonary edema. With time, however, ventricular function may deteriorate (ischemic insult, intrinsic dysfunction), causing the left ventricle to dilate. Left ventricular end-diastolic pressure may then rise sufficiently to raise mean left atrial pressure to levels greater than 20 mm Hg, and pulmonary edema ensues.

The hypertrophied left ventricular muscle mass, elevated systolic pressure, and prolonged ejection time increase myocardial oxygen consumption. At the same time, excessive intramyocardial systolic and diastolic tension may reduce myocardial blood flow by compression of the long, thin penetrating coronary artery branches. Therefore, the myocardium, particularly the subendocardium, is susceptible to ischemia, in both the presence or absence of coronary artery disease.

Important Clinical Implications in Caring for the Patient with Aortic Stenosis

The heart of the patient with aortic stenosis requires a very fine balance of preload and afterload to maintain cardiac output at acceptable levels while preventing pulmonary edema. Likewise, myocardial oxygen supply and demand are in a particularly precarious balance. Systemic vascular resistance must be sufficiently high to maintain mean arterial pressure and coronary blood flow but not so high as to excessively increase afterload and myocardial oxygen consumption. Ventricular filling volume and pressure (preload) must be high enough to maintain cardiac output but not so high as to produce pulmonary edema. Factors that may produce hemodynamic deterioration in the patient with aortic stenosis include:

A Reduction in Preload. The hypertrophied, noncompliant left ventricle in aortic stenosis requires a high filling pressure to maintain cardiac output although end-diastolic volume may be normal. Critical reductions in preload and cardiac output, therefore, may result from hemorrhage, excessive diuretic response, third space shifts, dehydration, venodilator agents, and/or vomiting and diarrhea. Since the atrial kick contributes significantly to left ventricular preload, loss of the atrial kick (atrial fibrillation, A–V dissociation, or ventricular pacing) may also produce critical reductions in end-diastolic pressure and cardiac output.

Arrhythmias. Myocardial oxygen consumption increases in proportion to increases in heart rate but tachyarrhythmias reduce coronary perfusion and ventricular filling (diastolic) time. Premature beats tend to poorly perfuse (if at all) the systemic and coronary circulation. Therefore, tachyarrhythmias or very frequent ectopy may predispose to myocardial ischemia and decreased pump function.

Extremes in Arterial Pressure. Systemic hypotension decreases coronary perfusion pressure but the stenotic valve continues to require a high systolic pressure of the left ventricle and consequent high oxygen demand. On the other hand, systemic hypertension further increases afterload and oxygen consumption for the left ventricle without producing proportionate increases in myocardial oxygen supply. There may also be critical reduction in stroke volume.

In summary, critical alterations in preload, afterload, heart rate, or rhythm, may push the previously stable patient "over the edge" by decreasing pump function or upsetting the delicate balance of myocardial oxygen supply and demand or both.

Hemodynamic Profile

In aortic stenosis, the hemodynamic profile does not relate to significant cardiovascular compromise until late in the course, when a critical reduction in the valve orifice size has developed and/or the left ventricle goes into failure. (See Table 16–2.)

Arterial Pressure. The arterial pressure may be maintained at normal levels until there is significant aortic stenosis. At that time the systolic pressure may decrease while the diastolic pressure is maintained. The cuff measurement of the arterial pressure may reveal an auscultatory gap between systolic and diastolic pressure, so care must be taken to estimate systolic pressure by palpation while inflating the cuff. See Chapter 7, Arterial Pressure Measurement; Indirect Methods—Auscultation. The arterial pressure waveform shows a slowed rate of rise to the systolic peak and an overall damped appearance due to the narrowed pulse pressure. It must be remembered that the left ventricular systolic pressure may be significantly higher than the systemic arterial systolic pressure and may reach levels as high as 260 to 300 mm Hg.

Systemic Vascular Resistance. Values are within normal limits until the volume of blood ejected from the left ventricle declines. At that time, systemic vascular resistance increases.

Pulmonary Vascular Resistance. This value is normal or slightly decreased until the advent of left ventricular failure and pulmonary edema. At that time, pulmonary vascular resistance increases.

CVP or Right Atrial Pressure. These values are within normal limits unless right-sided heart failure develops as a result of elevated pulmonary artery pressures secondary to left ventricular failure. The right atrial *a* wave may be prominent owing to reduced right ventricular compliance that results from hypertrophy of the ventricular septum.

Pulmonary Artery Pressure. These values remain normal until late in the disease when a critical aortic stenosis or left ventricular failure elevates mean left atrial pressure. Pulmonary artery systolic and diastolic pressures then rise proportionately.

Pulmonary Artery Wedge Pressure. This value, which reflects mean left atrial pressure, in a compensated state may be normal or slightly elevated due to the increased amplitude *a* waves that correlate with left ventricular end-diastolic pressure. The *a* waves may rise to 30 to 35 mm Hg, whereas the *v* waves are unremarkable. With the development of left ventricular failure, the mean PWP rises to levels that may produce pulmonary edema (greater than 18 to 20 mm Hg).

Cardiac Output. The cardiac output is normal at rest in most patients with severe aortic stenosis but fails to increase with physical stress (exercise, shivering, fever, sepsis). Late in the course of the disease, cardiac output fails, even at rest, as does the ejection fraction.

Mixed Venous Oxygen Saturation (SvO_2). With the advent of systemic underperfusion and/or pulmonary edema, this value falls.

Clinical Presentation

Most patients with mild to moderate aortic stenosis are asymptomatic until valve obstruction becomes severe. Clinical deterioration typically occurs when the aortic valve opening is reduced to one third to one fourth of its normal size. The patient then develops

1. *Syncope or lightheadedness,* which relates to decreased cerebral perfusion when cardiac output cannot increase commensurate to increased body need. This may occur with or immediately following physical exertion or when the patient suddenly assumes an upright position (orthostatic syncope).
2. *Angina pectoris* relates to the excessive oxygen needs of the myocardium and reduced oxygen delivery.

3. *Dyspnea and fatigue* relate to pulmonary edema and systemic underperfusion accompanying left ventricular failure at rest or failure of the left ventricle to step up output in response to exercise.

Mentation. The level of mentation is normal except for occasional episodes of giddiness, lightheadedness, or "fading out" spells. These symptoms relate to cerebral underperfusion.

Cutaneous. The skin is typically pale in the compensated state but may also appear cyanotic in severe disease. The skin is usually warm to touch, but the hands and feet may be cool.

Heart Rate and Rhythm. The patient may maintain a normal heart rate or slightly slower than normal in the compensated state, but heart rate increases as cardiac output falls. Irregularities in the pulse may occur due to transient arrhythmias, some of which predispose to sudden cardiac death. In fact, some syncopal episodes are thought to be due to transient ventricular fibrillation. Sudden death occurs in 15 to 20% of patients with aortic stenosis, and may be the first indication of disease.

Character of Pulse. The arterial pulse rises slowly and is small and sustained (pulsus parvus and tardus). Pulsus alternans is common with left ventricular failure, but obstruction of the aortic valve may prevent detection at a peripheral site.

Heart Sounds. The first heart sound is normal or soft. Paradoxical splitting of the second heart sound may occur due to the prolonged left ventricular systole and delayed aortic valve closure. Atrial and ventricular gallops are commonly heard in advanced disease. The murmur of aortic stenosis is systolic, harsh, and of varying intensity, with a crescendo-decrescendo (diamond-shaped) configuration. The murmur is loudest at the aortic area and is well transmitted to the neck, upper back, and the apex where it may have a musical quality. In barrel-chested persons, however, the murmur may be very faint or inaudible, particularly if they are in heart failure.

Palpation of the Precordium. The apical impulse is in the normal location if the patient is not in failure but is increased in force and duration. As the ventricle dilates in response to failure, the apical impulse becomes laterally and inferiorly displaced. A systolic thrill may be palpated over the aortic area and carotid arteries. A precordial *a* wave (the atrial thrust) may be visible and palpable.

Neck Veins. The external jugular veins are usually normal in appearance until left ventricular failure develops.

Respiratory Rate and Character of Breathing. These are unremarkable until the patient develops pulmonary edema.

Lung Sounds. Breath sounds are normal until pulmonary edema develops. At that time, diffuse crackles and wheezes are audible. The onset of pulmonary edema is generally an ominous sign and is associated with rapid clinical deterioration.

Acid/Base. The values are normal unless pulmonary edema and/or severe perfusion failure develops.

LABORATORY STUDIES

ECG. The ECG may be normal initially, but a pattern of left ventricular hypertrophy and strain gradually evolves. Conduction defects may be present, including left anterior hemiblock or left bundle branch block. Complete heart block is rare. P wave abnormalities signify left atrial enlargement. Atrial fibrillation is a late and ominous sign in aortic stenosis and is usually associated with concomitant mitral valve disease. Ventricular ectopy may also be noted.

Chest Radiograph. The chest film may be normal in the early stages of aortic stenosis. Cardiomegaly, due to left ventricular dilation and left atrial enlargement, are common late in the course of aortic stenosis. Aortic calcification may be noted as well as prominence of the ascending aorta. Radiographic evidence of pulmonary edema is a late and ominous sign.

Echocardiogram. This diagnostic procedure is useful in delineating valve structure and mobility as well as assessing left ventricular function. Left ventricular hypertrophy and chamber size can be quantified echocardiographically, as can valve and orifice size. The normal valve orifice size is 1.6 to 2.5 cm^2. A valve orifice less than 0.7 cm^2 is considered to be critically narrowed.

Cardiac Catheterization. This procedure is used to exclude or to assess the presence or severity of coronary artery disease and left ventricular function. The systolic pressure gradient between the left ventricle and aorta, left ventricular end-diastolic pressure, and the cross-sectional area of the valve can also be determined.

TREATMENT

Aortic stenosis with little obstruction requires no specific therapy. However, prophylactic antibiotic coverage is recommended prior to any dental or surgical procedure to protect against bacterial endocarditis.

Medical therapy generally is not justified in the symptomatic patient with aortic stenosis because once symptoms appear, the clinical course deteriorates rapidly. Without surgery, most patients are dead within 5 years. Some clinicians advocate surgery for asymptomatic patients who demonstrate aortic gradients greater than 50 mm Hg. Two surgical options are available.

Aortic Commissurotomy. This procedure may be effective in relieving the left ventricular outflow obstruction in younger patients who do not have calcified valves.

Aortic Valve Replacement. This procedure is recommended if valvular calcification exists. All patients with metal prosthetic valves require chronic anticoagulation.

Aortic Regurgitation

Aortic regurgitation is a valvular disorder in which incompetence of the aortic valve results in a reflux of blood from the aorta to the left ventricle during diastole. This disorder is also known as aortic insufficiency.

Causes and Pathophysiology

There are many causes of aortic regurgitation. *Syphilitic aortitis* causes loss of valvular support, *rheumatic fever* causes thickening and shortening of the valve cusps. *Infective endocarditis,* due to any microorganism, may cause progressive (days, weeks, or months) damage and distortion of the aortic valve cusps. *Dissecting aneurysm involving the aortic root* can produce regurgitation by displacement of one leaflet below the other; widening of the aortic root or loss of annular support may produce a flail leaflet. All abnormalities prevent the leaflets from meeting in diastole. *Blunt chest trauma,* which occurs during diastole when the ventricle is full of blood and the aortic valve is closed, can produce structural damage to a leaflet or leaflets. Various *systemic inflammatory diseases* or *cystic medial necrosis* of the aorta, as occurs with Marfan's syndrome, may also result in aortic insufficiency.

Hemodynamic Effects

The flow abnormality in aortic insufficiency occurs in diastole when the aortic valve should be closed. Since diastolic pressure in the aorta is approximately 70 to 80 mm Hg and the diastolic pressure in the left ventricle is approximately 4 to 12 mm Hg, a very large pressure gradient exists between the aorta and left ventricular chamber. Any opening in the aortic valve, therefore, will allow a large regurgitant stream into the left ventricle.

The magnitude of the regurgitant volume is determined by the size of the regurgitant orifice, the pressure difference between the aorta and left ventricle in diastole, and duration of diastole. In extreme cases the regurgitant volume may be as great as 60% of the systolic volume ejected. This retrograde blood flow results in diastolic volume overload of the left ventricle, since in diastole it now receives and accommodates blood entering normally from the left atrium as well as the regurgitant blood volume. This increased diastolic filling results in an increase in stroke volume that will be ejected rapidly into a poorly filled aorta. However, in the subsequent diastole, part of the blood reenters the left ventricle, thereby potentially decreasing effective systemic blood flow. The hemodynamic effects of compensated and decompensated chronic aortic regurgitation and acute regurgitation are presented in the following discussion. Between these extremes are many possible clinical gradations that relate to the preexisting state of the left ventricle, the presence or absence of coexisting disease, the size of the regurgitant orifice, and the time period over which the defect developed.

Chronic Aortic Regurgitation (Compensated). During the development of chronic aortic regurgitation, the regurgitant leak increases gradually. The left ventricle, therefore, has time to adapt to the progressive increase in end-diastolic volume by dilating and increasing compliance. These compensatory mechanisms allow the left ventricle to accommodate the increasing end-diastolic volume with little, if any, increase in end-diastolic pressure. The patient is thus protected from pulmonary edema. The ventricular wall also hypertrophies and is able to maintain a normal cardiac output by increasing stroke volume to levels much greater than normal. This is also associated with a compensatory decrease in systemic vascular resistance, which helps maintain forward flow to the periphery. The systolic pressure generated may be in excess of 200 mm Hg, and the diastolic pressure is typically low. To achieve this extraordinary functional state, the left ventricle may enlarge to exceed 1000 gm (normal: female, 244 gm; male, 328 gm), hence the name "ox heart" or "cor bovinum." This remarkably altered heart may maintain an adequate cardiac output even in exercise. In fact, at this level of disease, increased activity may be beneficial because exercise-induced tachycardia shortens diastolic (regurgitant) time and also further decreases systemic vascular resistance. Both effects decrease the regurgitant volume per beat.

Chronic Aortic Regurgitation (Decompensated). With time, the limits of ventricular compensation may be exceeded or there may be a gradual decline in the contractile state of the myocardium. This may be due to primary deterioration or to secondary factors such as ischemic disease. The patient with aortic regurgitation is particularly vulnerable to ischemic insult since aortic diastolic pressure, the primary determinant of coronary perfusion pressure, is reduced while at the same time myocardial oxygen requirements are increased. The progressive decreases in contractility result in a progressive decrease in forward stroke volume and a greater increase in the volume of blood remaining in the left ventricle at the end of systole and diastole. There is also a progressive decrease in ventricular distensibility. As a consequence of increased ventricular end-diastolic volume and decreased compliance, left ventricular end-diastolic pressure and pulmonary vascular pressure rise. This may ultimately lead to right ventricular failure. Thus, the once relatively efficient hyperdynamic circulation gradually deteriorates into one characterized by low cardiac output and congestive failure.

Acute Aortic Regurgitation. In acute aortic regurgitation (due to infective endocarditis, aortic dissection, trauma) the diastolic volume overload is suddenly imposed upon a left ventricle unable to dilate acutely to accommodate the regurgitant volume. Left ventricular end-diastolic pressure, left atrial pressure, and pulmonary capillary hydrostatic pressure rise abruptly to produce pulmonary edema. Since total stroke volume cannot suddenly increase markedly, cardiac output diminishes and systemic vascular resistance increases reflexively as a compensatory mechanism to maintain perfusion to core organs. The patient with sudden-onset severe aortic regurgitation presents with sudden-onset severe pulmonary edema and inadequate peripheral perfusion that can progress quickly to shock and death. Recognition is of critical importance because valve surgery is required to save the patient's life.

Hemodynamic Profile

There are significant variations between the hemodynamic profile seen in chronic compensated, decompensated, and acute aortic regurgitation (see Table 16–2). These differences are depicted in Table 16–7.

TABLE 16–7. Hemodynamic Profile in Chronic Compensated, Decompensated, and Acute Aortic Regurgitation

Hemodynamic Parameter	*Chronic Compensated Aortic Regurgitation*	*Chronic Decompensated Aortic Regurgitation*	*Acute Aortic Regurgitation*
Right atrial pressure	~	↑	~↑
Systemic vascular resistance	~↓	~↑	↑
Pulmonary vascular resistance	~	↑	↑
Pulmonary artery pressure	~	↑	↑
Pulmonary artery wedge pressure	~ or ↑	↑	↑
Cardiac output	~	↓	↓
Ejection fraction	~	↓	~↓
Mixed venous oxygen saturation	~	↓	↓

KEY: ↑ Increased; ↓ decreased; ~ no change.

Clinical Presentation

In the early phases of mild aortic regurgitation, the patient is asymptomatic, and physical examination is unremarkable except for the characteristic blowing decrescendo diastolic murmur, which is loudest along the left sternal border. Symptoms indicative of deterioration (dyspnea, arrhythmias, paroxysmal nocturnal dyspnea, and angina) usually develop in midlife, by which time significant ventricular dysfunction has occurred. Rest angina and nocturnal angina may occur and are likely due to the deleterious effects of bradycardia in aortic insufficiency. Patients may also be aware of their heart beat, especially when lying down, and may also complain of a pounding sensation in the head. Syncope and sudden death occasionally occur but are less common than with aortic stenosis.

Mentation. Mentation is normal, although the patient with severe acute aortic insufficiency who is in a state of cardiovascular collapse will be confused, agitated, or stuporous.

Cutaneous. In mild-to-moderate aortic regurgitation, the skin is typically flushed and diaphoretic, reflecting the hyperdynamic cardiovascular state. In severe decompensated or acute disease, the complexion is pale and cyanotic due to peripheral underperfusion.

Heart Rate and Character of Pulse. In a chronic, stable condition the heart rate is normal. The peripheral pulses are bounding and of the water-hammer quality, which is characterized by a quick upstroke followed by a rapid collapse (Corrigan's pulse). The pulse pressure may be greater than 100 mm Hg, and Korotkoff sounds may be audible to zero although true intraarterial pressure rarely falls below 30 mm Hg. The carotid pulse is accentuated with visible pulsations. Loud "pistol shot" systolic sounds may be heard over medium-sized arteries (Traube's sign). With ventricular decompensation, the pulse pressure progressively narrows and the force of the pulses weaken. In acute aortic insufficiency the blood pressure may be 90/50.

Heart Sounds. The characteristic murmur is high pitched, decrescendo, diastolic, and blowing in character and is best heard at the left sternal border at the third interspace. A ventricular gallop is also commonly audible. In acute aortic regurgitation, the regurgitant murmur may end in middiastole as left ventricular pressure rises to equal aortic pressure and thwarts further regurgitant flow. The murmur may also be so faint as to be inaudible.

Palpation of the Precordium. The position and character of the apex beat are important in assessing aortic regurgitation. The apex beat is not abnormally displaced nor hyperkinetic with mild disease. As the severity increases, the impulse becomes more forceful, lifting, and more sustained, and is displaced downward and to the left. With acute aortic regurgitation, the apex beat is in the normal position or moderately displaced and is not hyperkinetic.

Neck Veins. Distention of the external jugular veins will be present if the patient is in right ventricular failure.

Respirator Rate and Character of Breathing. The breathing pattern and rate are normal unless pulmonary edema is present. Tachypnea and dyspnea are therefore suggestive of a decompensated state.

Lung Sounds. Auscultatory findings are unremarkable unless pulmonary edema is present.

Acid/Base. In decompensated states, the patient will be hypoxemic and will have a mild respiratory alkalosis secondary to hyperventilation due to pulmonary edema. With severe perfusion failure, anaerobic metabolism is reflected by metabolic acidosis.

LABORATORY STUDIES

ECG. The ECG may be normal in mild-to-moderate aortic regurgitation, but a left ventricular hypertrophy and strain pattern are commonly seen in more severe aortic regurgitation. P wave abnormalities relating to left atrial enlargement may exist.

Chest Radiograph. Cardiac size relates to the duration and severity of the regurgitant flow and left ventricular function. In acute aortic regurgitation, there is little, if any, cardiac enlargement, but radiologic evidence of pulmonary edema is usually present. In chronic regurgitation, the enlarging heart assumes an ovoid, oblong shape, and signs of pulmonary venous congestion and edema are present with decompensation.

Echocardiogram. This test may be useful in determining the etiology of the regurgitant flow. For example, vegetations are evidence of infective endocarditis, whereas disruption of the valve cusps may be seen in aortic dissection. The regurgitant fraction can be approximated by echocardiogram. Increased left ventricular volume and chamber size are common findings.

Cardiac Catheterization. This procedure is used to assess left-sided heart function and ejection fraction. Any coexisting abnormalities, such as coronary artery lesions and concomitant valvular disease, can also be detected and quantified.

TREATMENT

The treatment protocol relates to patient symptoms as well as to the severity of aortic regurgitation. The asymptomatic patient with mild-to-moderate aortic regurgitation may lead a normal life with no exercise restrictions, but antibiotic coverage is necessary for dental, surgical, or instrumentation procedures.

The symptomatic patient with chronic aortic regurgitation should be instructed to avoid any strenuous activity. Digitalis and diuretics are used to treat symptoms of heart failure. Arterial vasodilators reduce left ventricular afterload, thereby reducing the volume of regurgitant flow and increasing the amount of blood ejected into the systemic circulation.

At the onset of symptoms, preparations should begin for aortic valve replacement while the patient is being managed medically. The results of valve replacement surgery are optimized, even if the patient is asymptomatic, if ventricular function has deteriorated.

The patient with acute, severe aortic regurgitation is treated with inotropic agents as well as diuretics and vasodilator agents while diagnostic tests and preparation for emergency aortic valve replacement are under way.

Cardiac Tamponade

Cardiac tamponade is a condition in which an abnormal accumulation of fluid within the pericardial space compresses the heart and impairs diastolic filling and cardiac function.

CAUSES AND PATHOPHYSIOLOGY

The accumulation of fluid, called a pericardial effusion, may result from:

1. *Infectious processes.* Viral, bacterial, or fungal pericarditis may lead to effusion and tamponade.

2. *Neoplasms.* Metastatic carcinoma of the breast or lung is a common cause of effusion.

3. *Trauma.* Gunshot wounds, stab wounds, catheter perforation, surgery, or blunt chest trauma may result in intrapericardial bleeding. Penetrating injury in the precordial area is generally regarded as a "hot spot" for tamponade; however *any* penetrating injury *anywhere* in the thorax or epigastrium should be suspect for possible tamponade.

4. *Nontraumatic Hemorrhage.* Ventricular rupture, leaking aneurysms, dissection of the ascending aorta, or anticoagulant therapy may result in effusion and tamponade.

5. *Other Causes.* Radiation pericarditis, connective tissue disease (rheumatoid arthritis, systemic lupus erythematosus), or uremic pericarditis may result in an accumulation of pericardial fluid.

The pericardium is a double-walled sac that completely encases the heart and attaches at its junctions to the great arteries and veins. The pericardial space normally contains approximately 20 to 30 ml of fluid that provide a friction-free surface for the beating heart. When intrapericardial volume and pressure increase, ventricular filling is restricted, and stroke volume decreases by the Starling effect. The amount of fluid required to produce cardiac dysfunction relates to the rapidity of fluid accumulation. For example, a sudden (minutes to hours) accumulation of as little as 100 to 200 ml may cause significant hemodynamic compromise. On the other hand, a slow accumulation of fluid of 1 to 2 liters over weeks may be fairly well tolerated because the pericardium stretches gradually.

Hemodynamic Effects

Normal intrapericardial pressure averages 3 to 5 mm Hg less than pressure in the central veins and right atrium. This pressure difference maintains slight distention of the right atrium and central veins. Central venous pressure averages approximately 3 to 5 mm Hg less than the pressure in the peripheral veins. This pressure gradient maintains continuous blood flow from the systemic veins to the right atrium. As pericardial fluid accumulates, intrapericardial pressure rises until it equilibrates with central venous and right atrial pressure. Further accumulation of intrapericardial fluid causes both pressures to rise together to the level of the left ventricular diastolic pressure, and as effusion worsens all pressures continue to rise together.

This equilibration of diastolic pressures is known as the diastolic plateau and is manifest when PWP (a correlate of left ventricular end-diastolic pressure), pulmonary artery diastolic pressure, and central venous pressure (a correlate of right ventricular end-diastolic pressure) equilibrate. This overall elevation in diastolic pressures relates to the external compression of the heart by the fluid-filled pericardium and is associated with two untoward hemodynamic effects.

- Both ventricles cannot distend and fill normally in diastole. In fact, ventricular end-diastolic volume may fall to as little as 25 to 30 ml, which is considerably less than a normal stroke volume. The end-diastolic volume/pressure relationship of both ventricles, therefore, is totally distorted, for as filling pressures rise, filling volumes fall.
- As the level of central venous pressure rises with intrapericardial pressure, venous return is progressively reduced. This results in systemic venous hypertension.

Arterial hypotension with concomitantly developing venous hypertension causes critical reductions in tissue perfusion. Three sympathetic nervous system–mediated mechanisms are quickly activated to compensate for these defects.

1. The ejection fraction increases from a normal range of 57 to 73% to 70 to 80%. Thus the heart empties more completely with each beat and the intraventricular diastolic suction may draw blood from the venous system.
2. The heart rate increases.

3. Systemic vascular resistance increases in skeletal muscle. This helps maintain mean arterial pressure and perfusion of the central organs.

As tamponade worsens, however, compensatory mechanisms are no longer able to maintain arterial pressure, and hypoperfusion of all organ systems ensues. Extreme tamponade is an absolute emergency because effective heart function and circulation may cease.

HEMODYNAMIC PROFILE

Individual hemodynamic responses to tamponade are modified by hypovolemia, hypervolemia, and the magnitude of the individual's sympathetic nervous system response (see Table 16–2).

Arterial Pressure. Initially, sympathetic nervous system stimulation may elevate the systolic pressure to levels as high as 150 mm Hg. More commonly, however, it is in the range of 90 to 100 mm Hg. Diastolic pressure is maintained by peripheral vasoconstriction, and the pulse pressure may be narrowed to 10 to 20 mm Hg, i.e., an arterial pressure of 100/80. The arterial pressure waveform has a damped appearance, and pulsus paradoxus gives a roller coaster appearance to the systolic peaks in a continuous arterial tracing (Fig. 16–11).

Systemic Vascular Resistance. This value increases with progressive reductions in stroke volume.

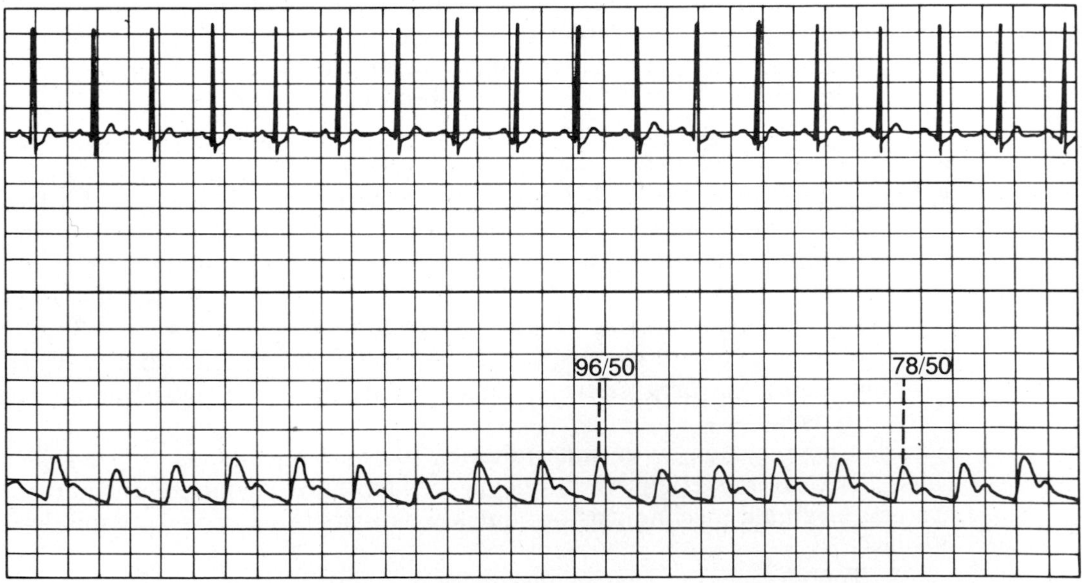

Pulsus paradoxus

FIGURE 16–11. Pulsus paradoxus. Note the cyclic variation in systolic pressure. An increased systolic pressure is associated with expiration and a decreased systolic pressure is associated with inspiration.

Pulmonary Vascular Resistance. This parameter will increase if hypoxemia or acidemia complicates the clinical picture.

CVP and Right Atrial Pressure. These values increase in proportion to and correlate with pressure in the pericardial space. The RA waveform may show a prominent *x* descent and a reduced or absent *y* descent. The mean RA pressure may be greater than 10 mm Hg in acute, severe tamponade.

Pulmonary Artery Pressure. The pulmonary artery systolic pressure is usually normal, and the pulmonary artery diastolic pressure is equal to right atrial pressure.

Pulmonary Artery Wedge Pressure. This value is elevated and closely approximates the aforementioned right atrial and pulmonary artery diastolic pressures.

Cardiac Output. Initially, compensatory mechanisms may maintain cardiac output within a normal range. With continued increases in intrapericardial volume, compensatory mechanisms are overwhelmed and cardiac output falls.

Mixed Venous Oxygen Saturation (SvO_2). This value falls with perfusion failure and/or hypoxemia.

Clinical Presentation

The symptoms of cardiac tamponade relate to the severity of circulatory compromise. The patient may be asymptomatic with minimal effusion or in a state of collapse with a large effusion producing tamponade. Symptoms include dizziness, a feeling of fullness in the head, dyspnea, retrosternal pain, or an oppressive feeling in the chest. Dysphagia, cough, or hiccoughs, as well as other symptoms that relate to the cause of the tamponade (pericarditis, trauma, aortic dissection) may also be present.

Mentation. The patient may be lucid and anxious in mild tamponade. This, then, may progress to restlessness, confusion, bizarre behavior, or stupor in severe tamponade.

Cutaneous. At first, the skin may be slightly pale and warm. With the development of severe circulatory failure, the skin is cool, pale, and moist with peripheral cyanosis.

Heart Rate and Character of Pulse. Tachycardia is an important compensatory mechanism to maintain cardiac output. In severe tamponade, bradycardia may usher in electrical-mechanical dissociation and death. *Pulsus paradoxus,* defined as a greater than 10 mm Hg inspiratory fall in systolic pressure, is a classic finding in tamponade. This produces a variation in amplitude of the peripheral pulses that diminishes in inspiration and strengthens on expiration (see Fig. 16–11). With severe cardiac tamponade, peripheral pulses are so weak that they may disappear totally during inspiration. This is known as total paradox and is commonly associated with combined cardiac tamponade and hypovolemia. Measurement with a sphygmomanometer may be useful for confirmation, but a *palpable paradoxus is a clinically significant paradoxus.* In a hemodynamically unstable patient, the time wasted attempting to confirm a numerical paradoxus by cuff technique may assume life or death significance for the patient. If the patient is *stable* and the situation is *not critical*, to determine the numerical paradoxus the clinician should first instruct the patient to breathe normally. The blood pressure cuff is inflated to 20 mm Hg above the systolic pressure and then gradually deflated. The point at which the first systolic sound is heard on expiration is noted—for example, 118 mm Hg. The cuff pressure should then be slowly released until Korotkoff sounds are heard equally well on inspiration and expiration—for example, 100 mm Hg. The difference between these two pressures is termed the paradox and should not normally exceed 10 mm Hg.

Heart Sounds. Heart sounds are muffled or totally inaudible—"the silent heart"—due to the damping effect of the pericardial fluid on the sounds.

Palpation of the Precordium. The apex beat is usually weak or may even be imperceptible.

Neck Veins. With severe tamponade, the external jugular veins may be distended up to the level of the jaw even with the patient sitting upright. If tamponade is accompanied by hypovolemia, jugular venous distention may be noted only after intravascular volume is restored to normal.

Respiratory Rate and Character of Breathing. The patient is typically tachypneic and dyspneic with significant tamponade and, if not hypotensive, prefers to sit upright, leaning forward slightly.

Lung Sounds. The chest is clear to auscultation.

Acid/Base. A respiratory alkalosis may dominate until severe perfusion failure results in lactic acidosis.

Laboratory Studies

ECG. The ECG often shows reduced QRS amplitude in the limb leads. Alternating amplitude of the QRS complexes (electrical alternans) or alternating amplitude of the entire PQRST sequence (total alternans) is a specific indicator of cardiac tamponade. This ECG phenomenon represents the swinging movement of the heart within the effusion, resulting in beat-to-beat changes in electrical axis. Typically, the patient is in sinus tachycardia; as mentioned earlier, sinus bradycardia is an ominous sign.

Chest Radiograph. Serial chest films may be helpful in detecting progressive enlargement of the cardiac silhouette. The shape of the heart may also be altered and appear globular. There are no specific signs on plain chest roentgenogram; however, patients with tamponade retain clear lung fields, which is helpful in distinguishing tamponade from heart failure.

Echocardiogram. This is one of the most sensitive tests for detecting pericardial fluid. It is extremely useful in the patient with actual or suspected tamponade and may be performed prior to pericardiocentesis if the patient's condition is sufficiently stable. The echocardiogram can document the presence and magnitude of pericardial fluid and can rapidly differentiate between cardiac tamponade and other causes of systemic venous hypertension and arterial hypotension, such as right ventricular infarction and constrictive pericarditis.

In some instances, the rapidly deteriorating hemodynamic status of the patient may obviate any laboratory tests, and the diagnosis is based solely on the history and physical examination.

TREATMENT

Medical therapy is directed at patient support, and maximizing cardiac function, is temporizing. The only definitive therapy in tamponade is to remove the pericardial effusion, thereby normalizing intrapericardial pressure and heart function. This can be accomplished either by pericardiocentesis or surgery.

Medical Therapy. Types of medical therapy include:

- Intravascular volume expanders—Colloids or Ringer's lactate is helpful in acute tamponade to maximize left ventricular filling and stroke volume.
- Isoproterenol (Isuprel)—This catecholamine is very useful in cardiac tamponade as it increases contractility and decreases systemic vascular resistance. Isoproterenol, however, is known to produce a marked increase in myocardial oxygen requirements and also predisposes to arrhythmia; therefore, continuous monitoring of the patient's hemodynamic parameters, ECG, and clinical status during administration of the drug is essential.
- Vasodilators—Hydralazine and nitroprusside have been shown experimentally to increase cardiac output in cardiac tamponade by reducing systemic vascular resistance.

Other medical therapy is related to the cause of the tamponade. For example, if warfarin-induced, vitamin K is prescribed.

Surgical Therapy. Surgery to treat cardiac tamponade includes:

- Pericardiocentesis—Needle aspiration of the pericardial fluid is used to relieve cardiac compression. Pericardiocentesis is usually reserved for serious cases that present with life-threatening symptoms, since the procedure carries the risk of ventricular puncture, ventricular arrhythmias, trauma to the myocardium, and coronary artery or pleural laceration. Elective pericardiocentesis is best performed in the operating room or in the cardiac catheterization laboratory; however, the emergency nature of the situation may require it be done "on the spot" such as in the emergency department.

  Pericardiocentesis is likely to be either complicated or unsuccessful in improving hemodynamics in patients with acute traumatic hemopericardium, small effusions of less than 200 ml, loculated effusions, or effusions that coexist with clot or fibrin.
- Surgical evacuation of pericardial fluid—This may be accomplished either by extensive pericardiectomy or by limited pericardiectomy. Total pericardiectomy is indicated when extensive exploration is required.

Dilated Cardiomyopathy

A cardiomyopathy is a disease involving the heart muscle that does not result from valvular, pericardial, hypertensive, congenital, or ischemic disease. Dilated cardiomyopathy (also known as congestive or hypodynamic cardiomyopathy) is a disease of the myocardium characterized by excessive ventricular dilatation and profoundly depressed systolic ejection.

As with all forms of heart disease, dilated cardiomyopathy may be present, progressing, and asymptomatic for years. The person so afflicted but undiagnosed may enter the hospital for elective or emergency surgery or other nonrelated illness. Under the stress of the primary problem, the patient may then exhibit signs and symptoms of heart disease such as heart failure or arrhythmia despite the absence of an apparent organic basis for the cardiac dysfunction. On the other hand, symptoms may develop gradually over an extended period of time, or recognition of the disorder may occur when cardiomegaly is detected on a routine chest x-ray film. Alcoholism is a well-known public health problem in industrialized society, and cardiomyopathy should be suspected in the alcoholic patient who suddenly, under the stress of other illness, shows signs of cardiac dysfunction.

Causes and Pathophysiology

The exact etiology of dilated cardiomyopathy is uncertain, but it is thought to be a multicausal disorder in which toxic, metabolic, or infectious insults to the myocardium result in a common pathophysiologic expression. Familial transmission is rare. The following conditions or factors appear to be related to or identified with dilated cardiomyopathy.

Alcohol Abuse. The chronic or excessive ingestion of alcoholic beverages is a major cause of dilated cardiomyopathy. Myocardial damage may be due to a direct toxic effect of ethanol on the myocardium; malnutrition, most commonly associated with a vitamin (particularly thiamine) deficiency; or toxic effects of additives in the alcoholic beverage, ie, cobalt in beer.

The amount or length of time of alcohol consumption required to produce dilated cardiomyopathy varies among individuals. Generally a large intake is necessary.

Hypertension. This appears to represent an unusual cardiac response to hypertension in which ventricular dilation rather than progressive hypertrophy occurs.

Pregnancy and the Puerperium. Some mothers in the last trimester of pregnancy develop cardiomyopathy. The reason is unknown, but it is most common in women over 30 years of age, multiparous women, those with a history of toxemia, and underprivileged, poorly nourished women.

Immunologic Factors. The venom of some snakes or hypersensitivity to drugs such as penicillin, sulfonamides, methyldopa, and tetracycline may predispose to cardiomyopathy.

Viral Infections. In some persons, following a viral illness (fever, fatigue, myalgias, rhinitis, cough) signs of cardiovascular deterioration surface in the subsequent weeks. It is postulated that the viral infection produces a state of altered cellular immunity, which then produces progressive myocardial damage.

Idiopathic. No cause can be determined.

Dilated cardiomyopathy is characterized by biventricular and atrial dilatation and impaired systolic performance. This will be manifest as a low ejection fraction and a large ventricular end-systolic and diastolic volume and possible functional mitral and tricuspid insufficiency due to dilatation of the valve annulus. The large end-systolic and diastolic volumes result in the stasis of blood and frequent thrombus formation within the ventricles, especially the apex. Hence, the patient is prone to pulmonary and systemic embolization. The heart valves are usually normal except for some occasional focal thickening of the mitral and tricuspid valve leaflets. The coronary arteries are usually normal.

Microscopic tissue examination reveals a variety of abnormalities, including myocardial cell degeneration, cellular hypertrophy and edema, and interstitial fibrosis.

Hemodynamic Effects

Initially, the reduction in stroke volume is compensated for by an increase in heart rate. Cardiac output, however, does not increase normally if the patient is stressed (sepsis, hypoxemia, hypercapnia, fever, strenuous activity) and ventricular end-diastolic pressures increase acutely. With the progression of time and the disease, as the ventricles become less contractile and dilated, there is also a greater increase in myocardial oxygen demand. Nevertheless, the ventricles may be dilated for a long time before an imbalance in myocardial oxygen supply and demand renders the patient symptomatic.

Hemodynamic Profile

The hemodynamic profile relates to global heart failure (see Table 16–2).

Arterial Pressure. The systolic values are usually in the normal range, but the pulse pressure is narrowed, reflecting the decreased stroke volume. The arterial pressure waveform shows a slow rate of rise, and the overall appearance of the waveform is damped.

Systemic Vascular Resistance. This value is usually elevated because the systemic arterioles are constricted as a compensatory measure to maintain mean arterial pressure despite a reduced stroke volume.

Pulmonary Vascular Resistance. This parameter is commonly slightly increased.

CVP or Right Atrial Pressure. The elevation of these values reflects the increased end-diastolic pressure of the right ventricle, which is in failure due to intrinsic right ventricular myocardial dysfunction. The *a* waves of the right atrial waveform may be prominent, and the *v* wave may be of increased amplitude if tricuspid regurgitation is present.

Pulmonary Artery Pressure. This value is usually modestly increased; markedly elevated values in the absence of acute pulmonary edema are uncommon. The waveform may additionally demonstrate a delayed rate of rise and damped appearance.

Pulmonary Artery Wedge Pressure. This value is elevated, reflecting the elevated end-diastolic pressure of the left ventricle. The ventricular end-diastolic pressure/volume correlation is good in this disorder as end-diastolic volumes of both ventricles are likewise increased. The *a* wave may be of increased amplitude and, if present, large *v* waves indicate mitral regurgitation.

Cardiac Output. This value may be normal or reduced relative to the severity of the disease and effectiveness of compensatory mechanisms. The ejection fraction is likewise reduced and, in severe disease, may be below 20%.

Mixed Venous Oxygen Saturation (SvO_2). In symptomatic patients, the severity of the reduction in oxygen saturation of mixed venous blood correlates with the severity of the perfusion deficit.

Clinical Presentation

The clinical manifestations of dilated cardiomyopathy relate to the degree of functional impairment of the heart. Unrecognized myocardial disease may exist for years and produce no symptoms. Sudden-onset arrhythmia (atrial fibrillation is common) may be the first indication of disease. Dyspnea on exertion is commonly the first symptom noticed by the patient. With progression of the disease, orthopnea, paroxysmal nocturnal dyspnea, fatigue, weakness, and chest pain are common complaints. Peripheral edema, enlargement of the liver, and ascites are late symptoms of severe disease.

Mentation. The patient is typically alert and lucid. However, previous cerebral embolization may produce varying degress of cerebral deficit.

Cutaneous. The skin is pale, cool at the extremities, and slightly cyanotic. Peripheral edema is an ominous sign.

Heart Rate and Character of Pulse. The patient tends to be tachycardic even at rest. The pulse is small in volume and pulsus alternans, if present, correlates with severe left ventricular failure. There may also be irregularities in the pulse relating to arrhythmias, which may predispose the patient to syncopal attack and sudden death.

Palpation of the Precordium. Because cardiomegaly is characteristic of the disease, the apex beat may be displaced as far left as the axilla and is diminished in force. A nonsustained right ventricular heave may be palpated along the left lower sternal border.

Heart Sounds. Atrial (S_4) and ventricular (S_3) gallop rhythms are common; if the patient is tachycardic, they may be heard as a summation gallop. The systolic murmurs of mitral and tricuspid regurgitation are also commonly auscultated in more advanced disease.

Neck Veins. Jugular venous distention is usually present in the symptomatic patient.

Respiratory Rate and Character of Breathing. Tachypnea and dyspnea, secondary to pulmonary congestion and/or edema, are present in the patient with symptomatic disease.

Lung Sounds. The lungs are clear to auscultation until clinically symptomatic pulmonary edema develops.

Acid/Base. Values are normal until severe overt disease produces hypoxemia as well as hypocapnia secondary to hyperventilation.

LABORATORY STUDIES

ECG. Sinus tachycardia is commonly present. Atrial fibrillation, which is seen in approximately 25% of patients with dilated cardiomyopathy, is an ominous sign because the loss of the atrial contribution to cardiac output usually leads to further deterioration in the patient's condition. Other arrhythmias—junctional rhythms, supraventricular tachycardia, varying degrees of heart block, ventricular tachycardia, and ventricular fibrillation—may also be seen. Q waves may be noted in the precordial leads and may be mistakenly interpreted as an old myocardial infarction.

Chest Radiograph. The chest roentgenogram generally reveals multichamber cardiac enlargement. Additionally, enlargement of the major pulmonary arteries and evidence of interstitial and alveolar pulmonary edema may be present.

Echocardiogram. Echocardiography is useful to assess the degree of impairment of ventricular function and to exclude valvular or pericardial disease. The echo reveals increased size of both ventricles, poor ventricular wall motion, and a reduced ejection fraction. Mural thrombi may also be detected echocardiographically.

Cardiac Catheterization. This invasive procedure may be used to exclude coronary artery disease (which typically is absent) as the cause of the patient's symptomatology. In fact, the coronary arteries are very commonly normal, smooth, and unobstructed or even widely dilated. Cardiac catheterization reveals enlarged heart chambers, generalized hypokinesis, and a low ejection fraction.

TREATMENT

The goals of therapy are to preserve the myocardium, maximize cardiac output, and eliminate the cause, if known.

Medical Therapy. Medical therapy is palliative, not curative, and includes

1. Oxygen therapy—In severe cases, oxygen therapy may be indicated to improve tissue oxygenation and relieve dyspnea.
2. Bed rest—In circumstances of severe symptomatic disease, bed rest may be required for prolonged periods of time to reduce myocardial work.
3. Salt and fluid restriction and diuretics—These therapeutic interventions help relieve the congestive symptoms of the disease. Care must be taken not to decrease ventricular filling pressures to levels that would further decrease stroke volume and cardiac output.

4. Inotropic agents—Digitalis may be used in the long term to maximize ventricular contractility and cardiac output. During the course of hospitalization, the more potent parenteral inotropic agents (dopamine, dobutamine) may be used.

5. Vasodilator agents—By reducing preload and afterload, these medications reduce heart work and increase stroke volume and tissue perfusion. Nitroprusside or intravenous nitroglycerin are used in the acute care setting. Captopril, hydralazine, prazosin, or nitrates are used over the long term.

6. Antiarrhythmic agents—This pharmacologic approach is indicated in life-threatening situations or when symptomatically disabling arrhythmias complicate the clinical picture. The patient should be observed closely for signs and symptoms of worsening heart failure because many antiarrhythmic agents have negative inotropic effects.

7. Corticosteroids or immunosuppressive agents—These agents may be helpful if the disease is associated with an inflammatory response but are not indicated in idiopathic cardiomyopathy.

Surgical Therapy. Surgical options include *replacement of atrioventricular valves* in circumstances of significant tricuspid or mitral regurgitation due to progressive cardiac enlargement. The overall benefit to the patient is not great because of the primary underlying myocardial dysfunction. *Cardiac transplant* is reserved for advanced dilated cardiomyopathy that is refractory to conventional therapy. Although this procedure offers a vastly improved survival rate (3-year survival is 70% in transplanted patients as compared with less than 5% survival in nontransplanted patients), the procedure is very costly, donor availability is a problem, and the risk of physical and emotional complications is high. For these reasons, candidates must be chosen carefully.

SUGGESTED READINGS

General

Chung E: *Quick Reference to Cardiovascular Disease,* 2nd ed. Philadelphia, JB Lippincott, 1983.

Hillis LD, Firth BG, Willerson JT: *Manual of Clinical Problems in Cardiology* 2nd ed. Boston, Little, Brown, 1984.

Horwitz DH, Berton MG: *Signs and Symptoms in Cardiology*. Philadelphia, JB Lippincott, 1985.

Ischemic Heart Disease

Akins C: Indications and results of surgery in unstable angina and Prinzmetal's variant angina. *In* McCarley K, Brest A (eds): *McGoon's Cardiac Surgery: An Inter-Professional Approach to Patient Care*. Philadelphia, FA Davis, 1985, pp 49–52, 61–64.

Borg N (ed): *Core Curriculum for Critical Care Nursing*. Philadelphia WB Saunders, 1981, pp 124–129.

Cohn P, Braunwald E: Chronic ischemic heart disease. *In* Braunwald E (ed): *Heart Disease: A Textbook of Cardiovascular Medicine*. Philadelphia, WB Saunders, 1984, pp 1334–1362.

Conti CR, Feldman R: Acute myocardial infarction: Thoughts about pathogenesis and treatment. *Mod Concepts Cardiovasc Dis* 1985; 54:35–38.

Daily E, Schroeder J: *Techniques in Bedside Hemodynamic Monitoring*. St. Louis, CV Mosby, 1981, pp 8–13, 132–147.

Forrester J, Chatterjee K, Jobin G: A new conceptual approach to the therapy of acute myocardial infarction. *Adv Cardiol* 1975: 15:111–123.

Huang S, Dasher L, Larson C, et al (eds): Myocardial infarction. *In Coronary Care Nursing.* Philadelphia, WB Saunders, 1983, pp 123–133.
Hutter A, DeSanctis R: The evaluation and management of patients with angina pectoris. *In* Johnson R, Haber E, Austen W (eds): *The Practice of Cardiology.* Boston, Little, Brown, 1980, pp 281–283.
Karliner J, Gregoratos G: *Coronary Care.* New York, Churchill Livingstone, 1981, pp 492–495, 559–570.
Kenner C, Guzzetta C, Dossey B: Acute myocardial infarction. *In Critical Care Nursing: Body—Mind—Spirit.* Boston, Little, Brown, 1981, pp 403–420.
Kirk E, Jennings R: Pathophysiology of myocardial ischemia. *In* Hurst JW (ed): *The Heart.* New York, McGraw-Hill, 1982, pp 976–988, 1002–1003.
Kloner R: Acute myocardial infarction. *In* Kligfield P (ed): *Cardiology Reference Book.* New York, CoMedica, 1984, pp 64–71.
Reuther M, Hansen C: Myocardial infarction. *In Cardiovascular Nursing.* New York, Medical Examination Publishing, 1985, pp 98–107.
Riegel B: The role of nursing in limiting myocardial infarct size. *Heart Lung* 1985, 14:247–254.
Stapleton J: Ischemic heart disease. *In* Essentials of Clinical Cardiology. Philadelphia, FA Davis, 1983, pp 251–271.
Underhill S: Diagnosis and treatment of the patient with coronary artery disease and myocardial ischemia. *In* Underhill S, Woods S, Silvarajan E, et al (eds): Philadelphia, JB Lippincott, 1982, pp 311–313, 328–331, 355–359.
Walsh R, O'Rourke R: The physical examination in acute uncomplicated and complicated myocardial infarction. *In* Harvey A, Johns R, Owens A, et al (eds): *The Principles and Practice of Medicine.* New York, Appleton-Century-Crofts, 1976, pp 177–182, 325–353.
Woods S: *Cardiovascular Critical Care Nursing.* New York, Churchill Livingstone, 1983, pp 41–42, 166–168.

Valvular Heart Disease

Borg N (ed): Physical examination. *In Core Curriculum for Critical Care Nursing.* Philadelphia, WB Saunders, 1981, pp 105–108.
Braunwald E: Valvular heart disease. *In Heart Disease: A Textbook of Cardiovascular Medicine,* Philadelphia, WB Saunders, 1984, pp 1064–1115.
Breu C: Valvular heart disease. *In* Hamilton H (ed): Diseases. Springhouse, PA, Intermed Communications, 1983, pp 1104–1108.
Daily E, Schroeder J: Monitoring the patient with acute myocardial infarction. *In Bedside Hemodynamic Monitoring,* St. Louis, CV Mosby, 1981, pp 141–142.
Ervin G, Long S: Waveforms and pressures. *In Memory Bank for Hemodynamic Monitoring.* Pacific Palisades, CA, Nurseco, Inc, 1984, pp 144–148.
Greenberg B, Rahimtoola S: Usefulness of vasodilator therapy in acute and chronic valvular regurgitation. *Curr Probl Cardiol* 1984; 9:4–31.
Grossman W: Profiles in valvular heart disease. *In Cardiac Catheterization and Angiography.* Philadelphia, Lea & Febiger, 1980, pp 305–321.
Harvey A, Jones R, Owens A, et al: Cardiovascular disease. *In The Principles and Practice of Medicine.* New York, Appleton-Century-Crofts, 1976, pp 276–277, 284–291.
Hurst JW: Valvular disease. *In The Heart.* New York, McGraw-Hill, 1982, pp 863–922.
Kenner C, Guzzetta C, Dorsey B: Cardiac surgery. *In Critical Care Nursing: Body—Mind—Spirit.* Boston, Little, Brown, 1981, pp 457–466.
O'Rourke R, Crawford M: Mitral valve regurgitation. *Curr Probl Cardiol* 1984; 9:8–52.
Pluth G: Mitral valve reconstruction versus prosthetic valve replacement. *In* McCauley K, Brest A (eds): *McGoon's Cardiac Surgery: An Inter-Professional Approach to Patient Care.* Philadelphia, FA Davis, 1985, pp 117–125.
Potter D: Cardiovascular system. *In Assessment.* Springhouse, PA, Intermed Communications, 1983, pp 368–371.
Reuther M, Hansen C: Valvular heart disease. *In Cardiovascular Nursing.* New York, Medical Examination Publishing, 1985, pp 126–135.
Stapleton, J: Valvular diseases. *In Essentials of Clinical Cardiology.* Philadelphia, FA Davis, 1983, pp 293–336.
Underhill S: Valvular disorders. *In Cardiac Nursing.* Philadelphia JB Lippincott, 1982, pp 635–650.
Waller B: Morphological aspects of valvular heart disease. Parts I and II. *Curr Probl Cardiol* 1984; 9:6–61.

Woods S (ed): *Cardiovascular Critical Care Nursing*. New York, Churchill Livingstone, 1983, pp 132–137.
Zschoche D: Clinical management of common cardiac abnormalities. *In Mosby's Comprehensive Review of Critical Care*. St. Louis, CV Mosby, 1981, pp 253–254.

Cardiac Tamponade

Hathaway R: Cardiac tamponade. *In* Hamilton H (ed): *Diseases*. Springhouse, PA, Intermed Communications, 1983, pp 1133–1134.
Huang S, Dasher L, Larson C, et al: *Coronary Care Nursing*. Philadelphia, WB Saunders, 1983, pp 248–249.
Karliner J, Gregoratos J: Sequellae of acute myocardial infarction. *In Coronary Care*. New York, Churchill Livingstone, 1981, pp 535–538.
Lorell B, Braunwald E: Pericardial disease. *In* Braunwald E (ed): *Heart Disease: A Textbook of Cardiovascular Medicine*. Philadelphia, WB Saunders, 1984, pp 1480–1488.
Reuther M, Hansen C: Cardiovascular pathologies. *In Cardiovascular Nursing*. New York, Medical Examination Publishing, 1985, pp 109–110.
Shabetai R: Pathophysiology of constrictive pericarditis and cardiac tamponade. *In* Hurst J (ed): *The Heart*. New York, McGraw-Hill, 1982, pp 1363–1389.
Shabetai R: *The Pericardium*. New York, Grune and Stratton, 1981.
Shabetai R, Fowler N, Guntheroth W: The hemodynamics of cardiac tamponade and constrictive pericarditis. *Am J Cardiol* 1970; 26:480–488.
Stapleton J: Diseases of the pericardium. *In Essentials of Clinical Cardiology*. Philadelphia, FA Davis, 1983, pp 373–374.
Underhill S, Woods S, Silvarajan E, et al: Cardiac Tamponade. *In Cardiac Nursing*. Philadelphia, JB Lippincott, 1982, pp 157–158, 407.
Vignola P, Johnson R, Scannel J: Pericardial diseases. *In The Practice of Cardiology*. Boston, Little, Brown, 1980, pp 669–674.

Cardiomyopathy

Abelmann W: Classification and natural history of primary myocardial disease. *Prog Cardiovasc Dis* 1984; 27:73–91.
Bohachick P, Rongaus A: Hypertrophic cardiomyopathy. *Am J Nurs* 1984; 40:320–326.
Braunwald E (ed): The cardiomyopathies and myocarditides. *In Heart Disease: A Textbook of Cardiovascular Medicine*. Philadelphia, WB Saunders, 1984, pp 1400–1423.
Grossman W: Profiles in congestive and hypertrophic cardiomyopathies. *In Cardiac Catheterization and Angiography*. Philadelphia, Lea and Febiger, 1980, pp 346–365.
Hamilton H (ed): *Diseases*. Springhouse, PA Intermed Communications, 1983, pp 1120–1125.
Harvey A, Johns R, Owens A, et al: Myocardial disease. *In The Principles and Practice of Medicine*. New York, Appleton-Century-Crofts, 1976, pp 251–255.
Huang S, Dasher L, Larson C, et al: Cardiomyopathy. *In Coronary Care Nursing*. Philadelphia, WB Saunders, 1983, pp 269–278.
Hurst JW (ed): Cardiomyopathy. *In The Heart*. New York, McGraw-Hill, 1982, pp 1299–1327.
Johnson R, Haber E, Austin W, (eds): Dilated cardiomyopathy and nonhypertrophic nondilated cardiomyopathy. *In The Practice of Cardiology*. Boston, Little, Brown, 1980, pp 603–618.
Lee W, Regan T: Clinical aspects of the cardiomyopathies: An update. *In Heart Failure*, 1985, pp 36–49.
McGurn W: Miscellaneous cardiac pathology. *In People with Cardiac Problems: Nursing Concepts*. Philadelphia, JB Lippincott, 1981, pp 373–380.
Reuther M, Hansen C: Cardiomyopathies. *In Cardiovascular Nursing*. New York, Medical Examination Publishing, 1985, pp 122–125.
Stapleton J: Cardiomyopathy. *In Essentials of Clinical Cardiology*. Philadelphia, FA Davis, 1983, pp 199–206.
Trobaugh G: Cardiomyopathies. *In Cardiac Nursing*. Philadelphia, JB Lippincott, 1982, pp 651–654.
Wingate S: Dilated cardiomyopathy, Part 1. Focus on Critical Care, 1984; 2:49–56.

Index

Note: Numbers in *italics* refer to illustrations; numbers followed by t refer to tables.